Pharmaceutics: Advanced Principles and Applications to Pharmacy Practice

Pharmaceutics: Advanced Principles and Applications to Pharmacy Practice

Editor: Jesse Hanson

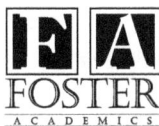

FA
FOSTER
ACADEMICS

www.fosteracademics.com

www.fosteracademics.com

FA
FOSTER
ACADEMICS

Cataloging-in-Publication Data

Pharmaceutics : advanced principles and applications to pharmacy practice / edited by Jesse Hanson.
    p. cm.
Includes bibliographical references and index.
ISBN 978-1-63242-833-2
1. Pharmacology. 2. Pharmacy. 3. Drugs. 4. Pharmaceutical industry. I. Hanson, Jesse.
RM300 .P43 2019
615--dc23

Foster Academics,
118-35 Queens Blvd., Suite 400,
Forest Hills, NY 11375, USA

ISBN 978-1-63242-833-2 (Hardback)

Contents

Preface

Pharmaceutics is a branch of pharmaceutical science. It is concerned with the process of converting old drugs or a new chemical entity into a new medication which can be used safely by the patients. It is also known as the science of dosage form design, as it deals with the conversion of a pure drug substance into a dosage form. Pharmaceutical formulation, pharmaceutical manufacturing, physical pharmacy, dispensing pharmacy, pharmaceutical technology and pharmaceutical jurisprudence are some of the branches of pharmaceutics. Pharmaceutical formulation is a process in which several chemical substances, including the active drug, are combined together for producing a final medicinal product. This book elucidates the concepts and innovative models around prospective developments with respect to pharmaceutics. It studies, analyzes and upholds the pillars of pharmaceutics and its utmost significance in modern times. This book will prove to be immensely beneficial to students and researchers in this field.

Significant researches are present in this book. Intensive efforts have been employed by authors to make this book an outstanding discourse. This book contains the enlightening chapters which have been written on the basis of significant researches done by the experts.

Finally, I would also like to thank all the members involved in this book for being a team and meeting all the deadlines for the submission of their respective works. I would also like to thank my friends and family for being supportive in my efforts.

Editor

Prediction of Drug-Drug Interactions with Bupropion and Its Metabolites as CYP2D6 Inhibitors Using a Physiologically-Based Pharmacokinetic Model

Caifu Xue [†], Xunjie Zhang [†] and Weimin Cai *

Department of Clinical Pharmacy and Pharmaceutical Management, School of Pharmacy, Fudan University, 826 Zhangheng Road, Shanghai 201203, China; 15111030045@fudan.edu.cn (C.X.); 12307120290@fudan.edu.cn (X.Z.)
* Correspondence: weimincai@fudan.edu.cn
† These authors contributed equally to this work.

Abstract: The potential of inhibitory metabolites of perpetrator drugs to contribute to drug-drug interactions (DDIs) is uncommon and underestimated. However, the occurrence of unexpected DDI suggests the potential contribution of metabolites to the observed DDI. The aim of this study was to develop a physiologically-based pharmacokinetic (PBPK) model for bupropion and its three primary metabolites—hydroxybupropion, threohydrobupropion and erythrohydrobupropion—based on a mixed "bottom-up" and "top-down" approach and to contribute to the understanding of the involvement and impact of inhibitory metabolites for DDIs observed in the clinic. PK profiles from clinical researches of different dosages were used to verify the bupropion model. Reasonable PK profiles of bupropion and its metabolites were captured in the PBPK model. Confidence in the DDI prediction involving bupropion and co-administered CYP2D6 substrates could be maximized. The predicted maximum concentration (C_{max}) area under the concentration-time curve (AUC) values and C_{max} and AUC ratios were consistent with clinically observed data. The addition of the inhibitory metabolites into the PBPK model resulted in a more accurate prediction of DDIs (AUC and C_{max} ratio) than that which only considered parent drug (bupropion) P450 inhibition. The simulation suggests that bupropion and its metabolites contribute to the DDI between bupropion and CYP2D6 substrates. The inhibitory potency from strong to weak is hydroxybupropion, threohydrobupropion, erythrohydrobupropion, and bupropion, respectively. The present bupropion PBPK model can be useful for predicting inhibition from bupropion in other clinical studies. This study highlights the need for caution and dosage adjustment when combining bupropion with medications metabolized by CYP2D6. It also demonstrates the feasibility of applying the PBPK approach to predict the DDI potential of drugs undergoing complex metabolism, especially in the DDI involving inhibitory metabolites.

Keywords: physiologically based pharmacokinetic model; drug-drug interactions; bupropion; hydroxybupropion; threohydrobupropion; erythrohydrobupropion; inhibitory metabolites

1. Introduction

Metabolized drug-drug interactions (mDDIs) have been one of the main reasons for the failure of new drug research and development; a variety of drugs have been forced to withdraw from the market due to serious DDIs [1–4]. With the increasing and development of new drugs and usage, clinical combination therapy has become very common and inevitably increases the probability of occurrence of DDI. Consequently, evaluation of a potential risk of mDDIs is essential to improve safety and minimize the clinical risks associated with drug interactions [5].

In general, metabolites are formed primarily via metabolic enzymes, which play an important role in pharmacological activity and toxicity. Compared to the parent drug, it is generally considered less likely to cause metabolized drug interactions due to more polarity. In vitro studies of parent drugs are sufficient to avoid DDI risks [6].

However, it has recently been found that some important metabolites of inhibitors also have inhibitory effects [6–8]. In the latest Food and Drug Administration (FDA) draft guidance [9], it is explicitly stated that metabolites should be studied in DDI if the metabolite's area under the plasma concentration-time curve (AUC) is greater than or equal to 25% of the parent AUC (AUCm/AUCp $\geq$ 0.25). The European Medicines Agency (EMA) further emphasizes that, for metabolites with AUCm/AUCp > 0.25 and represent >10% of total drug-related material [10], it is recommended to evaluate their DDI. In addition, regulators are also strongly proposing to predict and understand potential clinical DDI from the perspective of physiologically-based pharmacokinetic (PBPK), especially those complex DDIs [9–11]. The PBPK model provides a dynamic method for evaluation of DDI based on the physiological mechanism [12–15]. Compared with the static approach, it is reasonable to anticipate that the dynamic model is more accurate in the predication of DDIs, such as simultaneous inhibition and induction [16,17], the DDI of both substrate and inhibitory metabolites [15,18,19] and multiple DDIs. Recently, PBPK models have been widely applied in research and development, and even some good models are accepted by regulatory agencies and can be used to exempt some clinical trials [11,20–23].

Bupropion is widely used in the treatment of major depressive disorder and smoking cessation. As a classical probe substrate for CYP2B6, it is metabolized to hydroxybupropion. In human, carbonyl reductase also plays an important role in the metabolism of bupropion. Threohydrobupropion and erythrohydrobupropion are two major metabolites produced by the reduction of the carbonyl group [24–27] (Figure 1). Although bupropion is not a substrate for CYP2D6, it also inhibits CYP2D6 activity [27,28]. Clinical studies have shown that there is a significant increase in substrate exposure when bupropion was administered in combination with substrates for CYP2D6. For desipramine, a five-fold increase in exposure was caused [29]. However, in vitro studies have shown that bupropion and hydroxybupropion are weak CYP2D6 inhibitors (IC50 = 58 and 74 μM, respectively) [27]. Thus, bupropion was chosen as the model drug. To better understand the complex DDI, a PBPK model was taken in the present study.

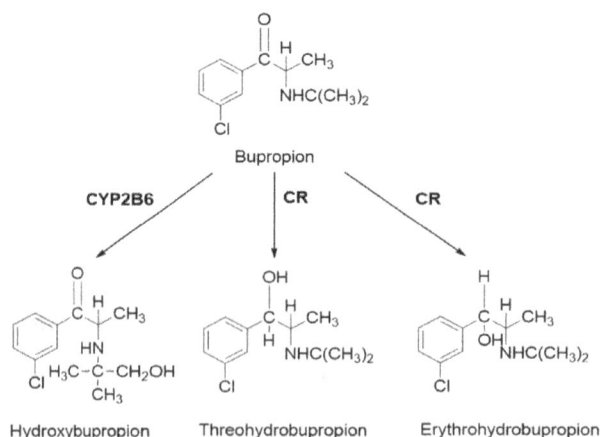

Figure 1. Bupropion and metabolism. Bupropion is metabolized by CYP2B6 to form hydroxybupropion and by carbonyl reductase to form the diastereoisomers threohydrobupropion and erythrohydrobupropion. CR: carbonyl reductase.

The objectives of the present work are (1) to build a PBPK model that can describe the PK profile of bupropion, hydroxybupropion, threohydrobupropion and erythrohydrobupropion; (2) to verify the bupropion PBPK model on the basis of the results of different-dose bupropion PK studies; and ultimately (3) to apply the PBPK model to predict the clinically observed DDIs with bupropion and its metabolites as the CYP2D6 inhibitors, and to better understand the involvement and impact of inhibitory metabolites for DDIs.

2. Materials and Methods

2.1. Physiologically-Based Pharmacokinetic (PBPK) Model Development

The Simcyp software package version 15 (Simcyp Limited, a Certara company, Sheffield, UK) was used to develop the PBPK model of bupropion and its metabolites. The absorption and distribution of bupropion was described by the first-order absoption and full PBPK model. For other metabolites, a minimal PBPK model were used to describe their distribution. To better predict the DDIs involving bupropion and its metabolites as CYP2D6 inhibitors, the model was first developed to simulate the PK of bupropion, hydroxybupropion, threohydrobupropion and erythrohydrobupropion when bupropion was given in different doses. Then, the verified model was used for the prediction of the involvement and impact of inhibitory metabolites in DDIs. Bufuralol, tolterodine, metoprolol, desipramine, and dextromethorphan as the CYP2D6 substrates from the Simcyp simulator library were used to simulate the DDIs. In addition, the PBPK model of venlafaxine was also built to simulate the DDI with bupropion. The observed clinical data were digitized from the graphs provided in literature using DigIt version 1.04 (Simulations Plus, Inc., Lancaster, CA, USA), a plot digitizer tool.

2.2. PBPK Model for Bupropion

The physicochemical properties of bupropion, including molecular weight, logP, pKa, blood-to-plasma ratio and fraction unbound in plasma were obtained from literature and in silico prediction as listed in Table 1. Bupropion binding to human plasma protein is 82% to 88%. Its absorption was described with a first-order absorption model. It has been reported that the absorption of bupropion is close to 100% [26]. A full PBPK model was used to describe the distribution of bupropion. The distribution of bupropion was predicted with Rogers method [30] based on the fitted K_p scalar to comparable to the observed value of 19 L/kg [31]. Bupropion is mainly metabolized by the liver and less than 1% of the parent drug is found in the urine [26,29]. According to the in vitro studies [27,32,33] with human liver microsomes, the enzyme kinetic parameters (V_{max} and K_m) of bupropion to form hydroxybupropion, threohydrobupropion and erythrohydrobupropion were integrated into the model. Considering the other metabolic pathways of bupropion, the formation of threohydrobupropion and erythrohydrobupropion were by carbonyl reductase. Therefore, in this model, we assumed that threohydrobupropion and erythrohydrobupropion were cleared likewise by CYP2B6. The $f_{u,mic}$ is used to correct the expression of carbonyl reductase to obtain the best simulation results closest to observed data.

Table 1. Parameters for bupropion used in physiologically-based pharmacokinetic (PBPK) modeling.

Parameter	Bupropion	
	Value	References/Comments
Mol weight (g/mol)	239.74	Drug bank
Log $P_{o:w}$	3.28	Drug bank
pKa	8.22	Drug bank
B/P	0.82	[29]
$f_{u,p}$	0.16	[28]
f_a	1	[26]
k_a (h^{-1})	0.8	[34]
T_{lag} (h)	0.8	[31]
K_p scalar	5.4	Simcyp best fit
V_{ss} (L/kg)	19	[31]
Enzyme	CYP2B6	Metabolite: hydroxybupropion
V_{max} (pmol/min per milligram)	3623	[27]
K_m (μM)	89	[27]

Table 1. *Cont.*

Parameter	Bupropion	
	Value	References/Comments
$f_{u,mic}$	0.16	Assumed = $f_{u,p}$
Enzyme	CYP2B6	Metabolite: threohydrobupropion
V_{max} (pmol/min per milligram)	98.4	[33]
K_m (μM)	186.3	[33]
$f_{u,mic}$	0.003	Simcyp best fit, correct expression of carbonyl reductase
Enzyme	CYP2B6	Metabolite: erythrohydrobupropion
V_{max} (pmol/min per milligram)	2.6	[33]
K_m (μM)	41.4	[33]
$f_{u,mic}$	0.003	Simcyp best fit, correct expression of carbonyl reductase

B/P, blood-to-plasma ratio; $f_{u,p}$, free fraction in plasma; f_a, fraction of dose absorbed; k_a, first-order absorption rate constant; T_{lag}, lag time; V_{ss}, steady-state volume of distribution; K_m, Michaelis constant; V_{max}, Maximum metabolic rate; $f_{u,mic}$, free fraction in liver microsome.

2.3. PBPK Model for Hydroxybupropion, Threohydrobupropion and Erythrohydrobupropion

The physicochemical properties of the three metabolites were obtained from in silico prediction. The distribution of metabolite hydroxybupropion, threohydrobupropion and erythrohydrobupropion were described by a minimal-PBPK distribution model with tissue partition coefficients predicted by the Rodgers method [30]. A single adjusting compartment in Simcyp optimized the V_{ss} of hydroxybupropion and threohydrobupropion. The elimination of all metabolites are fitted based on the corresponding observed clinical data. The corresponding parameters are listed in Table 2.

Table 2. Parameters for hydroxybupropion, threohydrobupropion and erythrohydrobupropion used in PBPK modeling.

Parameter	Hydroxybupropion		Threohydrobupropion		Erythrohydrobupropion	
	Value	References/Comments	Value	References/Comments	Value	References/Comments
Mol weight (g/mol)	255.74	ACD-ilab	241.757	ACD-ilab	241.757	ACD-ilab
Log $P_{o:w}$	2.03	ACD-ilab	2.88	ACD-ilab	2.88	ACD-ilab
pKa	7.4	ACD-ilab	7.4	ACD-ilab	9.6	ACD-ilab
B/P	0.82	Assigned using bupropion value	0.82	Assigned using bupropion value	0.82	Assigned using bupropion value
$f_{u,p}$	0.23	[28]	0.58	[28]	0.58	[28]
V_{sac} (L/kg)	0.5	Simcyp best fit	5.83	Simcyp best fit	N/A	
V_{ss} (L/kg)	2.15	Predicted with Rogers method	9.11	Predicted with Rogers method	1.47	Predicted with Rogers method
K_p scalar	1	Simcyp default value	1	Simcyp default value	2	Simcyp best fit
CL_{po} (L/h)	5.76	Simcyp best fit	21.15	Simcyp best fit	21.69	Simcyp best fit

B/P, blood-to-plasma ratio; $f_{u,p}$, free fraction in plasma; V_{sac}, volume of distribution of compartment; V_{ss}, steady-state volume of distribution; CL_{po}, oral clearance; N/A, not available. ACD-ilab, the online prediction engine from Advanced Chemistry Development, Inc.

2.4. PBPK Model for Venlafaxine

In addition, venlafaxine was also used as a CYP2D6 substrate to run the simulation with bupropion. To simulate the DDI between bupropion with venlafaxine, a PBPK model for venlafaxine was developed. The model of venlafaxine was built by a minimal PBPK model with tissue partition coefficients predicted by the Poulin and Theil method [35] combined with a first order absorption. The model parameters of venlafaxine are placed in Table 3. An oral absorption up to 92% was found. The K_p scalar of 2.3 was used to predict the V_{ss} comparable to the observed value of 7 L/kg [36–38]. The plasma protein binding of venlafaxine is low at 27% [37]. There is a consensus that the metabolic pathway of venlafaxine is mediated predominantly by CYP2D6. The CYP2C19, 2C9, and 3A4 isoforms also play a role in the metabolism of the drug, but to a lesser extent. The elimination of venlafaxine is fitted based on the corresponding observed clinical data. The intrinsic clearance (Clint) was calculated using retrograde model, assuming 80% Hep CL via CYP2D6 [39].

Table 3. Parameters for venlafaxine used in PBPK modeling.

Parameter	Venlafaxine	
	Value	References/Comments
Mol weight (g/mol)	277.402	[40]
Log $P_{o:w}$	2.8	[40]
pKa	9.4	[40]
B/P	1.17	[40]
$f_{u,p}$	0.73	[40]
f_a	0.92	[37]
k_a (h^{-1})	1.31	[38]
T_{lag} (h)	1.44	Simcyp best fit
K_p scalar	2.3	Predicted with Poulin and Theil method
V_{ss} (L/kg)	7	[38]
Enzyme	CYP2D6	
CLint (µL/min/pmol of isoform)	5.825	Retrograde calculation in Simcyp to account for 80% Hep CL from CYP2D6
CLint-additional (µL/min/mg protein)	11.65	Simcyp predicted

B/P, blood-to-plasma ratio; $f_{u,p}$, free fraction in plasma; f_a, fraction of dose absorbed; k_a, first-order absorption rate constant; T_{lag}, lag time; V_{ss}, steady-state volume of distribution.

2.5. Simcyp Simulation

The Simcyp software package version 15 (Simcyp Limited, a Certara company, Sheffield, UK) was used to build and develop the PBPK model of bupropion and its metabolites. The model parameters mentioned above were integrated into the PBPK model to simulate PK and DDI. The healthy volunteer population database in the Simcyp simulator is a powerful capability that allows us to assess the combined effects of variations in physiology and pharmacokinetics within populations, as well as formulate variables that are not precise values, but for which distributions of values can be estimated. Each subject is randomly ("Monte Carlo") generated to have a unique set of generic, anatomic, demographic, and tissue specific parameters, plasma protein binding, hepatic blood flow rate, and pharmacokinetic parameters. The default trial designed by Simcyp is selected to build the model of bupropion and its metabolites. A virtual population of 100 healthy volunteers (10 trials with 10 subjects each) aged 20–50 years with a female/male ratio of 0.5 was used in the simulation of PK following different single oral doses of bupropion (150, 75 and 100 mg).

2.6. Simulation of Drug-Drug Interaction (DDI)

In these DDI model, bufuralol, tolterodine, metoprolol, desipramine, and dextromethorphan from the Simcyp simulator library were selected as the CYP2D6 substrates to simulate the DDIs with bupropion and its metabolites. Venlafaxine, whose model was built by us, was also used in the simulation of DDIs. The detailed DDI parameters of bupropion and its metabolites are shown in Table 4.

Table 4. In vitro P450 inhibition parameters for bupropion and its metabolism.

Parameter	Bupropion	Hydroxybupropion	Threohydrobupropion	Erythrohydrobupropion
K_i (µM)	21	13	5.4	1.7

All data from [28]. K_i here are apparent values, and are corrected for free fraction in microsome ($f_{u,mic} = 0.01$) estimated in the Simcyp model.

Trials used in the DDI simulations were designed consistent with the reported clinical studies. The details of the trials were as follows:

(1)   The subjects (10 trials × 15 subject, aged 20–50, female/male ratio 0) received 150 mg bupropion or matching placebo orally twice daily for 10 days, and on day 11 the subjects received a single oral dose of 50 mg desipramine. Plasma concentrations of bupropion and desipramine were simulated during the drug treatment period.

(2)   The subjects (10 trials × 18 subject, aged 20–50, female/male ratio 0.5) received bupropion (at a daily dose of 150 mg/day) with venlafaxine (at a daily dose of 75 mg/day) for 8 weeks. Plasma concentrations of bupropion and venlafaxine were simulated during the drug treatment period.

(3)   The subjects (10 trials × 13 subject, aged 21–64, female/male ratio 0.5) received 150 mg bupropion or matching placebo orally twice daily for 17 days, and on day 18 the subjects received a single oral dose of 30 mg dextromethorphan. Plasma concentrations of bupropion and dextromethorphan were simulated during the drug treatment period.

(4)   The subjects (10 trials × 10 subject, aged 20–56, female/male ratio 0.5) received bupropion (at a twice daily dose of 150 mg) with metoprolol (at a twice daily dose of 75 mg) for 12 days. Plasma concentrations of bupropion and metoprolol were simulated during the drug treatment period.

(5)   The subjects (10 trials × 10 subject, aged 20–50, female/male ratio 0.5) received 150 mg bupropion or matching placebo orally twice daily for 2 weeks, and on day 15 the subjects received a single oral dose of 20 mg bufuralol or 2 mg tolterodine. Plasma concentrations of bupropion, bufuralol and tolterodine were simulated during the drug treatment period.

The fold-error was used to assess the success of model building and the accuracy of the predicted pharmacokinetic profile and data. Basically, two-fold-error was publicly recognized in the simulation [35,41–44]. The model was considered to have a goodness-of-fit when the fold-error was less than two. The fold-error was defined as observed/predicted or predicted/observed, where the numerator is greater than the denominator. The DDI effect, expressed as a ratio of AUC and C_{max} in the presence and absence of bupropion, was compared with observed data. The results are listed in Tables 5 and 6.

Table 5.   PBPK model-predicted drug-drug interactions (DDIs) between bupropion and desipramine/venlafaxine.

Inhibitors	AUC Ratio	C_{max} Ratio	T_{max} Ratio
Bupropion + Desipramine (observed)	5.2	1.9	2
Bupropion (predicted)	2.27	1.15	1.10
Hydroxybupropion (predicted)	4.58	1.76	1.84
Threohydrobupropion (predicted)	3.47	1.61	1.47
Erythrohydrobupropion (predicted)	2.83	1.45	1.47
Bup + H-Bup + T-Bup + E-Bup (predicted)	5.05	1.79	1.84
Bupropion + Venlafaxine (observed)	N/A	2.5	N/A
Bupropion (predicted)	1.30	1.27	1
Hydroxybupropion (predicted)	2.49	1.94	1
Threohydrobupropion (predicted)	2.14	1.80	1
Erythrohydrobupropion (predicted)	1.76	1.60	1
Bup + H-Bup + T-Bup + E-Bup (predicted)	3.03	2.24	1

Bup, Bupropion; H-Bup, Hydroxybupropion; T-Bup, Threohydrobupropion; E-Bup, Erythrohydrobupropion; AUC (concentration–time curve) ratio, AUC in the presence of inhibitor/AUC in the absence of inhibitor; C_{max} ratio, C_{max} in the presence of inhibitor/C_{max} in the absence of inhibitor; T_{max} ratio, T_{max} in the presence of inhibitor/T_{max} in the absence of inhibitor; N/A, not available.

Table 6. PBPK model-predicted DDIs between bupropion with other potential CYP2D6 substrates.

Substrate	AUC Ratio	C_{max} Ratio
Bufuralol	2.04	1.55
Tolterodine	2.91	2.17
Metoprolol	3.53	2.57
Dextromethorphan	4.06	3.05

AUC ratio, AUC in the presence of inhibitor/AUC in the absence of inhibitor; C_{max} ratio, C_{max} in the presence of inhibitor/C_{max} in the absence of inhibitor.

2.7. PBPK Model for Stereo-Selective Bupropion and Its Metabolites

The PBPK model for stereo-selective buproion and its metabolites were further developed based on the above model. The corresponding parameters are listed in Table 7. Other parameters not mentioned in Table 7 are similar to those of non-stereo selective buproion and its metabolites. The absorption and distribution of R-bupropion and S-bupropion were described by the first-order absoption and full PBPK model. For other metabolites, a minimal PBPK model were used to describe this distribution. The in vitro studies showed that R-bupropion was metabolized to form RR-hydroxybupropion via CYP2B6 2C19 and 3A4, respectively, RR-threohydrobupropion and SR-erythrohydrobupropion via carbonyl reductase, and R-4'-hydroxybupropion via CYP2C19; while the S-bupropion was metabolized to form SS-hydroxybupropion via CYP2B6 2C19 and 3A4, respectively, SS-threohydrobupropion and RS-erythrohydrobupropion via carbonyl reductase, and S-4'-hydroxybupropion via CYP2C19 [45]. We have integrated these metabolic pathways into our model. The CYP2J2 was used to define the carbonyl reductase. These corresponding intrinsic clearance rates are calculated by retrograde calculation in Simcyp to account for their proportion in the total clearance rate base on the in vitro study [46]. The total elimination of R-bupropion is divided into 34% hydroxybupropion, 50% threohydrobupropion, 8% erythrohydrobupropion and 8% 4'-hydroxybupropion. For S-bupropion, the proportion of these metabolites are 12% hydroxybupropion, 82% threohydrobupropion, 4% erythrohydrobupropion and 2% 4'-hydroxybupropion, respectively. The V_{ss} of SS-hydroxybupropion and RS-erythrohydrobupropion were predicted with Rogers method and Poulin and Theil method based on the optimized K_p value, respectively. The elimination of all metabolites are fitted based on the corresponding observed clinical data.

Table 7. Parameters for R-bupropion, S bupropion, RR-hydroxybupropion, SS-hydroxybupropion, RR-threohydrobupropion, SS-threohydrobupropion, SR-erythrohydrobupropion and RS-erythrohydrobupropion used in PBPK modeling.

Parameter	Value		References/Comments
R-BUP			
Clint (µL/min per pmol)			
CYP2B6 CYP2C19 CYP3A4	12 5.36 0.58	Metabolite: RR-OHBUP	Retrograde calculation in Simcyp to account for 34% of total CL [46]
CYP2J2	27	Metabolite: RR-TB	Retrograde calculation in Simcyp to account for 50% of total CL [46]
CYP2J2	4.24	Metabolite: SR-EB	Retrograde calculation in Simcyp to account for 8% of total CL [46]
CYP2C19	4.24	Metabolite: R-4'-OHBUP	Retrograde calculation in Simcyp to account for 8% of total CL [46]
S-BUP			
Clint (µL/min per pmol)			
CYP2B6 CYP2C19 CYP3A4	20.56 12.61 1.37	Metabolite: SS-OHBUP	Retrograde calculation in Simcyp to account for 12% of total CL [46]
CYP2J2	236.16	Metabolite: SS-TB	Retrograde calculation in Simcyp to account for 82% of total CL [46]
CYP2J2	11.52	Metabolite: RS-EB	Retrograde calculation in Simcyp to account for 4% of total CL [46]
CYP2C19	5.76	Metabolite: S- 4'-OHBUP	Retrograde calculation in Simcyp to account for 2% of total CL [46]
RR-OHBUP			
CL_{po} (L/h)	6.76		Simcyp best fit

Table 7. *Cont.*

Parameter	Value	References/Comments
SS-OHBUP		
V_{ss} (L/kg)	10.5	Predicted with Rogers method
K_p scalar	5	Simcyp best fit
CL_{po} (L/h)	305.8	Simcyp best fit
RR-TB		
V_{ss} (L/kg)	4.7	Predicted with Poulin and Theil method
K_p scalar	1	Simcyp default value
CL_{po} (L/h)	20	Simcyp best fit
SS-TB		
V_{ss} (L/kg)	4.7	Predicted with Poulin and Theil method
K_p scalar	1	Simcyp default value
CL_{po} (L/h)	120	Simcyp best fit
SR-EB		
V_{ss} (L/kg)	3.07	Predicted with Poulin and Theil method
K_p scalar	1	Simcyp default value
CL_{po} (L/h)	11.69	Simcyp best fit
RS-EB		
V_{ss} (L/kg)	9.08	Predicted with Poulin and Theil method
K_p scalar	3	Simcyp best fit
CL_{po} (L/h)	52	Simcyp best fit

R-BUP, R-Bupropion; S-BUP, S-Bupropion; RR-OHBUP, RR-Hydroxybupropion; SS-OHBUP, SS-Hydroxybupropion; RR-TB, RR-Threohydrobupropion; SS-TB, SS-Threohydrobupropion; SR-EB, SR-Erythrohydrobupropion; RS-EB, RS-Erythrohydrobupropion; R-4′-OHBUP, R-4′-Hydroxybupropion; S-4′-OHBUP, S-4′-Hydroxybupropion.

3. Results

3.1. Prediction of Bupropion and Its Metabolites Pharmacokinetics

The PBPK model of bupropion was successfully built based on the parameters in Table 1. The simulated PK profiles after oral doses of 150 mg bupropion are shown in Figure 2. There is a good match between predicted concentration profile and clinically observed data. The predicted C_{max}, AUC and T_{max} of bupropion were 136 ng/mL, 1402 ng·h/mL, and 1.8 h, respectively. All of them were within a two-fold error of the observed results (C_{max} = 143 ng/mL, AUC = 1161 ng·h/mL and T_{max} = 2.9 h) [47] (Figure 2A).

The simulated concentration-time profiles for hydroxybupropion, threohydrobupropion and erythrohydrobupropion are reasonably well consistent with the observed data based on the model parameters mentioned above (Figure 2B–D). The predicted PK parameters for hydroxybupropion were as follows: C_{max}, AUC and T_{max} were 457 ng/mL, 13,564 ng·h/mL, and 5.8 h, respectively. The observed C_{max}, AUC and T_{max} were 433 ng/mL, 16,651 ng·h/mL, and 7.7 h, respectively [47]. A fold error of less than two was simulated. The predicted C_{max} and AUC for threohydrobupropion were 96 ng/mL and 1358 ng·h/mL, respectively. The simulated C_{max} and AUC were also in good agreement with (<two-fold error) the observed results (C_{max} = 109 ng/mL, AUC = 1219 ng·h/mL) [34]. The predicted erythrohydrobupropion C_{max} and AUC were 12 ng/mL and 144 ng·h/mL, respectively. The simulated C_{max} and AUC were less than 2 fold error compared with the observed results (C_{max} = 15 ng/mL, AUC = 133 ng·h/mL) [34].

To verify the PBPK model, the PK profile of bupropion and its metabolites after oral different dose was also simulated and compared with reported data. Following a single oral doses of 75 mg bupropion to healthy subjects, the PK profiles of bupropion and its metabolites are shown in Figure 3. The predicted C_{max} (66 ng/mL), AUC (435 ng·h/mL) and T_{max} (1.9 h) less than 2 fold error compared with the observed data (C_{max} = 117 ng/mL, AUC = 456 ng·h/mL and T_{max} = 1.6 h, respectively) (Figure 3A) [48]. For the metabolites, the predicted PK parameters were as follows: C_{max}, AUC and T_{max} of hydroxybupropion were 222 ng/mL, 3827 ng·h/mL, and 5.8 h, respectively; C_{max}, AUC and

T_{max} of threohydrobupropion were 51 ng/mL, 719 ng·h/mL, and 4.6 h, respectively; C_{max}, AUC and T_{max} of erythrohydrobupropion were 7 ng/mL, 87 ng·h/mL, and 4.5 h, respectively. The simulated results compared reasonably well with the observed PK data (hydroxybupropion: C_{max} = 134 ng/mL, AUC = 2248 ng·h/mL, and T_{max} = 4.6 h; threohydrobupropion: C_{max} = 57 ng/mL, AUC = 647 ng·h/mL, and T_{max} = 1.9 h; erythrohydrobupropion: C_{max} = 7 ng/mL, AUC = 113 ng·h/mL, and T_{max} = 2.6 h, respectively) (Figure 3B–D) [48]. The simulated results compared reasonably well with the observed data: the predicted PK parameters were within a two-fold error of the observed data, whereas the T_{max} of threohydrobupropion was slightly overpredicted by two-fold error.

The PK profiles of bupropion and its metabolites after a single oral dose of 100 mg bupropion are shown in Figure 4. The predicted results were as follows: bupropion: C_{max} = 89 ng/mL, AUC = 586 ng·h/mL, and T_{max} = 1.9 h; hydroxybupropion: C_{max} = 299 ng/mL, AUC = 7764 ng·h/mL, and T_{max} = 5.8 h; threohydrobupropion: C_{max} = 68 ng/mL, AUC = 1329 ng·h/mL, and T_{max} = 4.6 h; erythrohydrobupropion: C_{max} = 9 ng/mL, AUC = 133 ng·h/mL, and T_{max} = 4.6 h, respectively. They were in agreement with (<two-fold error) the observed PK data (bupropion: C_{max} = 74 ng/mL, AUC = 360 ng·h/mL, and T_{max} = 1.7 h; hydroxybupropion: C_{max} = 281 ng/mL, AUC = 7468 ng·h/mL, and T_{max} = 4.2 h; threohydrobupropion: C_{max} = 73 ng/mL, AUC = 1354 ng·h/mL, and T_{max} = 3.0 h) [49]. However, no concentration-time profile data for erythrohydrobupropio from this study was available for direct comparison.

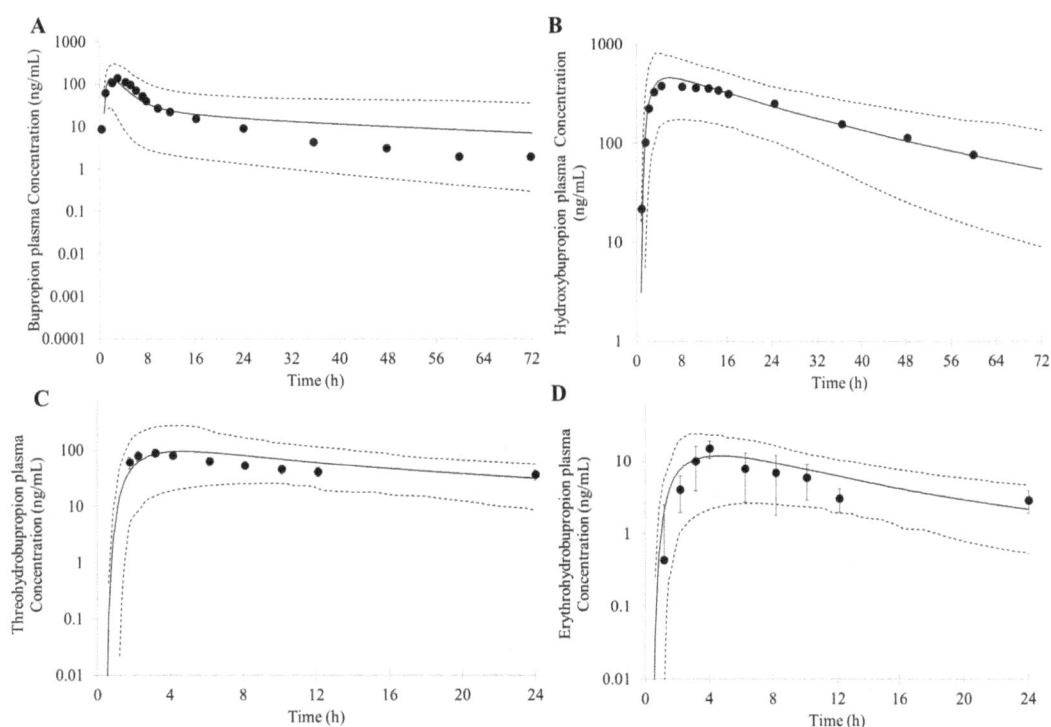

Figure 2. Predicted and observed mean plasma concentration-time profiles of bupropion (**A**); hydroxybupropion (**B**); threohydrobupropion (**C**) and erythrohydrobupropion (**D**) after a single oral dose of 150 mg bupropion. The solid lines represent the predicted mean. The dotted lines represent the 5th and 95th percentile of the predicted values for virtual population. Symbols represent mean observed data (*n* = 17) [34,47].

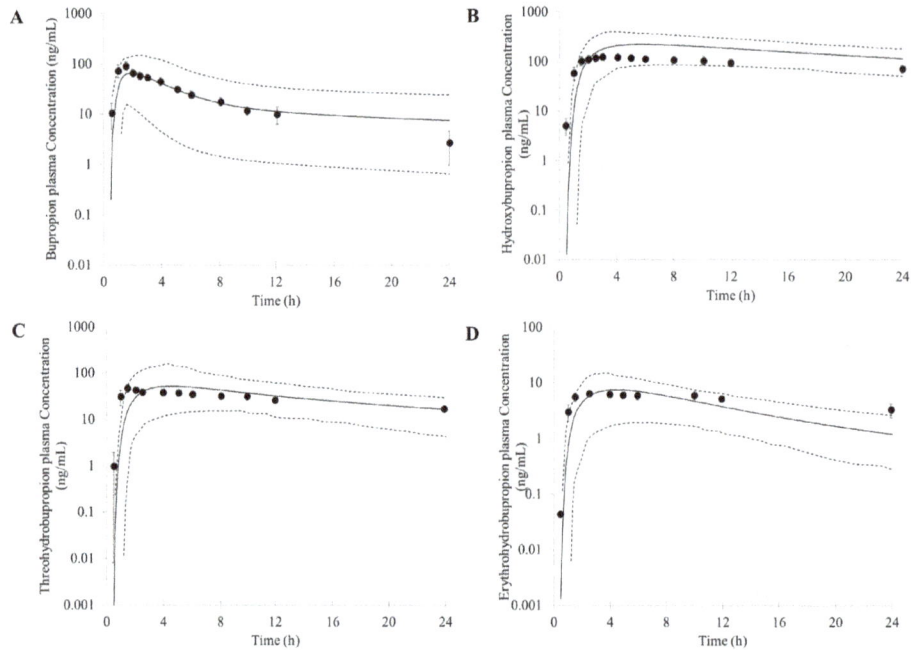

Figure 3. Predicted and observed mean plasma concentration–time profiles of bupropion (**A**); hydroxybupropion (**B**); threohydrobupropion (**C**) and erythrohydrobupropion (**D**) after a single oral dose of 75 mg bupropion. The solid lines represent the predicted mean. The dotted lines represent 5th and 95th percentile of the predicted values for virtual population. Symbols represent mean observed data ($n = 7$) [48].

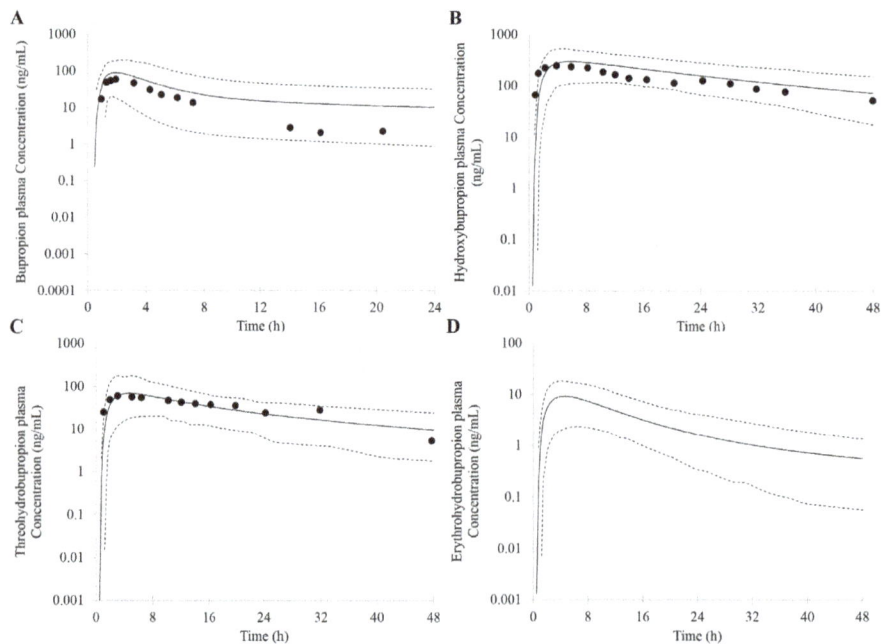

Figure 4. Predicted and observed mean plasma concentration–time profiles of bupropion (**A**); hydroxybupropion (**B**); threohydrobupropion (**C**) and erythrohydrobupropion (**D**) after a single oral dose of 100 mg bupropion. The solid lines represent the predicted mean. The dotted lines represent 5th and 95th percentile of the predicted values for virtual population. Symbols represent mean observed data ($n = 8$) [49].

3.2. Prediction of the Bupropion-Desipramine DDI

Desipramine is a substrate of CYP2D6. Although published in vitro data showed that bupropion and a major active metabolite, hydroxybupropion, were relatively weak CYP2D6 inhibitors (IC50 = 58 and 74 µM, respectively) [27], drug interactions resulting in increased exposure of CYP2D6-metabolized drugs following coadministration with bupropion were observed in clinic.

In this simulation, subjects were given a dose of 150 mg bupropion twice a day for 10 days before the administration of a single dose of 50 mg desipramine. The predicted and observed mean plasma concentration–time profiles of desipramine in the absence and presence of bupropion are shown in Figure 5. The predicted and observed pharmacokinetic parameter values are summarized in Table 5. The clinical interaction results showed a 5.2, 1.9 and 2.0-fold increase in the AUC, C_{max} and T_{max} of desipramine, respectively, when desipramine was codosed with bupropion [28]. The simulated results is reasonably well compared to the observed data when all of the inhibition from bupropion and its metabolites were integrated. The predicted AUC, C_{max} and T_{max} ratio were 5.05, 1.79 and 1.84-fold, respectively.

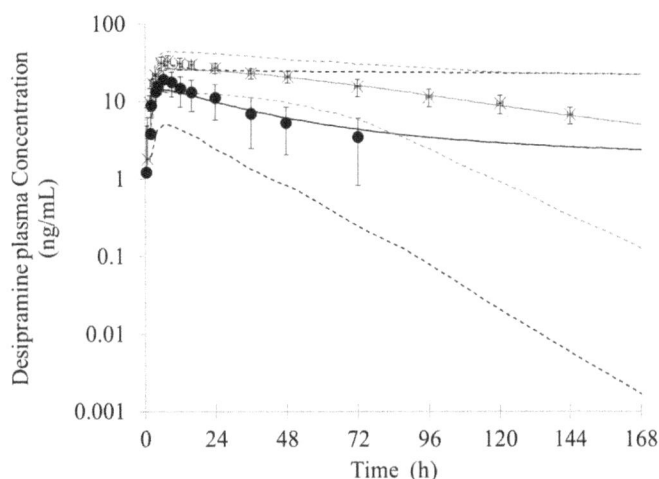

Figure 5. Predicted and observed mean plasma concentration-time profiles of desipramine after a single oral dose of 50 mg desipramine in the absence or presence of a twice-daily dose of 150 mg bupropion. The black solid lines represent the predicted mean concentrations when administered alone; the gray solid lines represent the predicted mean concentrations when co-administered with bupropion. The black and gray dotted lines represent 5th and 95th percentile of the predicted values for virtual population before and after co-administered with bupropion, respectively. Closed circles, observed plasma concentrations when administered alone (n = 15) [28]; Stars, observed plasma concentrations when co-administered with bupropion (n = 15) [28].

Simultaneously, the contribution of DDI for bupropion and its metabolites were simulated using the PBPK model. The model predicted a 2.27, 1.15 and 1.10-fold increase in desipramine AUC, C_{max} and T_{max}, respectively, when bupropion was considered alone as an inhibitor. If each of the metabolites were considered as the only inhibitor, the AUC, C_{max} and T_{max} ratio of metabolites were as follows: hydroxybupropion (4.58, 1.76 and 1.84-fold), threohydrobupropion (3.47, 1.61 and 1.47-fold), and erythrohydrobupropion (2.83, 1.45 and 1.47-fold), respectively. The results indicate that bupropion and its metabolites all are involved in the DDI between bupropion and desipramine. While the inhibition of bupropion is weaker than its metabolites, hydroxybupropion is a relatively strong CYP2D6 inhibitor.

3.3. Prediction of the Bupropion-Venlafaxine DDI

Venlafaxine is another substrate of CYP2D6. The clinical results showed inhibition of venlafaxine metabolism, resulting in a significant, 2.5-fold higher plasma venlafaxine concentration at steady state following co-adminstration of bupropion with venlafaxine [50]. To simulate the DDI, a PBPK model of venlafaxine was developed in the first place. The PBPK model of venlafaxine was successfully built based on the parameters in Table 3. Following a single dose of 75 mg venlafaxine to healthy subjects, the predicted C_{max} (50 ng/mL) and AUC (608 ng·h/mL) matched the observed data well (C_{max} = 34 ng/mL, AUC = 463 ng·h/mL) [51].

Then, a simulation of DDI was performed by the PBPK model. In the study, subjects received bupropion (at a daily dose of 150 mg/day) with venlafaxine (at a daily dose of 75 mg/day) for 8 weeks. The simulated results showed a 2.24-fold of C_{max} ratio when the inhibition from bupropion as well as its metabolites were considered. This model can reasonably predict the clinical DDI. The contribution of DDI for bupropion and its metabolites were also analyzed by this model. The predicted C_{max} ratio of bupropion, hydroxybupropion, threohydrobupropion and erythrohydrobupropion were 1.27, 1.94 1.80 and 1.60-fold. The result was similar to the DDI of bupropion on venlafaxine. There was a minimal effect on bupropion, whereas when the inhibition from hydroxybupropion, threohydrobupropion and erythrohydrobupropion were incorporated, significant DDI was captured (Table 5). In general, the inhibition from hydroxybupropion is the strongest, while bupropion has a relatively weak inhibitory effect.

3.4. Prediction of DDI between Bupropion with Other Potential CYP2D6 Substrates

The PBPK model was also used to predict more DDI of bupropion on other CYP2D6 substrates. The predicted interaction effect on different drugs was listed in Table 6. A simulation of bupropion inhibits dextromethorphan following a single oral dose of 30 mg dextromethorphan after 17 days of co-administration of bupropion (150 mg twice a day) was performed. According to the model, a 4.06 and 3.05-fold of AUC and C_{max} ratio was predicted, respectively. There are reports showed that interaction occurs when dextromethorphan is co-administered with bupropion in healthy volunteers, the mean dextromethorphan/dextrophan ratio was significantly increased in urine [52]. Even though no concentration-time profile data for the DDI study is available for direct comparison, a significant increase in exposure of dextromethorphan after co-administration of bupropion was predicted by our model.

In a case report, a severe bradycardia occurred between buproprion and metoprolol. It suggested that the serious adverse event might be attributed to the CYP2D6 inhibition of bupropion [53]. Following 12 days multiple oral administration of metoprolol 75 mg twice daily with and without coadministration of bupropion (150 mg twice a day), the predicted AUC and C_{max} ratio of metoprolol were 3.53 and 2.57-fold, respectively. This further confirms the need for caution when combining bupropion with metoprolol.

More drug interactions were studied based on the PBPK model. Following a single oral dose of 20 mg bufuralol or 2 mg tolterodine after 2 weeks of coadministration of bupropion (150 mg twice a day), the predicted AUC and C_{max} ratio of bufuralol were 2.04 and 1.55-fold respectively, and the predicted AUC and C_{max} ratio of tolterodine were 2.91 and 2.17-fold, respectively.

3.5. Prediction of Stereo-Selective Bupropion and Its Metabolites Pharmacokinetics and DDI

The above-established PBPK model of stereo-selective bupropion and its metabolites were used to simulate the PK profiles for the subject of 100 mg bupropion administered orally. The results showed that good PK profiles were captured by the PBPK model. All of the predicted C_{max} and AUC were within a two-fold error of the observed results and are shown in Table 8.

Table 8. Observed versus predicted PK data (AUC, C_{max} and T_{max}) of stereo-selective bupropion and its metabolites in the PBPK model of stereo-selective bupropion and its metabolites study.

PK Parameter	AUC (nM·h)		C_{max} (nM)	
	Predicted	Observed [54]	Predicted	Observed [54]
R-BUP	1343.68	1162	196.37	288
S-BUP	291.27	193	53.20	47
RR-OHBUP	37,777.63	37,421	1564.59	1240
SS-OHBUP	524.75	580	33.85	35.9
RR-TB	3228.59	3326	117.19	79.9
SS-TB	1813.4	1433	159.34	168
SR-EB	872.65	942	33.31	30.5
RS-EB	195.48	185	8.12	10.6

R-BUP, R-Bupropion; S-BUP, S-Bupropion; RR-OHBUP, RR-Hydroxybupropion; SS-OHBUP, SS-Hydroxybupropion; RR-TB, RR-Threohydrobupropion; SS-TB, SS-Threohydrobupropion; SR-EB, SR-Erythrohydrobupropion; RS-EB, RS-Erythrohydrobupropion.

On this basis, a DDI between bupropion with desipramine is further simulated following a dose of 150 mg bupropion twice a day for 10 days before the administration of a single dose of 50 mg desipramine. The simulated and observed DDI effect are listed in Table 9. The value of K_i was predicted base on IC50 from in vitro reports [55] in the Simcyp model. A 2.53, 1.21, and 1.47-fold of AUC, C_{max} and T_{max} ratio were predicted, respectively, when the inhibition from R-bupropion, RR-hydroxybupropion, threohydrobupropion and erythrohydrobupropion were integrated. Although the predicted DDI was lower than the observed clinical data. The results indicated that the RR-hydroxybupropion was a major coutribution to the inhibition of CYP2D6 from bupropion.

Table 9. PBPK model-predicted DDIs of between bupropion with desipramine.

Inhibitors	K_i	AUC Ratio	C_{max} Ratio	T_{max} Ratio
Bupropion + Desipramine (observed)		5.2	1.9	2
R-BUP + RR-OHBUP + EB + TB (predicted)		2.53	1.21	1.47
S-BUP + SS-OHBUP + EB + TB (predicted)		1.93	1.03	1.10
R-BUP (predicted)	12.5	1.83	0.96	1.10
S-BUP (predicted)	0.91	1.84	0.97	1.10
RR-OHBUP (predicted)	1.5	2.45	1.19	1.47
SS-OHBUP (predicted)	4.3	1.84	0.97	1.10
Threohydrobupropion (predicted)	3.97	1.88	0.99	1.10
Erythrohydrobupropion (predicted)	0.91	1.87	0.98	1.10

Bup, Bupropion; H-Bup, Hydroxybupropion; T-Bup, Threohydrobupropion; E-Bup, Erythrohydrobupropion; AUC ratio, AUC in the presence of inhibitor/AUC in the absence of inhibitor; C_{max} ratio, C_{max} in the presence of inhibitor/C_{max} in the absence of inhibitor; T_{max} ratio, T_{max} in the presence of inhibitor/T_{max} in the absence of inhibitor.

4. Discussion

It is common to think that the possibility of causing drug interactions for metabolites compared with the parent drug is low. However, recently, more and more studies have shown that the perpetrator drug's metabolites may also have a significant impact on CYP-mediated DDI. With the development of the PBPK model, it has been widely used in various stages of drug development, especially in evaluation of DDIs. The PBPK model can simulate a dynamic process which is closer to the in vivo behavior based on in vitro biotransformation and physicochemical parameters. Many studies have successfully evaluated drug interactions using PBPK model [12,56–58]. However, only a few studies have built a PBPK model to evaluate DDI caused by inhibitory metabolite [18,59–61]. Many compounds, such as bupropion, have an unexpected DDI in clinic, although in vitro study showed that bupropion was a weak CYP2D6 inhibitor. It is possible that the inhibition from metabolites contributes to the observed DDI. To better address this apparent discrepancy between in vitro and in vivo studies, bupropion was chosen as an example, and the PBPK model was employed to describe the complex drug interactions involving inhibitory metabolite.

First, an accurate simulation of PK profiles of both parent and metabolite is required to maximize the confidence in the DDI prediction. Therefore, in our study, many observed PK profiles of different doses were used to verify the bupropion model. A full PBPK distribution model and first order absorption model was used for a good description of bupropion PK profile. Bupropion is mainly metabolized by the liver, and less than 1% of the parent drug is found in the urine [26,29]. In addition to hydroxybupropion that are mediated by CYP enzymes, bupropion is also metabolized by 11β-HSD to form threohydrobupropion and erythrohydrobupropion [62,63]. To better describe and build the PBPK model, CYP2B6 instead of carbonyl reductase was set in Simcyp as the metabolic enzymes of formation of threohydrobupropion and erythrohydrobupropion, and a $f_{u,mic}$ was used to correct the expression of carbonyl reductase to obtain the best simulation results compared to observed data.

For those uncertain or unknown parameters, a sensitivity analysis is performed to assess the importance and effect of these parameters in human PK and DDI prediction. In the PBPK model of bupropion, the logP, pKa, and three $f_{u,mic}$ were considered for sensitivity analysis. According to the analysis, the logP, pKa and the $f_{u,mic}$ for formation of erythrohydrobupropion were not sensitive to the prediction of PK. However, $f_{u,mic}$ for formation of hydroxybupropion and threohydrobupropion has a certain impact on the prediction of PK and the $f_{u,mic}$ for formation of erythrohydrobupropion. Thus, the logP and pKa from the drug bank were inputted into the model. The $f_{u,mic}$ for formation of hydroxybupropion and threohydrobupropion were optimized at the 0.16 and 0.003, respectively. The erythrohydrobupropion and threohydrobupropion are formed via reduction of the carbonyl group. Thus, the same $f_{u,mic}$ is integrated into the model. The detailed sensitivity analysis results are shown in Supplementary Figure S1.

Based on the in vitro data and the mechanisms mentioned above, 1% of the fe (fraction of total body clearance via renal excretion) and geometric mean 174 (L/h) of CL were reasonably predicted by the PBPK model. Studies have shown that the CL for bupropion is in the range of 113 to 215 L/h [31,47,49,64–68]. For the PK profile of metabolites, the minimal PBPK distribution model or minimal PBPK distribution model + adjusting compartment distribution model have a good description based on in vitro data, in silico data and clinical PK data. More importantly, the developed PBPK model was well captured the PK profile after oral dose of 75 mg and 100 mg bupropion.

In the Simcyp, the user can only simultaneously select one specified inhibitor metabolite to simulate the interaction effects. To better describe the actual clinical DDI, metabolites were regarded as different inhibitors and combined with bupropion to simulate the complex DDI with other CYP2D6 substrates. A sensitivity analysis on the dosage of metabolites was conducted; the results predicted by the model were in good agreement with the observed PK profiles when doses of hydroxybupropion, threohydrobupropion and erythrohydrobupropion were assumed to be 90 mg, 30 mg and 4 mg, respectively. This indicates that the plasma concentration of metabolites formed by single oral 150 mg bupropion is equivalent to plasma levels in vivo after a single oral of 90 mg hydroxybupropion, 30 mg threohydrobupropion and 4 mg erythrohydrobupropion, respectively. (Figure 6). The predicted C_{max} (hydroxybupropion 443 ng/mL threohydrobupropion 107 ng/mL and erythrohydrobupropion 16 ng/mL) and AUC (hydroxybupropion 15,215 ng·h/mL, threohydrobupropion 1178 ng·h/mL and erythrohydrobupropion 185 ng·h/mL) were within 2-fold error of the observed values [34,47].

To sum up, dynamic PK process of bupropion and its metabolites were well characterized in PBPK models. The successful simulations of clinically observed PK profiles build confidence in the prediction and mechanistic understanding of the DDI caused by bupropion, and particularly the unexpected DDI potential contributed by its metabolites. On the basis of the above model, we then applied the PBPK model to predict the clinically observed DDIs involving bupropion and its metabolites as the CYP2D6 inhibitors. The result contribute to the understanding of the involvement and impact of inhibitory metabolites on DDIs observed in the clinic.

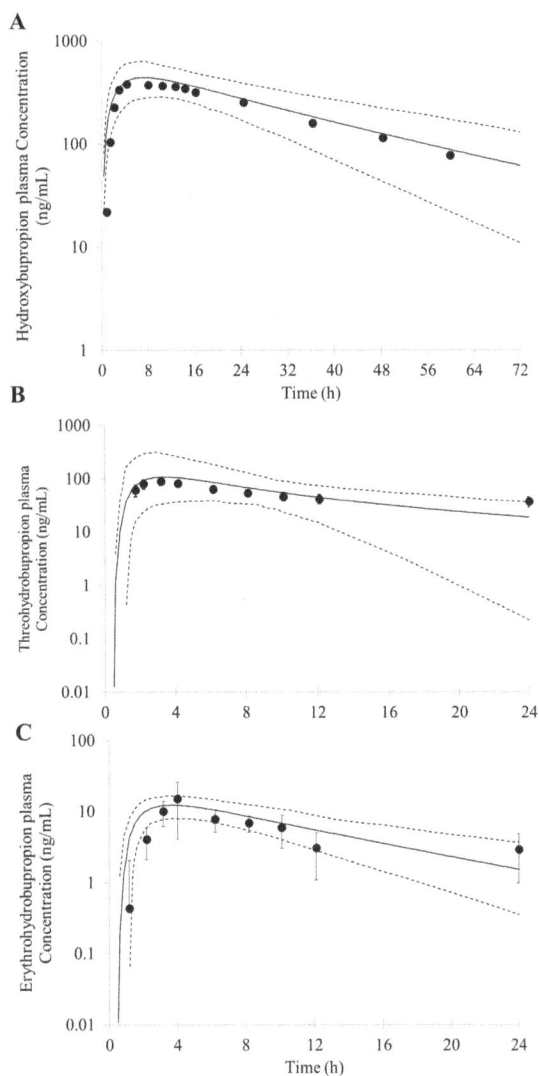

Figure 6. Predicted and observed mean plasma concentration–time profiles of hydroxybupropion with 90 mg (**A**); threohydrobupropion with 30 mg (**B**) and erythrohydrobupropion with 4 mg (**C**). The solid lines represents the predicted mean. The dotted lines represents 5th and 95th percentile of the predicted values for virtual population. Symbols represent mean observed data which is metabolized from a single oral dose of 150 mg bupropion (*n* = 17) [34,47].

In the simulation of bupropion-desipramine interaction, the addition of the inhibitory metabolites into the PBPK model resulted in more accurate prediction of DDIs (AUC and C_{max} ratio) compared with that when only the inhibition of P450 from the parent drug (bupropion) was taken into account. The simulation suggests that bupropion and its metabolites contribute to the DDI between bupropion and desipramin. Although in vitro study showed that the inhibitory potency from strong to weak were erythrohydrobupropion, threohydrobupropion, hydroxybupropion and bupropion, respectively, the simulation of in vivo DDI suggests that hydroxybupropion is the most potent competitive CYP2D6 inhibitor. It can be possible due to the greater exposure of hydroxybupropion. The plasma level of hydroxybupropion is five- to ten-fold higher than the parent drug [29,69–72]. The exposure of threohydrobupropion is similar to the parent drug; however, it has a stronger in vitro inhibition constant than parent drug and hydroxybupropion. For the erythrobupropion, it is predicted to have similar importance in in vivo DDIs as hydroxybupropion, despite the fact that its plasma concentration is much lower than hydroxybupropion. This may be related to its strongest inhibition constant. Conversely, even though the exposure of bupropion is similar to threohydrobupropion. The PBPK simulation shows bupropion is the weakest competitive CYP2D6 inhibitor. The result may attribute to the relatively weakest inhibition constant.

Consistently, a minimal effect of bupropion on venlafaxine was predicted if only the competitive inhibition from the parent drug was considered. With the addition of the inhibitory metabolites into the PBPK model, there was a more accurate prediction of DDIs. The inhibitory potency from strong to weak was hydroxybupropion, threohydrobupropion, erythrohydrobupropion, and bupropion, respectively.

In the DDI study of bupropion with other CYP2D6 substrates, the significant increase in exposure of dextromethorphan, metoprolol, bufuralol and tolterodine after coadministration of bupropion was predicted. These DDI predictions may explain the occurrence of severe sinus bradycardia after coadministration of bupropion and metoprolol and highlight the need for caution and dosage adjustment when combining bupropion with medications metabolized by CYP2D6.

To better understand the effect of stereo-selective bupropion and its metabolites on the DDI, a stereo-selective PBPK model for bupropion and its metabolites was further developed. The PBPK model considered multiple metabolic pathways including CYP2B6, 2C19, 3A4 and carbonyl reductase, and it is reasonable to describe the proportion of each metabolite in total clearance of bupropion. The simulated PK profile was a good match with the observed clinical data, although, in the simulation of DDI between bupropion with desipramine, the predicted DDI was lower than the observed. The results indicated that RR-hydroxybupropion was a major contributor to the inhibition of CYP2D6 from bupropion. The inhibitory effect of bupropion on CYP2D6 may be the result of synergistic production of all stereo-selective parent drugs and its metabolites. Currently, all inhibitors cannot be simultaneously integrated into the model for simulation. Only four inhibitors can be allowed to integrate into the model in Simcyp. In addition, the stereo-chemical threohydrobupropion and erythrohydrobupropion may have different inhibitory contributions compared to non-stereo-chemical, and the in vitro inhibition rate constants of the stereo-chemical threohydrobupropion and erythrohydrobupropion have not been reported. The PBPK model of stereo-selective bupropion and its metabolites still need to be further improved and optimized after obtaining more data in the future.

Overall, we successfully developed a PBPK model to describe the dynamic PK process of bupropion and its metabolites and understand the involvement and impact of inhibitory metabolites for DDIs observed in the clinic. The present bupropion PBPK model can be useful for predicting inhibition from bupropion in other clinical studies. However, the use of the PBPK model for a true prospective prediction of DDI caused by inhibitory metabolite is still very challenging, as the in vitro inhibition and human PK data for the metabolite are not routinely generated. To maximize confidence in the DDI prediction, more information is needed for the inhibitory potency of the metabolites towards the P450 enzymes.

Acknowledgments: This study was supported by a grant from the National Natural Science Foundation of China [Grant No. 81673501].

Author Contributions: Caifu Xue and Weimin Cai designed the research; Caifu Xue and Xuejie Zhang performed the research, analyzed the data and wrote the paper; Weimin Cai reviewed and revised the paper.

References

1.   Huang, S.M.; Lesko, L.J. Drug-drug, drug-dietary supplement, and drug-citrus fruit and other food interactions: What have we learned? *J. Clin. Pharmacol.* **2004**, *44*, 559–569. [CrossRef] [PubMed]
2.   Krayenbühl, J.C.; Vozeh, S.; Kondo-Oestreicher, M.; Dayer, P. Drug-drug interactions or new active substances; mibefradil example. *Eur. J. Clin. Pharmacol.* **1999**, *55*, 559–565. [PubMed]

3. Lee, S.Y.; Jang, H.; Lee, J.Y.; Kwon, K.I.; Oh, S.J.; Kim, S.K. Inhibition of cytochrome P450 by ethambutol in human liver microsomes. *Toxicol. Lett.* **2014**, *229*, 33–40. [CrossRef] [PubMed]

4. Wienkers, L.C.; Heath, T.G. Predicting in vivo drug interactions from in vitro drug discovery data. *Nat. Rev. Drug Discov.* **2005**, *4*, 825–833. [CrossRef] [PubMed]

5. Prueksaritanont, T.; Chu, X.; Gibson, C.; Cui, D.; Yee, K.L.; Ballard, J.; Cabalu, T.; Hochman, J. Drug-drug interaction studies: Regulatory guidance and an industry perspective. *AAPS J.* **2013**, *15*, 629–645. [CrossRef] [PubMed]

6. Callegari, E.; Kalgutkar, A.S.; Leung, L.; Obach, R.S.; Plowchalk, D.R.; Tse, S. Drug metabolites as cytochrome p450 inhibitors: A retrospective analysis and proposed algorithm for evaluation of the pharmacokinetic interaction potential of metabolites in drug discovery and development. *Drug Metab. Dispos.* **2013**, *41*, 2047–2055. [CrossRef] [PubMed]

7. Isoherranen, N.; Hachad, H.; Yeung, C.K.; Levy, R.H. Qualitative analysis of the role of metabolites in inhibitory drug-drug interactions: Literature evaluation based on the metabolism and transport drug interaction database. *Chem. Res. Toxicol.* **2009**, *22*, 294–298. [CrossRef] [PubMed]

8. Yeung, C.K.; Fujioka, Y.; Hachad, H.; Levy, R.H.; Isoherranen, N. Are circulating metabolites important in drug-drug interactions? Quantitative analysis of risk prediction and inhibitory potency. *Clin. Pharmacol. Ther.* **2011**, *89*, 105–113. [CrossRef] [PubMed]

9. US Department of Health and Human Services, Food and Drug Administration, Center for Drug Evaluation and Research (CDER). Drug Interaction Studies—Study Design, Data Analysis, Implications for Dosing, and Labeling Recommendations Draft Guidance. Available online: http://www.fda.gov/downloads/Drugs/GuidanceComplianceRegulatoryInformation/Guidances/ucm292362.pdf (accessed on 31 October 2017).

10. European Medicines Agency, Committee for Human Medicinal Products (CHMP). Guideline on the Investigation of Drug Interactions. Available online: http://www.ema.europa.eu/docs/en_GB/document_library/Scientific_guideline/2012/07/WC500129606.pdf (accessed on 31 October 2017).

11. Huang, S.M.; Rowland, M. The role of physiologically based pharmacokinetic modeling in regulatory review. *Clin. Pharmacol. Ther.* **2012**, *91*, 542–549. [CrossRef] [PubMed]

12. Fenneteau, F.; Poulin, P.; Nekka, F. Physiologically based predictions of the impact of inhibition of intestinal and hepatic metabolism on human pharmacokinetics of CYP3A substrates. *J. Pharm. Sci.* **2010**, *99*, 486–514. [CrossRef] [PubMed]

13. Jamei, M.; Marciniak, S.; Feng, K.; Barnett, A.; Tucker, G.T.; Rostami-Hodjegan, A. The Simcyp population-based ADME simulator. *Expert Opin. Drug Metab. Toxicol.* **2009**, *5*, 211–223. [CrossRef] [PubMed]

14. Kato, M.; Shitara, Y.; Sato, H.; Yoshisue, K.; Hirano, M.; Ikeda, T.; Sugiyama, Y. The quantitative prediction of CYP mediated drug interaction by physiologically based pharmacokineticmodeling. *Pharm. Res.* **2008**, *25*, 1891–1901. [CrossRef] [PubMed]

15. Vossen, M.; Sevestre, M.; Niederalt, C.; Jang, I.J.; Willmann, S.; Edginton, A.N. Dynamically simulating the interaction of midazolam and the CYP3A4 inhibitor itraconazole using individual coupled wholebody physiologically-based pharmacokinetic (WB-PBPK) models. *Theor. Biol. Med. Model.* **2007**, *4*, 13. [CrossRef] [PubMed]

16. Fahmi, O.A.; Maurer, T.S.; Kish, M.; Cardenas, E.; Boldt, S.; Nettleton, D. A combined model for predicting CYP3A4 clinical net drug-drug interaction based on CYP3A4 inhibition, inactivation, and induction determined in vitro. *Drug Metab. Dispos.* **2008**, *36*, 1698–1708. [CrossRef] [PubMed]

17. Rostami-Hodjegan, A.; Tucker, G.T. 'In silico' simulations to assess the 'in vivo' consequences of 'in vitro' metabolic drug-drug interactions. *Drug Discov. Today Technol.* **2004**, *1*, 441–448. [CrossRef] [PubMed]

18. Rowland Yeo, K.; Jamei, M.; Yang, J.; Tucker, G.T.; Rostami-Hodjegan, A. Physiologically basedmechanistic modeling to predict complex drug-drug interactions involving simultaneous competitive and time-dependent enzyme inhibition by parent compound and its metabolite in both liver and gut-the effect of diltiazem on the time-course of exposure to triazolam. *Eur. J. Pharm. Sci.* **2010**, *39*, 298–309. [PubMed]

19. Zhang, X.; Quinney, S.K.; Gorski, J.C.; Jones, D.R.; Hall, S.D. Semiphysiologically based pharmacokinetic models for the inhibition of midazolam clearance by diltiazem and its major metabolite. *Drug Metab. Dispos.* **2009**, *37*, 1587–1597. [CrossRef] [PubMed]

20. Huang, S.M. PBPK as a tool in regulatory review. *Biopharm. Drug Dispos.* **2012**, *33*, 51–52. [CrossRef] [PubMed]

21. Leong, R.; Vieira, M.L.; Zhao, P.; Mulugeta, Y.; Lee, C.S.; Huang, S.M.; Burckart, G.J. Regulatory experience with physiologically based pharmacokinetic modeling for pediatric drug trials. *Clin. Pharmacol. Ther.* **2012**, *91*, 926–931. [CrossRef] [PubMed]

22. Sinha, V.; Zhao, P.; Huang, S.M.; Zineh, I. Physiologically based pharmacokinetic modeling: From regulatory science to regulatory policy. *Clin. Pharmacol. Ther.* **2014**, *95*, 478–480. [CrossRef] [PubMed]

23. Zhao, P.; Rowland, M.; Huang, S.M. Best practice in the use of physiologically based pharmacokinetic modeling and simulation to address clinical pharmacology regulatory questions. *Clin. Pharmacol. Ther.* **2012**, *92*, 17–20. [CrossRef] [PubMed]

24. Faucette, S.R.; Hawke, R.L.; Lecluyse, E.L.; Shord, S.S.; Yan, B.; Laethem, R.M.; Lindley, C.M. Validation of bupropion hydroxylation as a selective marker of human cytochrome P450 2B6 catalytic activity. *Drug Metab. Dispos.* **2000**, *28*, 1222–1230. [PubMed]

25. Golden, R.N.; De Vane, C.L.; Laizure, S.C.; Rudorfer, M.V.; Sherer, M.A.; Potter, W.Z. Bupropion in depression. II. The role of metabolites in clinical outcome. *Arch. Gen. Psychiatry* **1988**, *45*, 145–149. [CrossRef] [PubMed]

26. Schroeder, D.H. Metabolism and kinetics of bupropion. *J. Clin. Psychiatry* **1983**, *44*, 79–81. [PubMed]

27. Hesse, L.M.; Nevkatakrishnan, K.; Court, M.H.; von Moltke, L.L.; Duan, S.X.; Shader, R.I.; Greenblatt, D.J. 2B6 mediates the in vitro hydroxylation of bupropion: Potential drug interactions with other antidipressants. *Drug Metab. Dispos.* **2000**, *28*, 1176–1183. [PubMed]

28. Reese, M.J.; Wurm, R.M.; Muir, K.T.; Generaux, G.T.; St John-Williams, L.; McConn, D.J. An in vitro mechanistic study to elucidate the desipramine/bupropion clinical drug-drug interaction. *Drug Metab. Dispos.* **2008**, *36*, 1198–1201. [CrossRef] [PubMed]

29. Jefferson, J.W.; Pradko, J.F.; Muir, K.T. Bupropion for major depressive disorder: Pharmacokinetic and formulation considerations. *Clin. Ther.* **2005**, *27*, 1685–1695. [CrossRef] [PubMed]

30. Rodgers, T.; Rowland, M. Physiologically based pharmacokinetic modelling 2: Predicting the tissue distribution of acids, very weak bases, neutrals and zwitterions. *J. Pharm. Sci.* **2006**, *95*, 1238–1257. [CrossRef] [PubMed]

31. Findlay, J.W.; Van Wyck Fleet, J.; Smith, P.G.; Butz, R.F.; Hinton, M.L.; Blum, M.R.; Schroeder, D.H. Pharmacokinetics of bupropion, a novel antidepressant agent, following oral administration to healthy subjects. *Eur. J. Clin. Pharmacol.* **1981**, *21*, 127–135. [CrossRef] [PubMed]

32. Kirchheiner, J.; Klein, C.; Meineke, I.; Sasse, J.; Zanger, U.M.; Mürdter, T.E.; Roots, I.; Brockmöller, J. Bupropion and 4-OH-bupropion pharmacokinetics in relation to genetic polymorphisms in CYP2B6. *Pharmacogenetics* **2003**, *13*, 619–626. [CrossRef] [PubMed]

33. Connarn, J.N.; Zhang, X.; Babiskin, A.; Sun, D. Metabolism of bupropion by carbonyl reductases in liver and intestine. *Drug Metab. Dispos.* **2015**, *43*, 1019–1027. [CrossRef] [PubMed]

34. Ketter, T.A.; Jenkins, J.B.; Schroeder, D.H.; Pazzaglia, P.J.; Marangell, L.B.; George, M.S.; Callahan, A.M.; Hinton, M.L.; Chao, J.; Post, R.M. Carbamazepine but not valproate induces bupropion metabolism. *J. Clin. Psychopharmacol.* **1995**, *15*, 327–333. [CrossRef] [PubMed]

35. Poulin, P.; Theil, F.P. Prediction of pharmacokinetics prior to in vivo studies. 1. Mechanism-based prediction of volume of distribution. *J. Pharm. Sci.* **2002**, *91*, 129–156. [CrossRef] [PubMed]

36. Ereshefsky, L.; Dugan, D. Review of the pharmacokinetics, pharmacogenetics, and drug interaction potential of antidepressants: Focus on venlafaxine. *Depress. Anxiety* **2000**, *12* (Suppl. 1), 30–44. [CrossRef]

37. Magalhães, P.; Alves, G.; LLerena, A.; Falcão, A. Clinical drug-drug interaction: Focus on venlafaxine. *Drug Metab. Pers. Ther.* **2015**, *30*, 3–17. [CrossRef] [PubMed]

38. Taft, D.R.; Iyer, G.R.; Behar, L.; DiGregorio, R.V. Application of a first-pass effect model to characterize the pharmacokinetic disposition of venlafaxine after oral administration to human subjects. *Drug Metab. Dispos.* **1997**, *25*, 1215–1218. [PubMed]

39. Fogelman, S.M.; Schmider, J.; Venkatakrishnan, K.; von Moltke, L.L.; Harmatz, J.S.; Shader, R.I.; Greenblatt, D.J. O-and N-demethylation of venlafaxine in vitro by human liver microsomes and by microsomes from cDNA-transfected cells: Effect of metabolic inhibitors and SSRI antidepressants. *Neuropsychopharmacology* **1999**, *20*, 480–490. [CrossRef]

40. Siccardi, M.; Marzolini, C.; Seden, K.; Almond, L.; Kirov, A.; Khoo, S.; Owen, A.; Back, D. Prediction of drug-drug interactions between various antidepressants and efavirenz or boosted protease inhibitors using a physiologically based pharmacokinetic modelling approach. *Clin. Pharmacokinet.* **2013**, *52*, 583–592. [CrossRef] [PubMed]

41. De Buck, S.S.; Sinha, V.K.; Fenu, L.A.; Gilissen, R.A.; Mackie, C.E.; Nijsen, M.J. The prediction of drug metabolism, tissue distribution, and bioavailability of 50 structurally diverse compounds in rat using mechanism-based absorption, distribution, and metabolism prediction tools. *Drug Metab. Dispos.* **2007**, *35*, 649–659. [CrossRef] [PubMed]

42. Jones, H.M.; Parrott, N.; Jorga, K.; Lavé, T. A novel strategy for physiologically based predictions of human pharmacokinetics. *Clin. Pharmacokinet.* **2006**, *45*, 511–542. [CrossRef] [PubMed]

43. Parrott, N.; Paquereau, N.; Coassolo, P.; Lave, T. An evaluation of the utility of physiologically based models of pharmacokinetics in early drug discovery. *J. Pharm. Sci.* **2005**, *94*, 2327–2343. [CrossRef] [PubMed]

44. Yamazaki, S.; Skaptason, J.; Romero, D.; Vekich, S.; Jones, H.M.; Tan, W.; Wilner, K.D.; Koudriakova, T. Prediction of oral pharmacokinetics of cMet kinase inhibitors in humans: Physiologically based pharmacokinetic model versus traditional one compartment model. *Drug Metab. Dispos.* **2011**, *39*, 383–393. [CrossRef] [PubMed]

45. Sager, J.E.; Price, L.S.; Isoherranen, N. Stereoselective metabolism of bupropion to OHbupropion, threohydrobupropion, erythrohydrobupropion, and 4′-OH-bupropion in vitro. *Drug Metab. Dispos.* **2016**, *44*, 1709–1719. [CrossRef] [PubMed]

46. Dash, R.P.; Rais, R.; Srinivas, N.R. Chirality and neuropsychiatric drugs: An update on stereoselective disposition and clinical pharmacokinetics of bupropion. *Xenobiotica* **2017**, *13*, 1–13. [CrossRef] [PubMed]

47. Hsyu, P.H.; Singh, A.; Giargiari, T.D.; Dunn, J.A.; Ascher, J.A.; Johnston, J.A. Pharmacokinetics of bupropion and its metabolites in cigarette smokers versus nonsmokers. *J. Clin. Pharmacol.* **1997**, *37*, 737–743. [CrossRef] [PubMed]

48. Hesse, L.M.; Greenblatt, D.J.; von Moltke, L.L.; Court, M.H. Ritonavir has minimal impact on the pharmacokinetic disposition of a single dose of bupropion administered to human volunteers. *J. Clin. Pharmacol.* **2006**, *46*, 567–576. [CrossRef] [PubMed]

49. Posner, J.; Bye, A.; Dean, K.; Peck, A.W.; Whiteman, P.D. The disposition of bupropion and its metabolites in healthy male volunteers after single and multiple doses. *Eur. J. Clin. Pharmacol.* **1985**, *29*, 97–103. [CrossRef] [PubMed]

50. Kennedy, S.H.; McCann, S.M.; Masellis, M.; McIntyre, R.S.; Raskin, J.; McKay, G.; Baker, G.B. Combining bupropion SR with venlafaxine, paroxetine, or fluoxetine: A preliminary report on pharmacokinetic, therapeutic, and sexual dysfunction effects. *J. Clin. Psychiatry* **2002**, *63*, 181–186. [CrossRef] [PubMed]

51. Jiang, F.; Kim, H.D.; Na, H.S.; Lee, S.Y.; Seo, D.W.; Choi, J.Y.; Ha, J.H.; Shin, H.J.; Kim, Y.H.; Chung, M.W. The influences of CYP2D6 genotypes and drug interactions on the pharmacokinetics of venlafaxine: Exploring predictive biomarkers for treatment outcomes. *Psychopharmacology* **2015**, *232*, 1899–1909. [CrossRef] [PubMed]

52. Kotlyar, M.; Brauer, L.H.; Tracy, T.S.; Hatsukami, D.K.; Harris, J.; Bronars, C.A.; Adson, D.E. Inhibition of CYP2D6 activity by bupropion. *J. Clin. Psychopharmacol.* **2005**, *25*, 226–229. [CrossRef] [PubMed]

53. McCollum, D.L.; Greene, J.L.; McGuire, D.K. Severe sinus bradycardia after initiation of bupropion therapy: A probable drug-drug interaction with metoprolol. *Cardiovasc. Drugs Ther.* **2004**, *18*, 329–330. [CrossRef] [PubMed]

54. Masters, A.R.; Gufford, B.T.; Lu, J.B.; Metzger, I.F.; Jones, D.R.; Desta, Z. Chiral plasma pharmacokinetics and urinary excretion of bupropion and metabolites in healthy volunteers. *J. Pharmacol. Exp. Ther.* **2016**, *358*, 230–238. [CrossRef] [PubMed]

55. Sager, J.E.; Tripathy, S.; Price, L.S.; Nath, A.; Chang, J.; Stephenson-Famy, A.; Isoherranen, N. In vitro to in vivo extrapolation of the complex drug-drug interaction of bupropion and its metabolites with CYP2D6; simultaneous reversible inhibition and CYP2D6 downregulation. *Biochem. Pharmacol.* **2017**, *123*, 85–96. [CrossRef] [PubMed]

56. Chenel, M.; Bouzom, F.; Cazade, F.; Ogungbenro, K.; Aarons, L.; Mentré, F. Drug-drug interaction predictions with PBPK models and optimal multiresponse sampling time designs: Application to midazolam and a phase I compound. Part 2: Clinical trial results. *J. Pharmacokinet. Pharmacodyn.* **2008**, *35*, 661–681. [CrossRef] [PubMed]

57. Jones, H.M.; Dickins, M.; Youdim, K.; Gosset, J.R.; Attkins, N.J.; Hay, T.L.; Gurrell, I.K.; Logan, Y.R.; Bungay, P.J.; Jones, B.C.; et al. Application of PBPK modelling in drug discovery and development at Pfizer. *Xenobiotica* **2012**, *42*, 94–106. [CrossRef] [PubMed]

58. Perdaems, N.; Blasco, H.; Vinson, C.; Chenel, M.; Whalley, S.; Cazade, F.; Bouzom, F. Predictions of metabolic drug-drug interactions using physiologically based modelling: Two cytochrome P450 3A4 substrates coadministered with ketoconazole or verapamil. *Clin. Pharmacokinet.* **2010**, *49*, 239–258. [CrossRef] [PubMed]

59. Chen, Y.; Mao, J.; Hop, C.E. Physiologically based pharmacokinetic modeling to predict drug-drug interactions involving inhibitory metabolite: A case study of amiodarone. *Drug Metab. Dispos.* **2015**, *43*, 182–189. [CrossRef] [PubMed]

60. Kudo, T.; Hisaka, A.; Sugiyama, Y.; Ito, K. Analysis of the repaglinide concentration increase produced by gemfibrozil and itraconazole based on the inhibition of the hepatic uptake transporter and metabolic enzymes. *Drug Metab. Dispos.* **2013**, *41*, 362–371. [CrossRef] [PubMed]

61. Varma, M.V.S.; Lai, Y.; Kimoto, E.; Goosen, T.C.; El-Kattan, A.F.; Kumar, V. Mechanistic modeling to predict the transporter- and enzyme-mediated drug-drug interactions of repaglinide. *Pharm. Res.* **2013**, *30*, 1188–1199. [CrossRef] [PubMed]

62. Loboz, K.K.; Gross, A.S.; Ray, J.; McLachlan, A.J. HPLC assay for bupropion and its major metabolites in human plasma. *J. Chromatogr. B Anal. Technol. Biomed. Life Sci.* **2005**, *823*, 115–121. [CrossRef] [PubMed]

63. Matsunaga, T.; Shintani, S.; Hara, A. Multiplicity of mammalian reductases for xenobiotic carbonyl compounds. *Drug Metab. Pharmacokinet.* **2006**, *21*, 1–18. [CrossRef] [PubMed]

64. Daviss, W.B.; Perel, J.M.; Rudolph, G.R.; Axelson, D.A.; Gilchrist, R.; Nuss, S.; Birmaher, B.; Brent, D.A. Steady-state pharmacokinetics of bupropion SR in juvenile patients. *J. Am. Acad. Child. Adolesc. Psychiatry* **2005**, *44*, 349–357. [CrossRef] [PubMed]

65. Loboz, K.K.; Gross, A.S.; Williams, K.M.; Liauw, W.S.; Day, R.O.; Blievernicht, J.K.; Zanger, U.M.; McLachlan, A.J. Cytochrome P450 2B6 activity as measured by bupropion hydroxylation: Effect of induction by rifampin and ethnicity. *Clin. Pharmacol. Ther.* **2006**, *80*, 75–84. [CrossRef] [PubMed]

66. Palovaara, S.; Pelkonen, O.; Uusitalo, J.; Lundgren, S.; Laine, K. Inhibition of cytochrome P450 2B6 activity by hormone replacement therapy and oral contraceptive as measured by bupropion hydroxylation. *Clin. Pharmacol. Ther.* **2003**, *74*, 326–333. [CrossRef]

67. Stewart, J.J.; Berkel, H.J.; Parish, R.C.; Simar, M.R.; Syed, A.; Bocchini, J.A., Jr.; Wilson, J.T.; Manno, J.E. Single-dose pharmacokinetics of bupropion in adolescents: Effects of smoking status and gender. *J. Clin. Pharmacol.* **2001**, *41*, 770–778. [CrossRef] [PubMed]

68. Worrall, S.P.; Almond, M.K.; Dhillon, S. Pharmacokinetics of bupropion and its metabolites in haemodialysis patients who smoke. A single dose study. *Nephron. Clin. Pract.* **2004**, *97*, c83–c89. [CrossRef] [PubMed]

69. Bondarev, M.L.; Bondareva, T.S.; Young, R.; Glennon, R.A. Behavioral and biochemical investigations of bupropion metabolites. *Eur. J. Pharmacol.* **2003**, *474*, 85–93. [CrossRef]

70. Damaj, M.I.; Carroll, F.I.; Eaton, J.B.; Navarro, H.A.; Blough, B.E.; Mirza, S.; Lukas, R.J.; Martin, B.R. Enantioselective effects of hydroxy metabolites of bupropion on behavior and on function of monoamine transporters and nicotinic receptors. *Mol. Pharmacol.* **2004**, *66*, 675–682. [CrossRef] [PubMed]

71. Damaj, M.I.; Grabus, S.D.; Navarro, H.A.; Vann, R.E.; Warner, J.A.; King, L.S.; Wiley, J.L.; Blough, B.E.; Lukas, R.J.; Carroll, F.I. Effects of hydroxymetabolites of bupropion on nicotine dependence behavior in mice. *J. Pharmacol. Exp. Ther.* **2010**, *334*, 1087–1095. [CrossRef] [PubMed]

72. Zhu, A.Z.; Cox, L.S.; Nollen, N.; Faseru, B.; Okuyemi, K.S.; Ahluwalia, J.S.; Benowitz, N.L.; Tyndale, R.F. CYP2B6 and bupropion's smoking-cessation pharmacology: The role of hydroxybupropion. *Clin. Pharmacol. Ther.* **2012**, *92*, 771–777. [CrossRef] [PubMed]

2

Magnetic Nanoparticles Conjugated with Peptides Derived from Monocyte Chemoattractant Protein-1 as a Tool for Targeting Atherosclerosis

Chung-Wei Kao [1,†], Po-Ting Wu [1,†], Mei-Yi Liao [2], I-Ju Chung [3], Kai-Chien Yang [4,*], Wen-Yih Isaac Tseng [3,5,*] and Jiashing Yu [1,5,*] (ID)

[1] Department of Chemical Engineering, National Taiwan University, Taipei 10617, Taiwan; r04524101@ntu.edu.tw (C.-W.K.); r05524112@ntu.edu.tw (P.-T.W.)

[2] Department of Applied Chemistry, National Pingtung University, Pingtung 90003, Taiwan; myliao@mail.nptu.edu.tw

[3] Department and Graduate Institute of Pharmacology College of Medicine, National Taiwan University, Taipei 10617, Taiwan; r05458006@ntu.edu.tw

[4] Institute of Medical Device and Imaging, National Taiwan University, Taipei 10617, Taiwan

[5] Molecular Imaging Center, National Taiwan University, Taipei 10617, Taiwan

* Correspondence kcyang@ntu.edu.tw (K.-C.Y.); wytseng@ntu.edu.tw (W.-Y.I.T.); jiayu@ntu.edu.tw (J.Y.)

† These authors contributed equally to this work.

Abstract: Atherosclerosis is a multifactorial inflammatory disease that may progress silently for long period, and it is also widely accepted as the main cause of cardiovascular diseases. To prevent atherosclerotic plaques from generating, imaging early molecular markers and quantifying the extent of disease progression are desired. During inflammation, circulating monocytes leave the bloodstream and migrate into incipient lipid accumulation in the artery wall, following conditioning by local growth factors and proinflammatory cytokines; therefore, monocyte accumulation in the arterial wall can be observed in fatty streaks, rupture-prone plaques, and experimental atherosclerosis. In this work, we synthesized monocyte-targeting iron oxide magnetic nanoparticles (MNPs), which were incorporated with the peptides derived from the chemokine receptor C-C chemokine receptor type 2 (CCR2)-binding motif of monocytes chemoattractant protein-1 (MCP-1) as a diagnostic tool for potential atherosclerosis. MCP-1-motif MNPs co-localized with monocytes in in vitro fluorescence imaging. In addition, with MNPs injection in ApoE knockout mice (ApoE KO mice), the well-characterized animal model of atherosclerosis, MNPs were found in specific organs or regions which had monocytes accumulation, especially the aorta of atherosclerosis model mice, through in vivo imaging system (IVIS) imaging and magnetic resonance imaging (MRI). We also performed Oil Red O staining and Prussian Blue staining to confirm the co-localization of MCP-1-motif MNPs and atherosclerosis. The results showed the promising potential of MCP-1-motif MNPs as a diagnostic agent of atherosclerosis.

Keywords: iron oxide magnetic nanoparticle; monocytes; MCP-1; atherosclerosis

1. Introduction

Atherosclerosis, the primary cause of cardiovascular diseases, is a chronic inflammatory disorder in the walls of large arteries or the medium and intima of large arteries. Inflammation is the immune system's response to injury and has been implicated in the pathogeneses of aortas. After lipid-rich plaques and cholesterol particles accumulate within the artery wall, endothelial cell dysfunction/activation is then triggered by the accumulation of low-density lipoprotein (LDL) and other lipoproteins. Afterward, the inflamed endothelial cells and oxidized lipids induce the excretion of chemokines, cytokines, and mediators of inflammation into the bloodstream for monocytes and other immune cells recruitment to the site. As the monocytes migrate into the aorta wall, they differentiate into dendritic cells, macrophages, or foam cells [1,2]. At the same time, the continued recruitment and accumulation of leukocytes is associated with the development of vulnerable plaques. The plaques can become unstable and thus rupture, leading to thrombosis, myocardial infarction, or stroke. In addition, the invasion and accumulation of white blood cells create atheromatous plaques, which make the artery walls lose their flexibility and obstruct blood circulation [3,4]. Also, the inflammation hypothesis has recently been proved by genetic evidence. The latest research has shown the relation between coronary artery disease and the transendothelial pathway by genetic evidence [5,6].

Chemokines play important roles in atherosclerotic vascular disease. They are also expressed by cells of the vessel wall [7]. As endothelial cells undergo inflammatory activation, the increased expression of cell adhesion molecules, such as vascular cell adhesion molecule-1 and intercellular adhesion molecule-1, promotes the adherence of monocytes. Furthermore, the monocytes migration is controlled by the concentration gradient of monocytes chemoattractant protein-1, a chemokine that binds to the C-C chemokine receptor named CCR2. Then, monocytes transmigrate into the innermost layer of the arterial wall, pass between the endothelial cells to differentiate into macrophages, and transform into foam cells [8,9].

In atherosclerotic arteries and atheromatous plaques, MCP-1 can be found in endothelial cells, macrophages, and vascular smooth muscle cells. MCP-1 recruits monocytes into the subendothelial cell layer and thus advances the development of atherosclerosis [10,11].

Due to the internal filters in the human body such as the liver, kidneys, and lymph nodes, site-specific delivery by the conjugation of the modification of ligands can provide stable routes to avoid damaging normal tissue and enhance therapeutic efficiency. Pan et al. developed VCAM-1-targeting nanocarriers with a four-fold aggregation in the aortas of atherosclerosis model mice compared to control model mice [12]. Chung et al. developed peptide amphiphile micelles incorporated with the chemokine receptor CCR2-binding motif of MCP-1 for atherosclerosis targeting. The results showed that MCP-1 peptide amphiphile micelles (PAMs) bind with monocytes in vitro and can be detected in early-stage atherosclerotic aortas [13].

Nanoparticles have been used for various applications in the biomedical field. The increasing permeability allows more small sized particles to migrate into the intimal layer, resulting in enhanced permeability and retention (EPR) effect [14,15]. When atherosclerosis lesions develop, endothelial cells are prone to be leaky and fragile, which enhances the EPR effect.

Iron oxide magnetic nanoparticles possess superior physical and chemical properties, such as superparamagnetism and the quantum tunneling of magnetization. Additionally, iron oxide magnetic nanoparticles (MNPs) are also non-toxic, biocompatible, and easy to separate under external magnetic fields. Owing to their unique properties, such as superparamagnetism, high surface area, large surface-to-volume ratio, low toxicity, and easy separation under external magnetic fields, iron oxide MNPs have enormous potential in fields such as magnetic resonance imaging (MRI), bioseparation, environmental treatment, fluorescence labeling, and biomedical and bioengineering usage [16,17].

Although Fe_3O_4 MNP is a promising drug carrier, there are still drawbacks to its use, such as aggregation and oxidation to γ-Fe_2O_3. Therefore, polymer coatings are usually applied to modify its surface characteristics [18]. In recent years, the common reagents employed for the modification of iron oxide MNPs have included surfactants, polymers, and natural dispersants [19–22]. Nevertheless, the most used modification for medical applications is dextran, a biocompatible derivative. In aqueous solutions, dextran interacts with metals and covers its surface, yielding aggregates with hydrodynamic diameters between 20 nm and 150 nm [23,24].

In this work, iron oxide MNPs and MCP-1-motif iron oxide MNPs were stained with Cyanine 5 (Cy5) in fluorescence microscopy. The properties of MNPs were characterized. For in vitro cell experiments, cell viability was measured by the MTT assay and Live/Dead staining. To test the spatial distribution of cells and MCP-1-motif iron oxide MNPs, two types of cells, including 3T3 cells and WEHI 274.1 monocytes [13], were cultivated with iron oxide MNPs.

Apolipoprotein E-knockout (ApoE KO) mice, which are the most commonly used and well-characterized animal model of atherosclerosis, were treated with a high-fat diet for further plaque development and the monocytes accumulation was continuous and proportional to disease progression [25–27].

Through the in vivo test, ApoE KO mice fed a high-fat diet and C57BL/6 wild-type mice fed a normal diet for four weeks made up the atherosclerosis model and control group, respectively. Mice were injected with iron oxide MNPs through the tail vein and the nanoparticle distribution was observed by magnetic resonance imaging (MRI) and in vivo imaging system (IVIS). Figure 1 gives a representative scheme of this research.

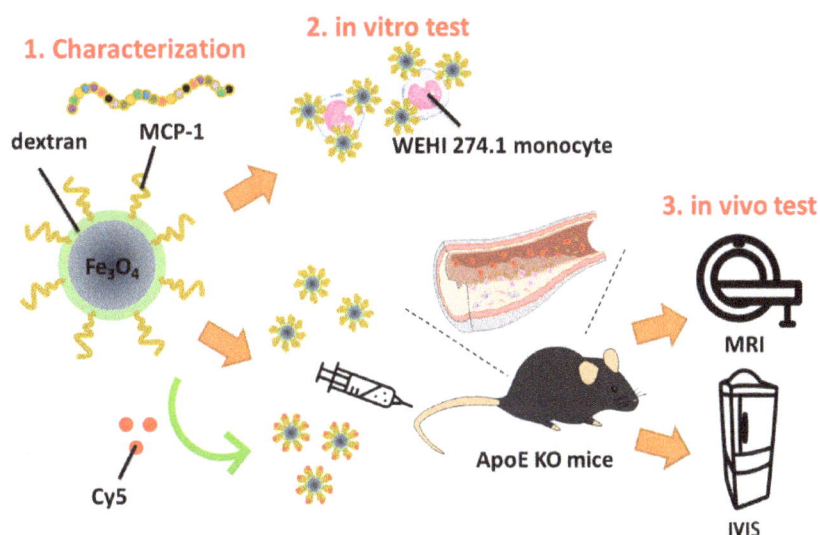

Figure 1. Scheme of the experiment.

2. Materials and Methods

2.1. Materials

MCP-1 peptides (YNFTNRKISVQRLASYRRITSSK) were purchased from Yao-Hong Biotechnology (New Taipei, Taiwan). Iron oxide nanoparticles and the conjugation of MCP-1 peptides and iron nanoparticles were obtained from MagQu (Taipei, Taiwan). 3T3 cells and WEHI 274.1 monocytes were purchased from American Type Culture Collection (ATCC). Cyanine 5 NHS Ester were purchased from Lumiprobe (Hunt Valley, MD, USA). Dulbecco's modified Eagle's medium-high glucose (DMEM-HG), 2-mercaptoethanol (β-ME), thiazolyl blue tetrazolium bromide (MTT solvent), and Oil Red O were purchased from Thermo (Waltham, MA, USA). Fetal bovine serum (FBS) and antibiotic antimycotic solution (penicillin/streptomycin/amphotericinβ) were purchased from Biological (Cromwell, CT, USA).

2.2. Characterization of Iron Oxide MNPs

The structure of iron oxide MNPs were characterized by scanning electron microscopy (SEM) (J NanoSEM 230, Nova, Pallini, Greece) and transmission electron microscopy (TEM) (H-7650, Hitachi, Tokyo, Japan). Particle size and zeta potential were measured in a Zetasizer nanosystem (Zetasizer Nano, Malvern, UK). Iron oxide MNPs solution was stored at $-20\ °C$ overnight and then moved to a freeze dryer overnight to remove all water. The iron oxide MNPs powders were investigated by X-ray photoelectron spectroscopy (XPS) (Theta Probe, Thermo Scientific, Waltham, MA, USA) for composition synthesis (carbon, nitrogen, and oxygen) and by a magnetometer (MPMS7, Quantum Design, San Diego, CA, USA) for magnetic hysteresis loop.

2.3. Cell Culture

WEHI 274.1 monocytes (ATCC, Manassas, VA, USA) were cultured in DMEM-HG culture medium supplemented with 10% fetal bovine serum, 1% antibiotic-antimycotic solution, and 0.05 mM 2-mercaptoethanol for in vitro testing. The cells were cultured on a T75 flask at 37 °C in a humidified incubator under 5% CO_2. After two days of cultivation, the medium with suspended monocytes was moved to a centrifuge tube and centrifuged at 100 relative centrifugal force (rcf) for 5 min. Then the supernatant was removed to eliminate the wastes and the monocytes were resuspended in culture medium. To estimate the number of the cells, trypan blue was used to mark the dead cells and hemocytometer was used to evaluate the number of viable cells. The suspended cells were prepared for the use of the following experiments.

3T3 cells were cultured in DMEM-HG culture medium with 10% FBS and 1% antibiotic-antimycotic solution for in vitro testing. First, the cells were seeded on a 10-cm culture dish at 37 °C in a humidified incubator under 5% CO_2. After washing with PBS, trypsin-EDTA was added and incubated with cells for 4 min at 37 °C to detach cells from the culture plate. Then, culture medium was added to the dish. The medium with suspended cells was centrifuged at 100 rcf for 5 min. Then the supernatant was removed and the cells were resuspended in culture medium. To estimate the number of the cells, trypan blue was used to mark the dead cells and hemocytometer was used to evaluate the number of viable cells. The suspended cells were prepared for the use of the following experiments.

2.4. Cell Viability Evaluation

2.4.1. MTT Assay

3T3 cells were cultivated with different concentrations (0.1, 0.2, and 0.3 mg Fe/mL culture medium) of iron oxide MNPs for four days. Cell viability was investigated on days 1 and 4 via MTT assay. Prior to use, MTT stock solution was diluted to 0.5 mg/mL with cell culture medium. After removing the original medium and PBS buffer washing, 500 μL MTT working solution was added to each well and the mixture was placed in an incubator for 3 h. Finally, the MTT solution was replaced with the same volume of DMSO and the mixture was shaken for 30 min. The absorbance value of the product solution was observed at 570 nm. The whole process was operated without light exposure.

2.4.2. Live/Dead Assay

After WEHI 274.1 monocytes and 3T3 cells were cultivated with different concentrations (0.1, 0.2, and 0.3 mg Fe/mL culture medium) of iron oxide MNPs for four days, the samples were stained by Live/Dead dye to check cell viability. Live cells were stained fluorescent green due to reveal intracellular esterase activity that deacetylated fluorescein diacetate to a green fluorescent product. Dead cells were stained fluorescent red, as their compromised membranes were permeable to nucleic acid stain (propidium iodide). Photos were taken by an inverted fluorescence microscope (Olympus, IX-71, Tokyo, Japan).

2.5. In Vitro Imaging of Nanoparticles

First of all, MCP-1-motif iron oxide MNPs were stained with Cy5 fluorescence and the composition of the reaction was as follows: 2 μL MCP-1-motif iron oxide MNPs solution (8.2 mg Fe/mL), 10 μL Cy5 solution (1 mg/mL), and 90 μL sodium bicarbonate solution (0.1 M, pH 8.3). The reaction occurred at 4 °C refrigerator overnight with shaking. After the reaction, the solution was centrifuged 110 rcf for 10 min and the supernatant was removed in order to remove excess Cy5 fluorescence. The process was repeated twice to avoid excess Cy5 reacting with cells. The Cy5-MCP-1-motif iron oxide MNPs were refilled in PBS for future use.

Thirty thousand monocytes were cultured in 48-well plates and incubated with Cy5-MCP-1-motif iron oxide MNPs suspension for 1 h at 37 °C in a humidified incubator under 5% CO_2. Finally, DAPI was used for nucleus staining and the results were achieved with an inverted fluorescence microscope. 3T3 cells with same quantities were used for control cells.

2.6. Animal Model

ApoE KO mice (male, 7 weeks old) and C57BL/6 wild-type mice (male, 7 weeks old) were given a high-fat diet (HFD, 45% fat, 35% carbohydrate, 20% protein) and/or a normal diet (ND, 10% fat, 70% carbohydrate, 20% protein) in National Yang-Ming University, Taipei, Taiwan (for MRI) and Laboratory Animal Center, National Taiwan University College of Medicine, Taipei, Taiwan (for IVIS). The animal protocol was approved by National Taiwan University College of Medicine Laboratory Animal Center (#20160214) (Effective dates: 2016/07/01 ~2020/06/30).

The high-fat diet and gene deficiency promoted atherosclerosis plaque progression. Mice were shaved and the tail veins were dilated and sterilized with 70% ethanol before iron oxide nanoparticles injection (10 µg/g mice). The injection detail and mice choice are shown in Tables 1 and 2.

Table 1. Experimental design of animal model for magnetic resonance imaging (MRI).

Mice	Diet	Nanoparticle Injection
Wild-type	Four weeks ND	MCP-1-motif MNPs
ApoE KO	Four weeks ND	MCP-1-motif MNPs
ApoE KO	Two weeks ND and two weeks HFD	MCP-1-motif MNPs
ApoE KO	Four weeks HFD	MCP-1-motif MNPs

Normal diet (ND), High fat diet (HFD), monocytes chemoattractant protein-1 (MCP-1), magnetic nanoparticles (MNP).

Table 2. Experimental design of animal model for in vivo imaging system (IVIS).

Mice	Diet	Nanoparticle Injection
Wild-type	Four weeks ND	PBS
Wild-type	Four weeks ND	MNPs
Wild-type	Four weeks ND	MCP-1-motif MNPs
ApoE KO	Four weeks HFD	PBS
ApoE KO	Four weeks HFD	MNPs
ApoE KO	Four weeks HFD	MCP-1-motif MNPs

2.7. Nuclear Magnetic Resonance Imaging (MRI)

All of the mice were anesthetized by ether and were measured using a T2*-contrast (axial view) FLASH sequence 7.0 T imaging (BRUKER BIOSPEC 70/30 MRI, Billerica, MA, USA) for every 2-mm sectioning thickness. (Repetition time (TR) = 200 ms, Echo time (TE) = 5 ms, Matrix 256 × 256 pixel, Field of view (FOV) = 4 × 4 cm, Flip angle = 30°) Images were acquired at 40 h after nanoparticles injection [28].

2.8. Non-Invasive In Vivo Imaging System (IVIS)

For IVIS, iron oxide MNPs all had been modified with Cy5 fluorescence and the imaging time spots of IVIS were 0, 2, 8, 24, 48, 72 h after nanoparticles injection [29]. Mice were anesthetized with 2.5% isoflurane in O_2 and whole-body fluorescence imaging was conducted by IVIS. The emission at 680 nm was measured with an optimal excitation wavelength of 640 nm (FOV: 12.5, f2, 0.75 s). Mice were then euthanized via CO_2 overdose and the aorta, heart, liver, spleen, lung, and kidney were harvested. The aorta and organs fluorescence were also conducted using IVIS. After imaging, all were immersed in 5% formaldehyde for fixation and preservation [13].

2.9. Histology Staining

Freshly dissected tissues were covered with enough O.C.T for a few minutes in a labeled small weigh boat. Then the prepared sample was placed in a metal beaker filled 2/3 full with isopentane and subsequently placed in a Dewar of liquid nitrogen. Samples (6–8 μm) were cryosectioned and stained with hematoxylin for 1 min, or Prussian Blue staining for iron oxide MNPs for 30 min, or Oil Red O staining for atherosclerosis for 5 min, depending on the investigation [30–33].

2.10. Statistical Analysis

All data are expressed as means ± standard deviation. A comparison of different groups was determined using Student's t-test and significant difference was assumed at p-value ≤ 0.05. The statistical data was analyzed using ORIGIN® 8.6 (OriginLab Corp., Northampton, MA, USA).

3. Results and Discussion

3.1. Characterization of Iron Oxide MNPs

TEM and SEM images were employed to observe the structures of iron oxide MNPs and MCP-1-motif MNPs. The SEM images reveal that most of the nanoparticles are quasi-spherical and attempt to aggregate in the solid state because of their high surface energy [34] (Figure S1). Due to peptide surface modification, peptides derived from MCP-1 might have physical, such as Van der Waals force, and chemical interactions, such as NH· · ·OH-bonds, with each other and thus impede nanoparticles dispersion [35,36].

Also, the TEM images show the size and the structure of the iron oxide MNPs (Figure 2). Comparing the size of two types of MNPs, MCP-1-motif MNPs formed a larger morphology and shape that is more irregular. The diameter of MCP-1-motif MNPs and MNPs were approximately 20 ± 3 nm and 10 ± 3 nm in a spherical shape, respectively.

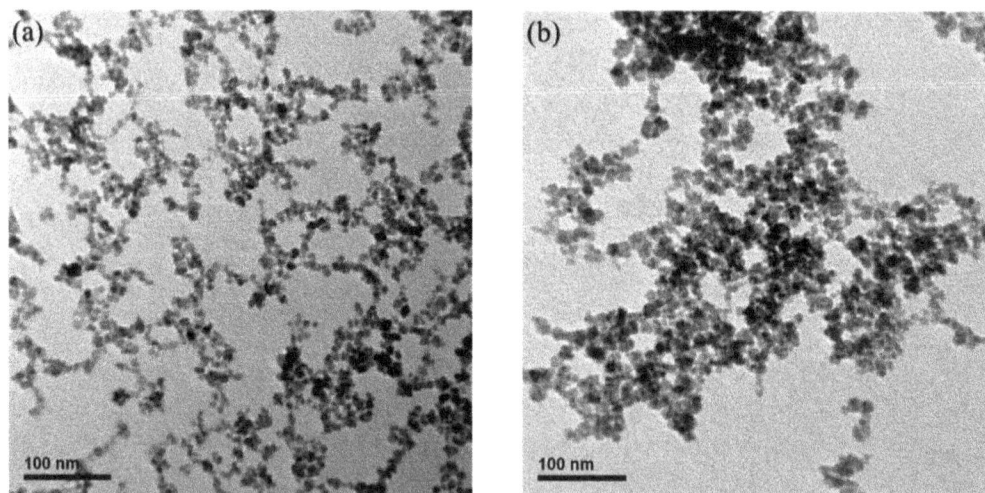

Figure 2. Characterization of (**a**) magnetic nanoparticles (MNPs) and (**b**) monocytes chemoattractant protein-1 (MCP-1)-motif MNPs using TEM.

Moreover, the hydrodynamic diameter of the iron oxide MNPs was measured by the dynamic light scattering (DLS) method to test aqueous properties (Table 3). In the results of DLS, the peaks of the diameter were approximately 90 nm and 300 nm (Figure S2). The higher value in particle size determined by the DLS method compared to the TEM image was attributed to the interaction of water molecules in the aqueous solution [37]. Furthermore, the zeta potential value of MNPs (−14.1 mV) and MCP-1-motif MNPs (−17.6 mV) were higher than −20 mV, which indicated that the dispersion was relatively stable [38]. Therefore, the nanoparticles solution would be sonicated before the experiment.

Table 3. Dynamic light scattering (DLS) results of MNPs and MCP-1-motif MNPs ($n = 3$).

Nanoparticles	Zeta Potential (mV)	Hydrodynamic Diameter (nm)
MNPs	-14.1 ± 0.16	90.0 ± 4.90
MCP-1-motif MNPs	-17.6 ± 0.25	323.8 ± 12.17

XPS measurements were made to quantify the element composition of nanoparticles, and the results are shown in Figure 3. Three bands of the XPS survey spectrum at around 285, 397.5, and 532.5 eV represented C1s, N1s, and O1s, respectively. In Figure 3a,b, the C1s XPS spectra had a large peak at 284.5 eV, corresponding to sp^2 hybridized carbon (C-C bonds), as well as two small peaks at 286.0 and 288.0 eV, which could be ascribed to C-O bonds and C=O bonds [39,40]. On the other hand, the N1s XPS spectra in Figure 3c,d all exhibited a major peak at around 400.0 eV. The binding energies at 398.8 and 400.0 eV, respectively, were attributed to N atoms bonded with sp^3-hybridized C atoms (N-sp^3C, N(H)-C bonds) and N atoms bonded with sp^2-hybridized C atoms (N-sp^2C, N(C)-C bonds) [41,42]. Figure 3e,f show the O1s XPS spectra of iron oxide MNPs and the two major peaks were located at around 530.0 and 535 eV. The O1s peaking at 532.0 and 533.3 eV could be assigned to oxygen in the form of O=C bonds and C-O bonds. In addition, the binding energies at 529.7 eV and 535.3 eV represented Fe_3O_4 and H_2O, respectively [43,44].

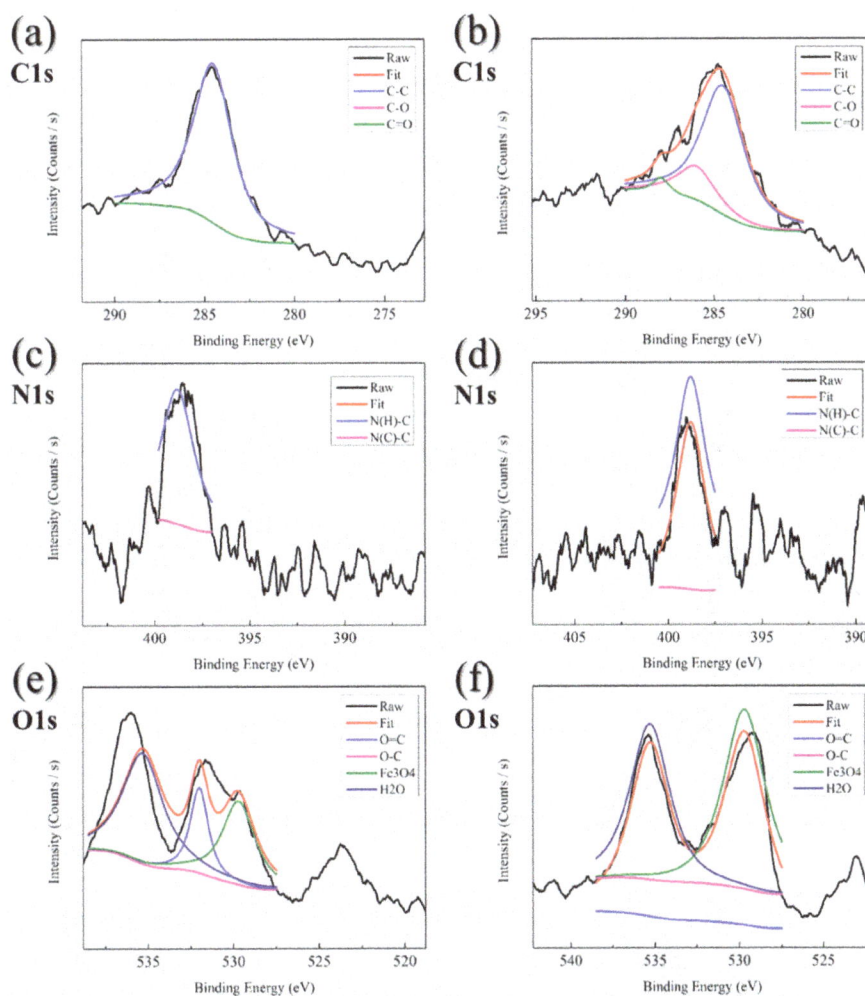

Figure 3. X-ray photoelectron spectroscopy (XPS) spectra of (**a,c,e**) MNPs and (**b,d,f**) MCP-1-motif MNPs.

Tables 4 and S1 show the compositions of different kinds of bonds and the chemical elements of iron oxide MNPs. MNPs only had dextran shell modification, which had a large quantity of C-C bonds. Moreover, the hydroxyl bond was replaced with an amine bond, so no signal (C-O bonds) could be found in the C1s XPS spectrum of MNPs. Also, we observed that the C1s XPS spectrum of MCP-1-motif MNPs had peaks at the C-O bonds and C=O bonds because of the peptide sequence. According to the description above, the amine bond was the major composition in the MNPs consistent with the N1s XPS spectrum. On the other hand, both N(C)-C bonds and N(H)-C bonds could be found in the results of MCP-1-motif MNPs. Through the oxygen analysis, two kinds of nanoparticles presented Fe_3O_4 and H_2O. With the C=O bonds existing on the shell of the nanoparticles, the ratio of Fe_3O_4 and H_2O decreased compared to the control group.

Table 4 shows the chemical element composition of two iron oxide MNPs. MNPs had dextran shells, a kind of organic compound, so carbon was the major element in the composition. On the other hand, the peptides sequence and iron oxide core presented oxygen, so the ratio of oxygen was higher than those of the other two elements.

Table 4. Chemical element composition ratio of iron oxide MNPs.

	MNPs	MCP-1-Motif MNPs
C1s	54.25%	40.32%
N1s	5.44%	2.14%
O1s	40.31%	57.55%

3.2. Magnetic Measurements

To make sure that the magnetic properties remained after dextran coating and peptide grafting, a superconducting interference magnetometer was applied. Figure 4 shows the M-H Curve/Hysteresis Loop of MNPs (2.2 mg) and MCP-1-motif MNPs (9.0 mg). The operation temperature was 310 K and the magnetic field range was ±7.0 Tesla.

The hysteresis loops were normal and tight with no remnant magnetization, indicating a typical superparamagnetic behavior. In general, iron oxide MNPs, whose size was smaller than 20 nm, were supposed to be superparamagnetic at room temperature. Hence, from Figure 4, we could observe that the saturation magnetization values of MNPs and MCP-1-motif MNPs were 15.5 and 31.0 emu/g, respectively, due to the size difference of the two types of nanoparticles [45–47].

Paramagnetic materials had unpaired electrons, such as atomic or molecular orbitals. Therefore, superparamagnetic nanoparticles were free to align their magnetic moment in any direction. When an external magnetic field was applied, these magnetic moments would tend to align themselves in the same direction as the applied field. In addition, peptides derived from MCP-1 also contained free electrons and might enhance the magnetic moments in the applied magnetic field, promoting high saturation magnetization values [48].

3.3. Cytotoxicity

The MTT assay was conducted with 3T3 cells incubated with different concentrations of MCP-1-motif MNPs for one day and four days. The result is shown in Figure 5a and could estimate the cytotoxicity of the nanoparticles. The normal Fe concentration of the injection solution was 0.2 mg Fe/mL. The lower and higher Fe concentrations were also investigated in the MTT assay. The percentages were calculated by comparing the 3T3 cells without iron oxide MNPs. The cytotoxicity of MCP-motif MNPs under three concentrations did not have a negative effect on cell proliferation. Even after four days of incubation, the cell viability still reached around 100%.

Figures 5b, S3 and S4 are the Live/Dead staining images. The counting results are shown in Figure S5. WEHI 274.1 monocytes and 3T3 cells were also incubated with different concentrations of MCP-1-motif MNPs for one day and four days. The monocytes all maintained a round shape and the quantities were consistent with the control group. Similarly, 3T3 cells were still in elongation and proliferated stably in all groups.

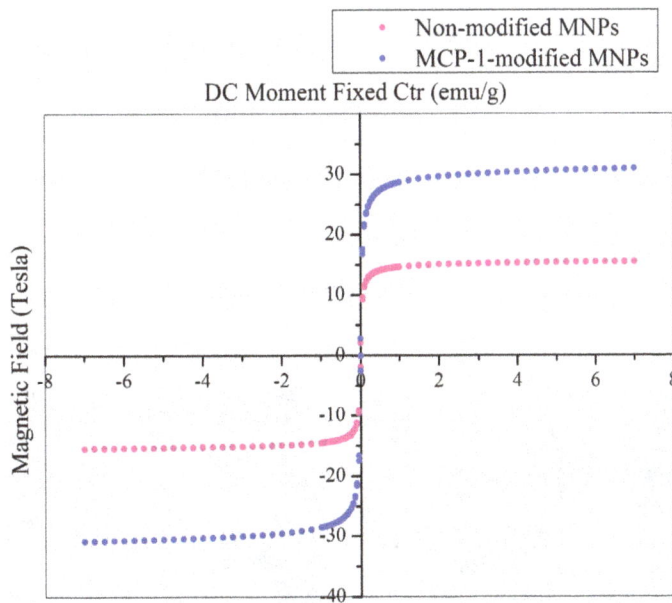

Figure 4. M-H curve/hysteresis loop of iron oxide MNPs.

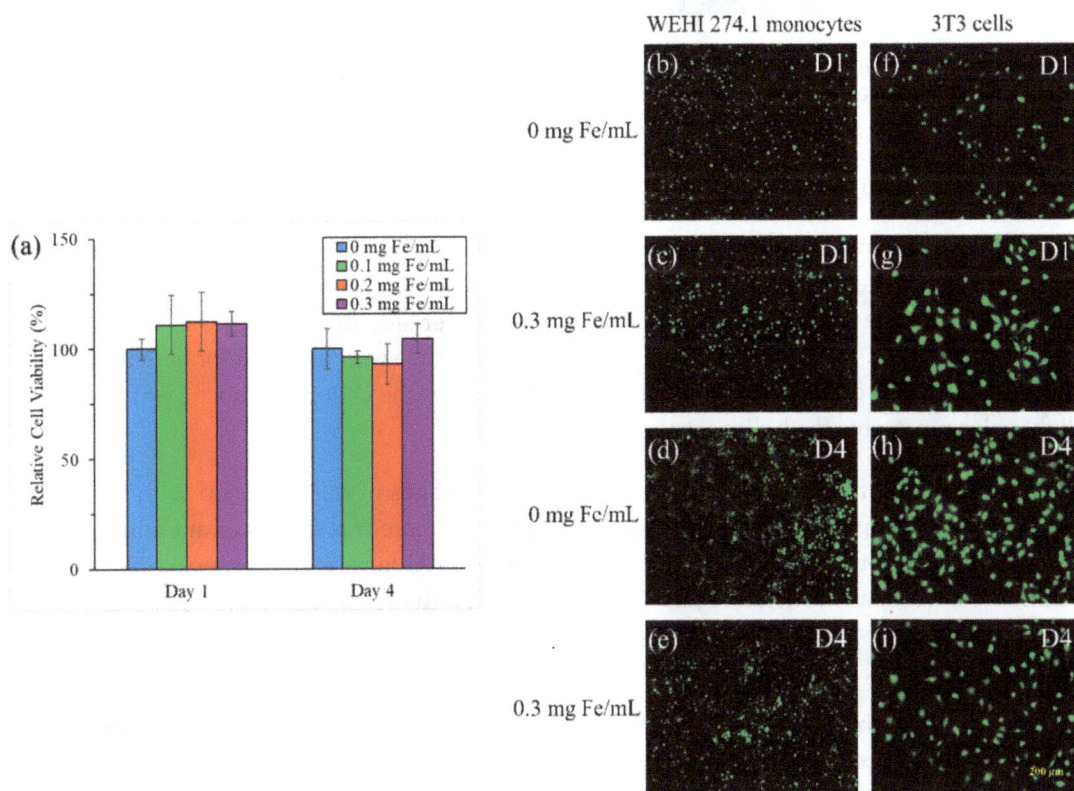

Figure 5. (a) MTT assay of 3T3 cells with different concentration of MCP-1-motif MNPs; **(b–i)** Live/Dead staining of WEHI 274.1 monocytes **(b–e)**, and 3T3 cells **(f–i)** in 0 and 0.3 mg Fe/mL at day 1 (D1) **(b,c,f,g)** and day 4 (D4) **(d,e,h,i)** ($n = 4$).

3.4. In Vitro Imaging of MCP-1-Motif MNPs

Figure S6a is the fluorescence image of Cy5-MCP-1-motif MNPs; the further conformation can be observed through the merged image in Figure S6b. WEHI 274.1 monocytes were cultured with Cy5-MNPs or Cy5-MCP-1-motif MNPs after 1 h and stained with DAPI (Figure 6). After cultivation, the nanoparticles in solution were removed by centrifugation. Whether in the fluorescence or the bright image, there was no Cy5 signal, which represented MNPs co-localized with WEHI 274.1 monocytes. However, monocytes stained by DAPI (blue) had a spherical shape and the surfaces were overlapped with Cy5-MCP-1-motif MNPs (red), indicating the potential affinity to monocytes of peptides derived from MCP-1. Moreover, 3T3 cells were also cultured with MCP-1-motif MNPs, but no nanoparticle seemed to attach on the cell surface (Figure S7). Therefore, we could conclude that the binding ability of MCP-1 was preserved and MCP-1-motif MNPs had the ability to target monocytes.

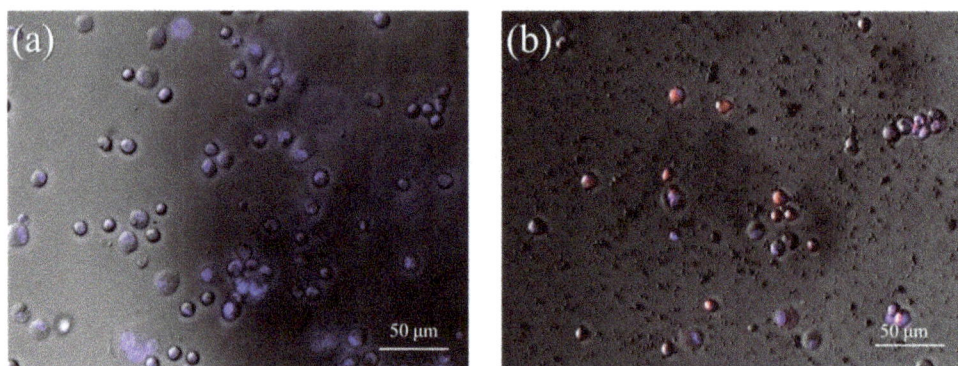

Figure 6. Overlaid image (fluorescence and bright) of WEHI 274.1 monocytes cultured with (**a**) Cy5-MNPs or (**b**) Cy5-MCP-1-motif MNPs.

3.5. Nuclear Magnetic Resonance Imaging (MRI)

Magnetic resonance microscopy permitted to us obtain high-resolution images of the aorta in mice at the level of the abdominal aorta. Figure 7a–h show the MRI abdomen axial cross-sectional anatomy of wild-type mice and ApoE KO mice. The upper side of the images is anterior and the lower side is posterior. Before the nanoparticle injection, all mice were scanned for baseline, which are recorded in Figure 7a–d. The red arrowhead symbol indicates the abdominal aortic walls of mice and the light color represents the hollow structure.

Figure 7e–h are the images of magnetic resonance images of mice injected with MCP-1-motif MNPs after 40 h. Bright aortic lumen and wall indicated that there was no significant iron oxide MNPs accumulation in wild-type mice (Figure 7e). Besides, ApoE KO mice with four weeks of high-fat diet had dark aorta walls, as shown in Figure 7h, indicating that the aorta was full of MCP-1-motif MNPs. The degree of darkness in the aorta was more obvious when mice were fed a high-fat diet for a longer period of time [49–51].

Figure 7i shows the pixel density of aorta (area = 41.31 mm^2), which stood for the degree of light color. The values of pixel density of all groups decreased because of the existence of iron oxide MNPs. The ratio of pixels decreased after injections: 25.43% (wild-type mice ND4), 26.51% (ApoE KO mice ND4), 38.14% (ApoE KO mice ND2 + HFD2), 40.86% (ApoE KO mice HFD4). This indicated that MCP-1-motif MNPs in the blood flow obviously attached to the monocytes during the formation of atherosclerosis plaques in ApoE mice compared to the other three groups. The MRI results concluded that the MCP-1-motif MNPs would accumulate in the aorta in the atherosclerosis model.

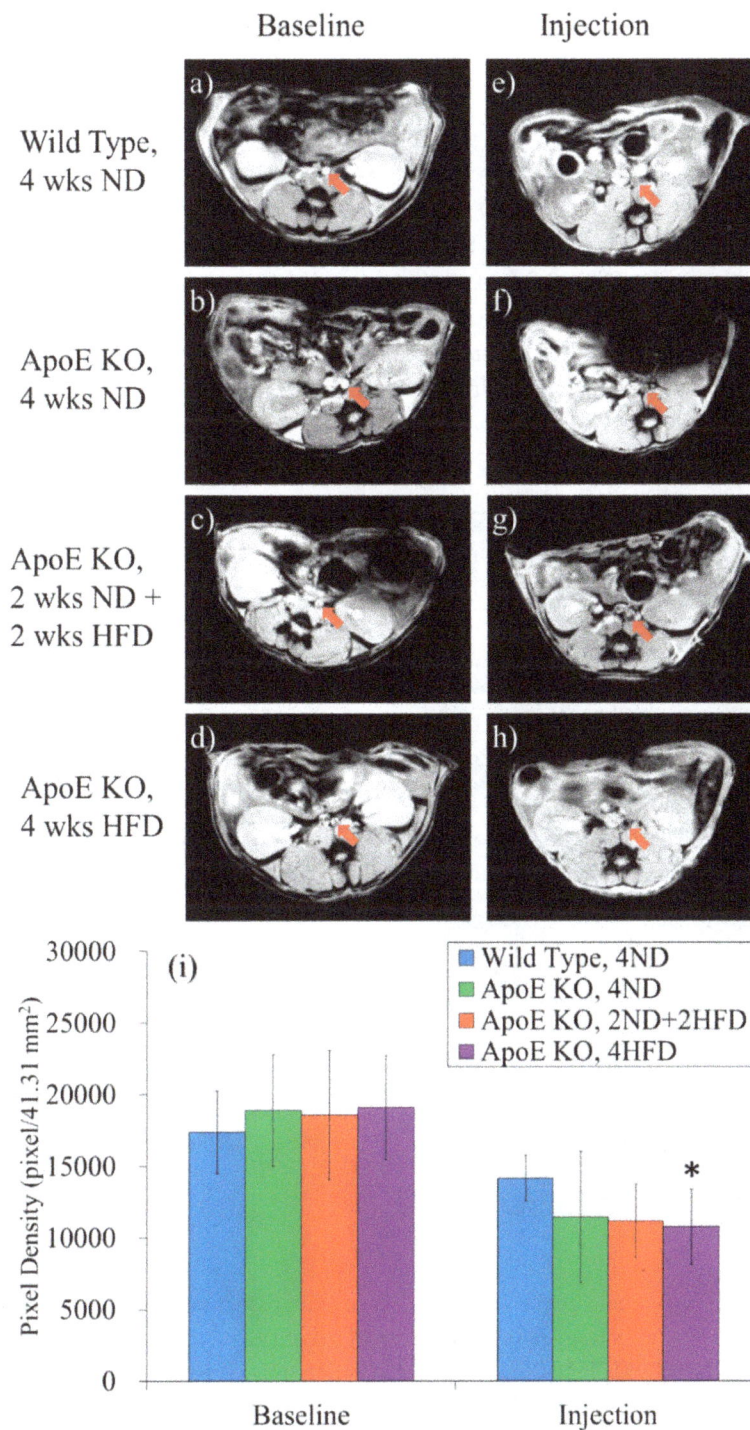

Figure 7. (**a–h**) Magnetic resonance images of mice injected with MCP-1-motif MNPs before and after experiments (wks = weeks); (**i**) Diagram of pixel density throughout the aorta area ($n = 3$) (* $p < 0.05$, compared to the same group of baseline).

3.6. Non-Invasive In Vivo Imaging System

The IVIS spectrum system confirmed the existence of Cy5 MNPs and Cy5-MCP-1-motif MNPs in the bloodstream of mice in 72 h through a background level of fluorescence throughout the body. Figures 8 and S8 show the body fluorescence images of ApoE mice as well as wild-type mice injected with iron oxide MNPs, respectively. Body fluorescence decreased due to nanoparticles being excreted when the time reached 48 or 72 h. The fluorescence distribution in MCP-1-motif MNPs (Figure 8) tended to accumulate at the backbone of the body, which might indicate the aggregation of iron oxide MNPs in the aorta. Compared to the experimental groups, MNPs distributed randomly throughout the body.

Figure 8e shows the backbone fluorescence at any time point compared to the 0-h backbone fluorescence. The fluorescence of ApoE KO mice with MCP-1-motif MNPs still maintained over 90% at 2 h compared to the other test groups. On the other hand, the fluorescence of MNPs in the two types of mice all reduced to under 80% at 2 h, and the two wild-type groups were significantly different from the ApoE KO mice with the injection of MCP-1-motif MNPs. This might result from the retention ability of MCP-1-motif MNPs in the atherosclerosis model. After the 24-h injection, the signals all decreased to about 30–40%, and they declined to under 20% in 72 h [52].

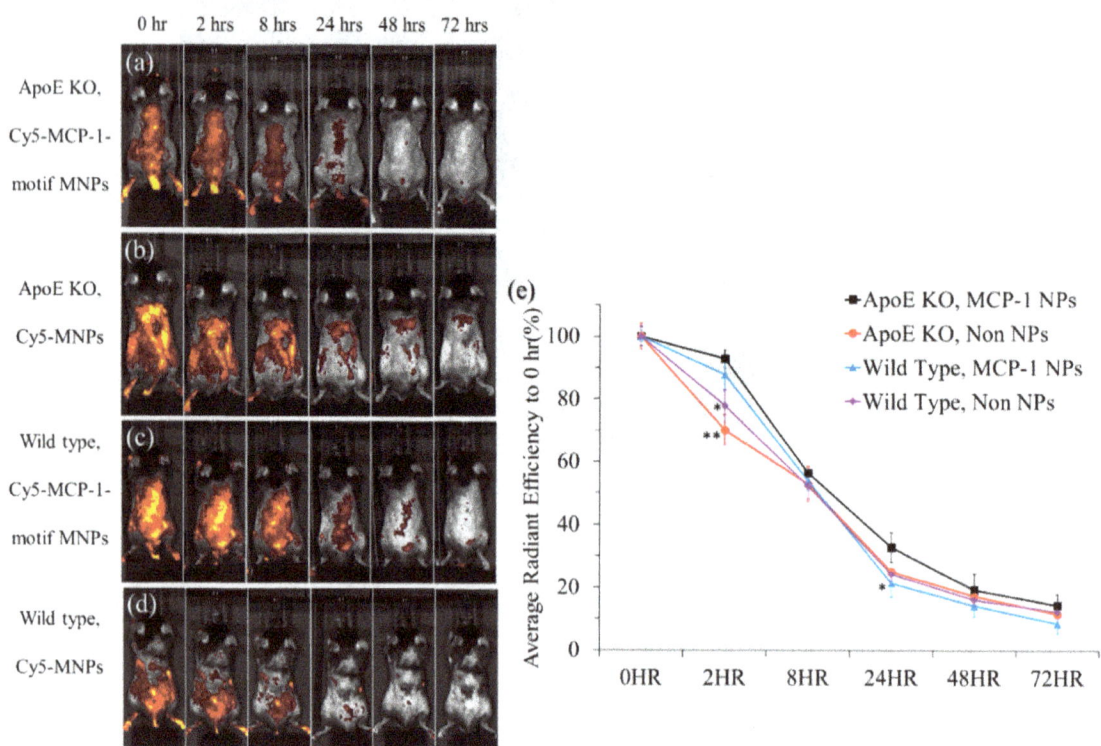

Figure 8. (**a–d**) IVIS body fluorescence of ApoE KO mice, wild-type mice injected with Cy5-MCP-1-motif MNPs and Cy5-MNPs; (**e**) average radiant efficiency at 0 h of IVIS body fluorescence ($n = 3$) (* $p < 0.05$ compared with ApoE KO, MCP-1 NPs at the same injection time; ** $p < 0.01$ compared with ApoE KO, MCP-1 NPs at the same injection time).

After the 72-h injection, mice were sacrificed and the aorta, heart, liver, spleen, lung, and kidney were harvested. The aorta and organs fluorescence conducted by IVIS are shown in Figure 9. From the results of different organs, the presence of iron oxide MNPs was detected in the kidney of all types of mice, indicating that mice would excrete the nanoparticles in urine through the kidney and the bladder. However, the aorta of the atherosclerosis model injected with MCP-1-motif MNPs had notable fluorescence signals, confirming the longer retention time of MCP-1-motif MNPs to atherosclerosis plaque in the aorta.

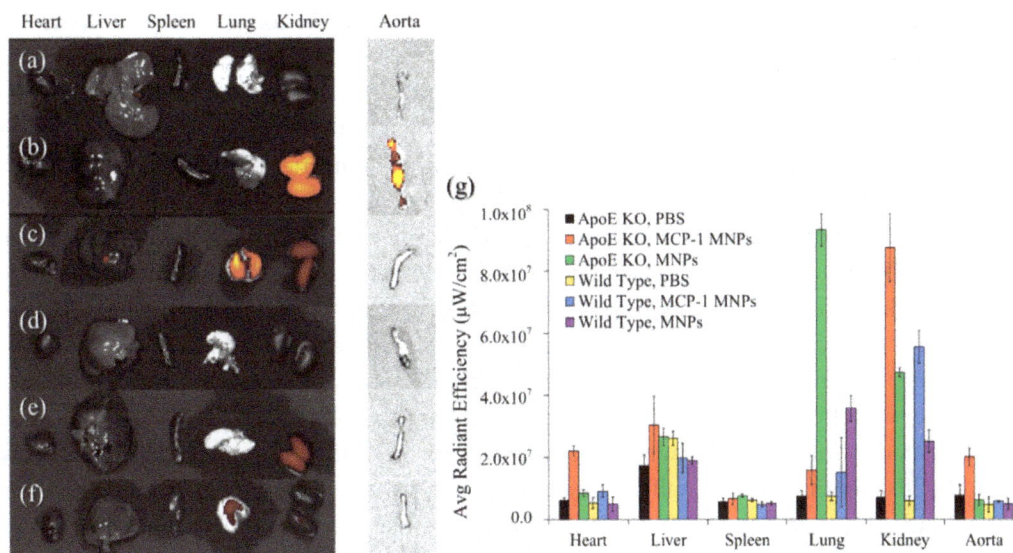

Figure 9. IVIS organ fluorescence of ApoE KO mice injected with (**a**) PBS; (**b**) MCP-1-motif MNPs; (**c**) MNPs, and wild-type mice injected with (**d**) PBS; (**e**) MCP-1-motif MNPs; (**f**) MNPs. (**g**) Average radiant efficiency diagram of IVIS organ fluorescence (n = 3).

3.7. Iron and Oil Drops in Specific Organs

After in vivo imaging, kidneys were cut into 6–8 μm cross-sections and the tissue sections were stained with hematoxylin and Prussian Blue (Figure S9). Blue precipitation found in the kidney tissue due to the injection of iron oxide MNPs confirmed that the kidney was the major organ employed for excreting nanoparticles [31]. For further confirmation of MCP-1-motif MNPs in the atherosclerosis model, the vessel wall of aorta was stained with Oil Red O, which illustrated atherosclerotic lesions, and Prussian Blue, which illustrated precipitations of iron oxide MNPs (Figure 10). The staining results showed the co-localization of MCP-1-motif MNPs and plaques. Oil drops and Prussian Blue are all observed in Figure 10c, indicating the potential affinity of MCP-1-motif MNPs in the atherosclerosis model [53–55].

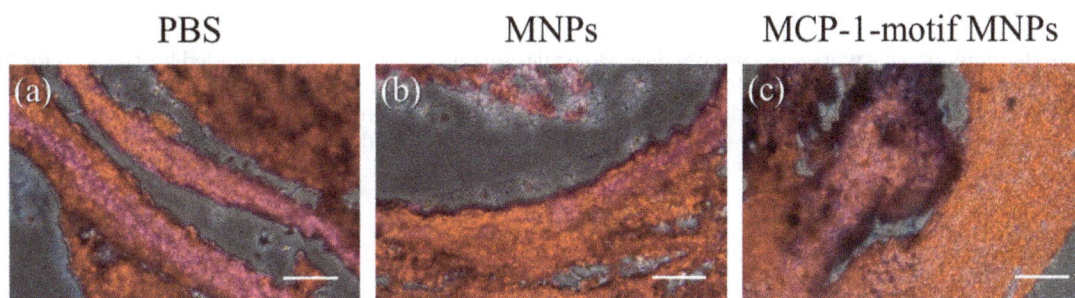

Figure 10. Prussian Blue and Oil Red O staining of the aorta of ApoE KO mice with injection of (**a**) PBS, (**b**)MNPs, and (**c**) MCP-1-motif MNPs (scale bar = 50 μm).

4. Conclusions

In this work, the characteristics of iron oxide MNPs were measured and analyzed. Electron microscope images showed the quasi-spherical shape of nanoparticles and XPS spectra further confirmed that the MCP-1 peptides conjugated on the iron oxide MNPs. They were relatively stable in aqueous solution and dispersive when stirred.

Then, the following in vitro experiment was examined. We developed the cell viability process of iron oxide MNPs, including an MTT assay and a Live/Dead assay. Whether in WEHI 274.1 monocytes or 3T3 cells, MCP-1-motif MNPs exhibited a cell viability around 100% compared to the control group. Next, we successfully attached Cy5 fluorescence to iron oxide MNPs using an amine-ester reaction. With different types of cells incubated with iron oxide MNPs for 1 h, we observed that MCP-1-motif MNPs co-localized with WEHI 274.1 monocytes, indicating a potential tool for tracking early-stage atherosclerosis lesions in aorta, usually aggregated with large quantities of monocytes.

Next, iron oxide MNPs were injected into wild-type mice, for the control group, and ApoE KO mice, a widely-used atherosclerosis model, and in vivo imaging was performed. First, MRI showed that MCP-1-motif MNPs were obviously accumulated in the abdomen aorta of ApoE KO mice fed a high-fat diet for four weeks compared to other experimental groups. Second, we also found that the average radiant efficiency of Cy5-MCP-1-motif MNPs nearby the backbone of the atherosclerosis model mice was still 90% after 2 h. In addition, organs harvested after 72 h showed that nanoparticles accumulated in the kidney for excretion in all mice injected with nanoparticles. Above all, Cy5-MCP-1-motif MNPs largely aggregated in the aorta of atherosclerosis model mice, confirming the co-localization of aorta plaque and MCP-1-motif MNPs. Finally, vital organs tissues were stained with Prussian Blue and Oil Red O, which identified that the MCP-1-motif MNPs have the potential ability to track aorta lesions and can be a promising targeting tool for early-stage atherosclerosis.

In conclusion, from the in vitro test and in vivo test, we observed that MCP-1-motif MNPs could interact with monocytes and accumulate in the aorta of an atherosclerosis model, indicating a potential targeting tool for early-stage atherosclerosis.

Author Contributions: C.-W.K. and P.-T.W. conducted the experiments and wrote the manuscript. M.-Y.L. provided technical support for the nanoparticles characterization. I.-J.C. assisted on the data curation of MRI imaging. K.-C.Y. and W.-Y.I.T. provided the disease model and supervision of the in vivo study. J.Y. designed and investigated the study.

Funding: This research was funded by Molecular Imaging Center, National Taiwan University, Taipei, Taiwan.

Acknowledgments: This work was supported by Molecular Imaging Center, which is funded by The Aim for The Top University Project, Ministry of Education, Taiwan. We would like to acknowledge the useful discussion and technical service and assistance provided by the NTU Instrumentation Center, Technology Commons, College of Life Science, and Department of Biochemical Science and Technology, National Taiwan University.

References

1. Woollard, K.J.; Geissmann, F. Monocytes in atherosclerosis: Subsets and functions. *Nat. Rev. Cardiol.* **2010**, *7*, 77–86. [CrossRef] [PubMed]
2. Moss, J.W.E.; Ramji, D.P. Cytokines: Roles in atherosclerosis disease progression and potential therapeutic targets. *Future Med. Chem.* **2016**, *8*, 1317–1330. [CrossRef] [PubMed]
3. Libby, P.; Ridker, P.M.; Maseri, A. Inflammation and Atherosclerosis. *Circulation* **2002**, *105*, 1135–1143. [CrossRef] [PubMed]
4. Mlinar, L.B.; Chung, E.J.; Wonder, E.A.; Tirrell, M. Active targeting of early and mid-stage atherosclerotic plaques using self-assembled peptide amphiphile micelles. *Biomaterials* **2014**, *35*, 8678–8686. [CrossRef] [PubMed]
5. Klarin, D.; Zhu, Q.M.; Emdin, C.A.; Chaffin, M.; Horner, S.; McMillan, B.J.; Leed, A.; Weale, M.E.; Spencer, C.C.A.; Aguet, F.; et al. Genetic analysis in UK Biobank links insulin resistance and transendothelial migration pathways to coronary artery disease. *Nat. Genet.* **2017**, *49*, 1392. [CrossRef] [PubMed]

6. Howson, J.M.M.; Zhao, W.; Barnes, D.R.; Ho, W.-K.; Young, R.; Paul, D.S.; Waite, L.L.; Freitag, D.F.; Fauman, E.B.; Salfati, E.L.; et al. Fifteen new risk loci for coronary artery disease highlight arterial-wall-specific mechanisms. *Nat. Genet.* **2017**, *49*, 1113. [CrossRef] [PubMed]

7. Zernecke, A.; Weber, C. Chemokines in Atherosclerosis. *Proc. Resumed* **2014**, *34*, 742–750. [CrossRef]

8. Libby, P. Current Concepts of the Pathogenesis of the Acute Coronary Syndromes. *Circulation* **2001**, *104*, 365–372. [CrossRef] [PubMed]

9. Szmitko, P.E.; Wang, C.-H.; Weisel, R.D.; de Almeida, J.R.; Anderson, T.J.; Verma, S. New Markers of Inflammation and Endothelial Cell Activation: Part I. *Circulation* **2003**, *108*, 1917–1923. [CrossRef] [PubMed]

10. Deshmane, S.L.; Kremlev, S.; Amini, S.; Sawaya, B.E. Monocyte chemoattractant protein-1 (MCP-1): An overview. *J. Interferon Cytokine Res.* **2009**, *29*, 313–326. [CrossRef] [PubMed]

11. Taub, D.D. Chemokine-leukocyte interactions. The voodoo that they do so well. *Cytokine Growth Factor Rev.* **1996**, *7*, 355–376. [CrossRef]

12. Pan, H.; Myerson, J.W.; Hu, L.; Marsh, J.N.; Hou, K.; Scott, M.J.; Allen, J.S.; Hu, G.; San Roman, S.; Lanza, G.M.; et al. Programmable nanoparticle functionalization for in vivo targeting. *FASEB J.* **2013**, *27*, 255–264. [CrossRef] [PubMed]

13. Chung, E.J.; Nord, K.; Sugimoto, M.J.; Wonder, E.; Tirrell, M.; Mlinar, L.B.; Alenghat, F.J.; Fang, Y. Monocyte-Targeting Supramolecular Micellar Assemblies: A Molecular Diagnostic Tool for Atherosclerosis. *Adv. Healthc. Mater.* **2015**, *4*, 367–376. [CrossRef] [PubMed]

14. Zhang, J.; Zu, Y.; Dhanasekara, C.S.; Li, J.; Wu, D.; Fan, Z.; Wang, S. Detection and treatment of atherosclerosis using nanoparticles. *Wiley Interdiscip. Rev. Nanomed. Nanobiotechnol.* **2017**, *9*. [CrossRef] [PubMed]

15. Kim, Y.; Lobatto, M.E.; Kawahara, T.; Lee Chung, B.; Mieszawska, A.J.; Sanchez-Gaytan, B.L.; Fay, F.; Senders, M.L.; Calcagno, C.; Becraft, J.; et al. Probing nanoparticle translocation across the permeable endothelium in experimental atherosclerosis. *Proc. Natl. Acad. Sci. USA* **2014**, *111*, 1078–1083. [CrossRef] [PubMed]

16. Popescu, R.C.; Andronescu, E.; Grumezescu, A.M. In vivo evaluation of Fe_3O_4 nanoparticles. *Rom. J. Morphol. Embryol.* **2014**, *55*, 1013–1018. [PubMed]

17. Bietenbeck, M.; Florian, A.; Faber, C.; Sechtem, U.; Yilmaz, A. Remote magnetic targeting of iron oxide nanoparticles for cardiovascular diagnosis and therapeutic drug delivery: Where are we now? *Int. J. Nanomed.* **2016**, *11*, 3191–3203. [CrossRef]

18. Jadhav, N.V.; Prasad, A.I.; Kumar, A.; Mishra, R.; Dhara, S.; Babu, K.R.; Prajapat, C.L.; Misra, N.L.; Ningthoujam, R.S.; Pandey, B.N.; et al. Synthesis of oleic acid functionalized Fe_3O_4 magnetic nanoparticles and studying their interaction with tumor cells for potential hyperthermia applications. *Colloids Surf. B Biointerfaces* **2013**, *108*, 158–168. [CrossRef] [PubMed]

19. Chen, L.; Xu, Z.; Dai, H.; Zhang, S. Facile synthesis and magnetic properties of monodisperse Fe_3O_4/silica nanocomposite microspheres with embedded structures via a direct solution-based route. *J. Alloys Compd.* **2010**, *497*, 221–227. [CrossRef]

20. Yang, J.; Zou, P.; Yang, L.; Cao, J.; Sun, Y.; Han, D.; Yang, S.; Wang, Z.; Chen, G.; Wang, B.; et al. A comprehensive study on the synthesis and paramagnetic properties of PEG-coated Fe_3O_4 nanoparticles. *Appl. Surf. Sci.* **2014**, *303*, 425–432. [CrossRef]

21. Lüdtke-Buzug, K.; Biederer, S.; Sattel, T.; Knopp, T.; Buzug, T.M. Preparation and Characterization of Dextran-Covered Fe_3O_4 Nanoparticles for Magnetic Particle Imaging. In Proceedings of the 4th European Conference of the International Federation for Medical and Biological Engineering: ECIFMBE, Antwerp, Belgium, 23–27 November 2008; Vander Sloten, J., Verdonck, P., Nyssen, M., Haueisen, J., Eds.; Springer: Berlin/Heidelberg, Germany, 2009; pp. 2343–2346.

22. Xu, J.K.; Zhang, F.F.; Sun, J.J.; Sheng, J.; Wang, F.; Sun, M. Bio and nanomaterials based on Fe_3O_4. *Molecules* **2014**, *19*, 21506–21528. [CrossRef] [PubMed]

23. Bautista, M.C.; Bomati-Miguel, O.; Zhao, X.; Morales, M.P.; González-Carreño, T.; Alejo, R.P.d.; Ruiz-Cabello, J.; Veintemillas-Verdaguer, S. Comparative study of ferrofluids based on dextran-coated iron oxide and metal nanoparticles for contrast agents in magnetic resonance imaging. *Nanotechnology* **2004**, *15*, S154. [CrossRef]

24. Carmen Bautista, M.; Bomati-Miguel, O.; del Puerto Morales, M.; Serna, C.J.; Veintemillas-Verdaguer, S. Surface characterisation of dextran-coated iron oxide nanoparticles prepared by laser pyrolysis and coprecipitation. *J. Magn. Magn. Mater.* **2005**, *293*, 20–27. [CrossRef]

25. Nakashima, Y.; Plump, A.S.; Raines, E.W.; Breslow, J.L.; Ross, R. ApoE-deficient mice develop lesions of all phases of atherosclerosis throughout the arterial tree. *Arterioscler. Thromb.* **1994**, *14*, 133–140. [CrossRef] [PubMed]

26. Swirski, F.K.; Pittet, M.J.; Kircher, M.F.; Aikawa, E.; Jaffer, F.A.; Libby, P.; Weissleder, R. Monocyte accumulation in mouse atherogenesis is progressive and proportional to extent of disease. *Proc. Natl. Acad. Sci. USA* **2006**, *103*, 10340–10345. [CrossRef] [PubMed]

27. Li, Y.; Zhang, G.C.; Wang, X.H.; Liu, D.H. Progression of atherosclerosis in ApoE-knockout mice fed on a high-fat diet. *Eur. Rev. Med. Pharmacol. Sci.* **2016**, *20*, 3863–3867. [PubMed]

28. Wen, S.; Liu, D.F.; Cui, Y.; Harris, S.S.; Chen, Y.C.; Li, K.C.; Ju, S.H.; Teng, G.J. In vivo MRI detection of carotid atherosclerotic lesions and kidney inflammation in ApoE-deficient mice by using LOX-1 targeted iron nanoparticles. *Nanomedicine* **2014**, *10*, 639–649. [CrossRef] [PubMed]

29. Wu, S.C.; Chen, Y.J.; Wang, H.C.; Chou, M.Y.; Chang, T.Y.; Yuan, S.S.; Chen, C.Y.; Hou, M.F.; Hsu, J.T.; Wang, Y.M. Bispecific Antibody Conjugated Manganese-Based Magnetic Engineered Iron Oxide for Imaging of HER2/neu- and EGFR-Expressing Tumors. *Theranostics* **2016**, *6*, 118–130. [CrossRef] [PubMed]

30. Liu, D.; Chen, C.; Hu, G.; Mei, Q.; Qiu, H.; Long, G.; Hu, G. Specific targeting of nasopharyngeal carcinoma cell line CNE1 by C225-conjugated ultrasmall superparamagnetic iron oxide particles with magnetic resonance imaging. *Acta Biochim. Biophys. Sin.* **2011**, *43*, 301–306. [CrossRef] [PubMed]

31. Koiwaya, H.; Sasaki, K.; Ueno, T.; Yokoyama, S.; Toyama, Y.; Ohtsuka, M.; Nakayoshi, T.; Mitsutake, Y.; Imaizumi, T. Augmented neovascularization with magnetized endothelial progenitor cells in rats with hind-limb ischemia. *J. Mol. Cell. Cardiol.* **2011**, *51*, 33–40. [CrossRef] [PubMed]

32. Andres-Manzano, M.J.; Andres, V.; Dorado, B. Oil Red O and Hematoxylin and Eosin Staining for Quantification of Atherosclerosis Burden in Mouse Aorta and Aortic Root. *Methods Mol. Biol.* **2015**, *1339*, 85–99. [CrossRef] [PubMed]

33. Mohanta, S.; Yin, C.; Weber, C.; Hu, D.; Habenicht, A.J.R. Aorta Atherosclerosis Lesion Analysis in Hyperlipidemic Mice. *Bio Protocol.* **2016**, *6*, e1833. [CrossRef] [PubMed]

34. Khalkhali, M.; Rostamizadeh, K.; Sadighian, S.; Khoeini, F.; Naghibi, M.; Hamidi, M. The impact of polymer coatings on magnetite nanoparticles performance as MRI contrast agents: A comparative study. *DARU J. Pharm. Sci.* **2015**, *23*, 45. [CrossRef] [PubMed]

35. Adhikari, U.; Scheiner, S. Preferred Configurations of Peptide–Peptide Interactions. *J. Phys. Chem. A* **2013**, *117*, 489–496. [CrossRef] [PubMed]

36. Vallee, A.; Humblot, V.; Pradier, C.-M. Peptide Interactions with Metal and Oxide Surfaces. *Acc. Chem. Res.* **2010**, *43*, 1297–1306. [CrossRef] [PubMed]

37. Souza, T.G.F.; Ciminelli, V.S.T.; Mohallem, N.D.S. A comparison of TEM and DLS methods to characterize size distribution of ceramic nanoparticles. *J. Phys. Conf. Ser.* **2016**, *733*, 012039. [CrossRef]

38. Bhattacharjee, S. DLS and zeta potential—What they are and what they are not? *J. Controll. Release* **2016**, *235*, 337–351. [CrossRef] [PubMed]

39. Li, G.; Sun, J.; Hou, W.; Jiang, S.; Huang, Y.; Geng, J. Three-dimensional porous carbon composites containing high sulfur nanoparticle content for high-performance lithium–sulfur batteries. *Nat. Commun.* **2016**, *7*, 10601. [CrossRef] [PubMed]

40. Liu, Y.; Williams, M.G.; Miller, T.J.; Teplyakov, A.V. Nanoparticle layer deposition for highly controlled multilayer formation based on high- coverage monolayers of nanoparticles. *Thin Solid Films* **2016**, *598*, 16–24. [CrossRef] [PubMed]

41. Zhao, M.; Cao, Y.; Liu, X.; Deng, J.; Li, D.; Gu, H. Effect of nitrogen atomic percentage on N($^+$)-bombarded MWCNTs in cytocompatibility and hemocompatibility. *Nanoscale Res. Lett.* **2014**, *9*, 142. [CrossRef] [PubMed]

42. Liu, Y.; Yu, H.; Quan, X.; Chen, S.; Zhao, H.; Zhang, Y. Efficient and durable hydrogen evolution electrocatalyst based on nonmetallic nitrogen doped hexagonal carbon. *Sci. Rep.* **2014**, *4*, 6843. [CrossRef] [PubMed]

43. Gharbi, A.; Legigan, T.; Humblot, V.; Papot, S.; Berjeaud, J.-M. Surface functionalization by covalent immobilization of an innovative carvacrol derivative to avoid fungal biofilm formation. *AMB Express* **2015**, *5*, 9. [CrossRef] [PubMed]

44. Wang, Q.; Zhang, C.; Shen, G.; Liu, H.; Fu, H.; Cui, D. Fluorescent carbon dots as an efficient siRNA nanocarrier for its interference therapy in gastric cancer cells. *J. Nanobiotechnol.* **2014**, *12*, 58. [CrossRef] [PubMed]

45. Liang, P.C.; Chen, Y.C.; Chiang, C.F.; Mo, L.R.; Wei, S.Y.; Hsieh, W.Y.; Lin, W.L. Doxorubicin-modified magnetic nanoparticles as a drug delivery system for magnetic resonance imaging-monitoring magnet-enhancing tumor chemotherapy. *Int. J. Nanomed.* **2016**, *11*, 2021–2037. [CrossRef]

46. Bumb, A.; Brechbiel, M.W.; Choyke, P.L.; Fugger, L.; Eggeman, A.; Prabhakaran, D.; Hutchinson, J.; Dobson, P.J. Synthesis and characterization of ultra-small superparamagnetic iron oxide nanoparticles thinly coated with silica. *Nanotechnology* **2008**, *19*, 335601. [CrossRef] [PubMed]

47. Ho, D.; Sun, X.; Sun, S. Monodisperse Magnetic Nanoparticles for Theranostic Applications. *Acc. Chem. Res.* **2011**, *44*, 875–882. [CrossRef] [PubMed]

48. Mohapatra, J.; Mitra, A.; Bahadur, D.; Aslam, M. Surface controlled synthesis of MFe_2O_4 (M = Mn, Fe, Co, Ni and Zn) nanoparticles and their magnetic characteristics. *CrystEngComm* **2013**, *15*, 524–532. [CrossRef]

49. Yao, Y.; Wang, Y.; Zhang, Y.; Li, Y.; Sheng, Z.; Wen, S.; Ma, G.; Liu, N.; Fang, F.; Teng, G.-J. In Vivo Imaging of Macrophages during the Early-Stages of Abdominal Aortic Aneurysm Using High Resolution MRI in ApoE$^{-/-}$ Mice. *PLoS ONE* **2012**, *7*, e33523. [CrossRef] [PubMed]

50. Kitagawa, T.; Kosuge, H.; Uchida, M.; Iida, Y.; Dalman, R.L.; Douglas, T.; McConnell, M.V. RGD targeting of human ferritin iron oxide nanoparticles enhances in vivo MRI of vascular inflammation and angiogenesis in experimental carotid disease and abdominal aortic aneurysm. *J. Magn. Reson. Imaging* **2017**, *45*, 1144–1153. [CrossRef] [PubMed]

51. Salinas, B.; Ruiz-Cabello, J.; Lechuga-Vieco, A.V.; Benito, M.; Herranz, F. Surface-Functionalized Nanoparticles by Olefin Metathesis: A Chemoselective Approach for In Vivo Characterization of Atherosclerosis Plaque. *Chem. A Eur. J.* **2015**, *21*, 10450–10456. [CrossRef] [PubMed]

52. Braidwood, L.; Learmonth, K.; Graham, A.; Conner, J. Potent efficacy signals from systemically administered oncolytic herpes simplex virus (HSV1716) in hepatocellular carcinoma xenograft models. *J. Hepatocell. Carcinoma* **2014**, *1*, 149–161. [PubMed]

53. Langheinrich, A.C.; Kampschulte, M.; Scheiter, F.; Dierkes, C.; Stieger, P.; Bohle, R.M.; Weidner, W. Atherosclerosis, inflammation and lipoprotein glomerulopathy in kidneys of apoE$^{-/-}$/LDL$^{-/-}$ double knockout mice. *BMC Nephrol.* **2010**, *11*, 18. [CrossRef] [PubMed]

54. Yoo, M.-K.; Park, I.-K.; Lim, H.-T.; Lee, S.-J.; Jiang, H.-L.; Kim, Y.-K.; Choi, Y.-J.; Cho, M.-H.; Cho, C.-S. Folate–PEG–superparamagnetic iron oxide nanoparticles for lung cancer imaging. *Acta Biomater.* **2012**, *8*, 3005–3013. [CrossRef] [PubMed]

55. Lee, B.-S.; Choi, J.Y.; Kim, J.Y.; Han, S.H.; Park, J.E. Simvastatin and losartan differentially and synergistically inhibit atherosclerosis in apolipoprotein e($^{-/-}$) mice. *Korean Circ. J.* **2012**, *42*, 543–550. [CrossRef] [PubMed]

3

Orally Disintegrating Tablets Containing Melt Extruded Amorphous Solid Dispersion of Tacrolimus for Dissolution Enhancement

Poovizhi Ponnammal [1,2], Parijat Kanaujia [1,*], Yin Yani [1] (ID), Wai Kiong Ng [1,3] and Reginald B. H. Tan [1,2,*]

[1] Institute of Chemical and Engineering Sciences, 1, Pesek Road Jurong Island, Singapore 627833, Singapore; poovizhi1387@gmail.com (P.P.); yinyani@gmail.com (Y.Y.); ng_wai_kiong@ices.a-star.edu.sg (W.K.N.)
[2] Department of Chemical and Biomolecular Engineering, National University of Singapore, Singapore 117585, Singpore
[3] Department of Pharmacy, National University of Singapore, Singapore 117559, Singpore
*   Correspondence: parijat_kanaujia@ices.a-star.edu.sg (P.K.); reginald_tan@ices.a-star.edu.sg (R.B.H.T.)

Abstract: In order to improve the aqueous solubility and dissolution of Tacrolimus (TAC), amorphous solid dispersions of TAC were prepared by hot melt extrusion with three hydrophilic polymers, Polyvinylpyrrolidone vinyl acetate (PVP VA64), Soluplus® and Hydroxypropyl Cellulose (HPC), at a drug loading of 10% w/w. Molecular modeling was used to determine the miscibility of the drug with the carrier polymers by calculating the Hansen Solubility Parameters. Powder X-ray diffraction and differential scanning calorimetry (DSC) studies of powdered solid dispersions revealed the conversion of crystalline TAC to amorphous form. Fourier transform Infrared (FTIR) spectroscopy results indicated formation of hydrogen bond between TAC and polymers leading to stabilization of TAC in amorphous form. The extrudates were found to be stable under accelerated storage conditions for 3 months with no re-crystallization, indicating that hot melt extrusion is suitable for producing stable amorphous solid dispersions of TAC in PVP VA64, Soluplus® and HPC. Stable solid dispersions of amorphous TAC exhibited higher dissolution rate, with the solid dispersions releasing more than 80% drug in 15 min compared to the crystalline drug giving 5% drug release in two hours. These stable solid dispersions were incorporated into orally-disintegrating tablets in which the solid dispersion retained its solubility, dissolution and stability advantage.

Keywords: melt extrusion; amorphous solid dispersion; dissolution enhancement; tacrolimus; orally-disintegrating tablets

1. Introduction

Tacrolimus (TAC) is a potent immunosuppressive drug widely used to prevent organ rejection of liver and kidney transplants and less frequently in heart, lung and heart lung transplants. TAC acts by engaging an immunophilin, FK506-binding protein-12 (FKBP12) and forming a complex which inhibits calcineurin with much more potency than cyclosporine [1,2]. TAC is a highly hydrophobic drug with aqueous solubility of 0.7–2 µg/mL [3,4]. It falls under class 2 of the Biopharmaceutics Classification System (BCS) for drugs and permeability of TAC has been reported to be approximately 1.4×10^{-4} cm/s [5,6]. TAC is marketed as a capsule (Prograf®) containing solid dispersion of drug with hydroxypropyl methylcellulose in order to improve dissolution and bioavailability [4,7] and extended release tablet (Envarsus XR®) prepared by melt agglomeration technology [8]. It exhibits low bioavailability (10–25%) and significantly variable pharmacokinetics due to its poor aqueous solubility, extensive metabolism by intestinal and hepatic cytochrome P450 3A4 enzyme [9] along with the effects of P glycoprotein efflux in the intestine [5,10,11]. TAC has a narrow therapeutic window (5–20 ng/mL) and overexposure increases the risk of nephrotoxicity and neurotoxicity [12,13] whereas low level can lead to graft rejection.

Several attempts have been made to improve the dissolution rate of TAC using solid dispersion formulation with various hydrophilic excipients. Solid dispersions of TAC with poloxamer 407, polyvinyl alcohol and sodium dodecyl sulfate were prepared using ultra-rapid freeze-drying. Upon dissolution in acidic media, these solid dispersions formed supersaturated solution and the solid dispersion with poloxamer 407 showed 1.5 fold improvement in oral bioavailability [14]. Effect of the formulation method on the dissolution rate was studied by preparing solid dispersions by spray drying with solvent evaporation/solvent wetting/surface attach method with water. The formulations prepared by solvent evaporation method produced amorphous dispersion which showed a 15 fold increase in dissolution [3]. TAC was formulated as solid dispersion with amino alkyl methacrylate copolymer (Eudragit E®) with hydrochloric acid. The solubility and dissolution of the drug was improved several fold with no re-precipitation of drug for up to 24 h [15,16]. Solubility and dissolution enhancing effect of different types of cyclodextrins was studied by complexing TAC with cyclodextrins [17]. Proliposomes for TAC were formulated using various lipids by the thin film hydration method. In Vitro studies show that the drug release from the optimized proliposome formulation was significantly higher than that of the pure drug, this has also been correlated to in vivo studies which showed promising results [18].

These formulation approaches were based on increasing dissolution rate of TAC and lack in preventing or reducing the effect of intestinal enzymatic degradation and p-glycoprotein efflux pump on bioavailability of TAC. An inhalable formulation of TAC was developed by spray drying TAC with lung lipids like DPPC and DPPG at 100 °C in a molar ration of 3:1 to mimic the lung surfactant layer [19]. In a clinical study, 17 heart and lung transplant patients were given TAC sublingually twice a day by administering contents of marketed capsuled below the tongue for 15 min and patients were advised to not to swallow the saliva during this 15 min period. The sublingual delivery of TAC was able to generate therapeutic levels of TAC in blood without initial spike in blood levels. The sublingual TAC administration was found to be effective in replacing intravenous injection [20]. A fast disintegrating tablet containing solid dispersion of TAC was prepared and evaluated for dissolution and stability. The solid dispersion was prepared by solvent removal method with three different stabilizers namely inulin 1.8 kDa, inulin 4 kDa and PVP K 30. The tablet prepared from solid dispersion containing 10% of TAC showed optimal results and inulin 1.8 kDa tablet showed excellent stability and retention of fast dissolution property [21].

In this research work, an attempt was made to stabilize TAC in amorphous form by preparing solid dispersions with different polymeric excipients using melt extrusion and incorporating into orally-disintegrating tablets (ODTs). Melt extrusion is a continuous and industrially feasible process which does not involve the use of solvents. It is easily scalable and has few processing steps [22]. This work shows the development of formulations of TAC, their characterization and a study of their dissolution profiles and storage stability. The advantages of the amorphous state, the method of production and the dosage form have been harnessed to produce formulations by synergizing the benefits.

2. Materials and Methods

2.1. Materials

TAC was purchased from Concord Biotech Ltd., Ahmedabad, India. PVP VA64 (Kollidon VA 64) and Soluplus® were kindly gifted by BASF, Ludwigshafen, Germany. Hydroxypropyl Cellulose (HPC, LF grade) was received as sample from Ashland (Ashland Inc. Covington, KY, USA) Micro Crystalline cellulose (Avicel PH101), Mannitol, Magnesium stearate and other chemicals used were purchased from

Sigma Aldrich (Sigma, St. Louis, MO, USA). HPLC grade methanol and acetonitrile were purchased from Fischer Scientific (Fischer Scientific Pte. Ltd, Pandan Cres., Singapore).

2.2. Hansen Solubility Parameter and Excipient Selection

Molecular dynamics (MD) simulations were carried out using the Materials Studio Version 7.0.100 (Accelrys Software Inc, San Diego, CA, USA) for TAC [23]. The crystal structure (Figure 1A) was obtained from the Cambridge Structural Database, Ver. 5.26 (Cambridge Crystallographic Data Centre Cambridge, UK). The space group of the crystal is P212121 (orthorhombic with the unit cell dimensions of a = 10.939 Å, b = 15.878 Å, c = 27.184 Å, and Z = 4). The crystal structure was extended to $3 \times 3 \times 2$ unit cells (72 TAC molecules). The COMPASS [24] (condensed-phase optimized molecular potentials for the atomistic simulation studies) force field was used to model the atomic interactions for TAC molecules. COMPASS force field model gives densities of 1.104 g/cm^3 for pure TAC. The integration time step used was 1 fs. Ewald summation was used to enable the long-range interactions. A cutoff radius of 12.5 Å was used for both non-bonded and electrostatic interactions. Simulation in the NPT (constant number of particle, constant pressure, and constant temperature) ensemble was conducted at 298 K for 2 ns to ensure that TAC system reaches equilibration condition. The equilibrated amorphous cell of TAC is shown in Figure 1B. Equilibration was determined by observing the change in the thermodynamic properties (energies, temperatures, and densities) as a function of time. The system was concluded to have reached equilibration condition if these properties showed sufficiently small variations over time. The required time was less than 100 ps. The Nose/Hoover thermostat [25] and Berendsen barostat [26] were used to control the temperature and pressure, respectively. The production run was done by choosing three different trajectories (at time step of 1 ns, 1.5 ns, and 2 ns) from the equilibrated system. Energy minimization was then performed for the three sets of data, followed by MD simulation in NVT (isothermal) ensemble at 298 K for 100 ps. The final 50 ps were used to calculate the Hansen solubility parameter. The three data sets were then averaged to obtain the solubility parameter for TAC. The solubility parameters of the polymers were taken from literature.

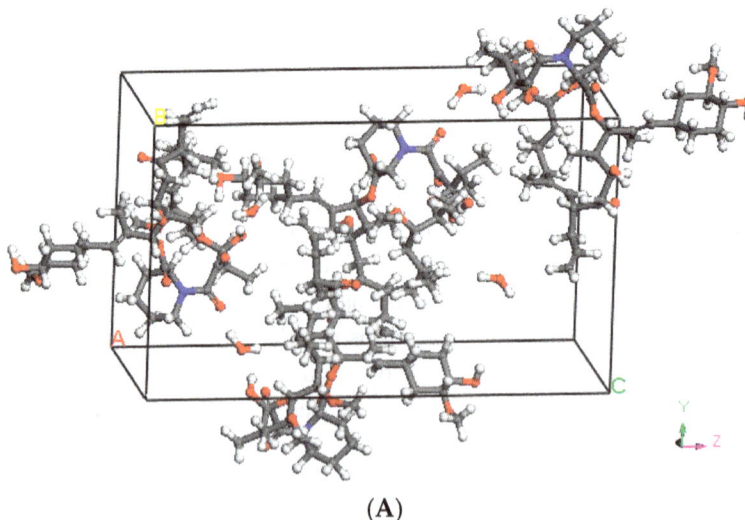

(A)

Figure 1. *Cont.*

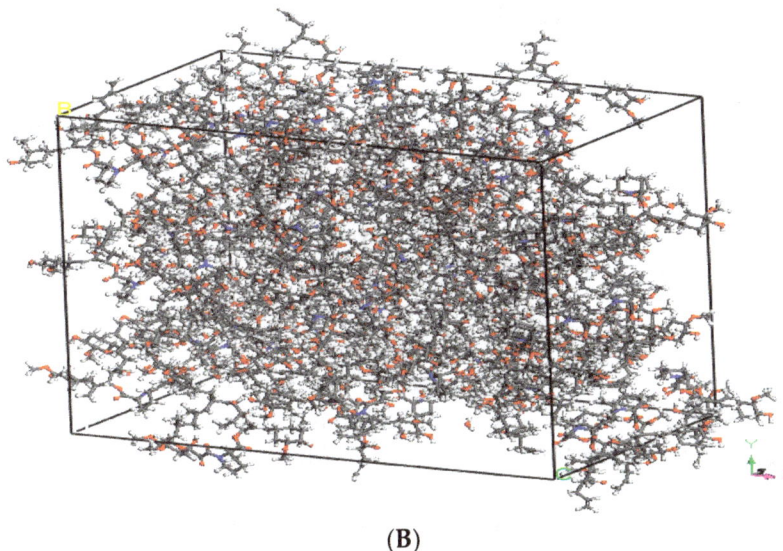

(B)

Figure 1. (**A**) Crystal structure of tacrolimus (TAC) (**B**) equilibrated amorphous cell of TAC (72 molecules).

2.3. Thermogravimetric Analysis

In order to study the thermal stability of TAC alone and in combination with polymers, thermogravimetric analysis (TGA) was performed using a TGA Q500 V6.7 build 203 (TA Instruments, New Castle, DE, USA). Alumina crucibles were used and the sample weight ranged from 5–15 mg. The sample was heated from 25 to 200 °C at the rate of 10 °C/min and weight loss was recorded.

2.4. Differential Scanning Calorimetry

A hyper differential scanning calorimetry (DSC) (PerkinElmer instruments, Shelton, CT, USA) was used to record the thermogram. The enthalpic response was calibrated with Indium and zinc. An empty sealed pan was used as reference. The samples were kept under isothermal condition at 25 °C for 10 min in sealed standard aluminum pans. DSC study was performed at 10 °C min^{-1} from 25 to 160 °C under a nitrogen flow rate of 20 mL min^{-1}. A second reheating step at 10 °C/min to 160 °C after cooling to -50 °C was added to DSC of pure TAC to determine the glass transition temperature (T_g). The data treatment and integration were done by Pyris Analysis (PerkinElmer, instruments, Shelton, CT, USA).

2.5. Preparation of Solid Dispersions by Hot Melt Extrusion (HME)

The physical mixtures were prepared by geometric mixing of the individually weighed polymers and drug. The physical mixture was placed in a powder mixer (Alphie powder mixer, Hexagon product development, Vadodara, Gujarat, India) for 20 min to ensure homogeneity. A preheated co-rotating twin screw melt extruder (Prism Eurolab 16 Melt extruder from Thermo Scientific, Karlsruhe, Germany) having a horizontally split barrel with length to diameter ratio of 25:1 and 15.6 mm diameter screws was used for the extrusion. About 30–40 g of the physical mixture containing 10% w/w of TAC was manually fed to preheated twin-screw extruder rotating at a speed of 200 rpm. In order to reduce the residence time in the heated barrel, the physical mixture was fed from zone 3. The temperatures used in the different zones are shown below.

Barrel Zone	1	2	3	4	5	6	Rod die
Temperature (°C)	not used	not used	70	125	135	140	135

A rod die with a 2 mm orifice was used for the extrusion of solid dispersion in the shape of cylindrical strands. A small (40 cm) conveyor belt was used to collect and air-cool the extrudates. Extrudes were stored in screw-capped glass bottles at room temperature (25 °C) under low humidity (25% relative humidity).

The extrudates were milled (MM 200 Retsch GmbH, Haan, Germany) for 2 min at a frequency of 30 Hz in a stainless-steel ball mill using a 1.5-cm diameter stainless steel ball. The powdered solid dispersions were sieved and 50–250 μm fraction was collected and stored in screw-capped glass bottles in dry cabinet (25% RH) at room temperature. The sieved fraction of solid dispersion was used for the characterization and analysis.

2.6. High Performance Liquid Chromatography (HPLC) Analysis

The analysis of the drug was done using an Agilent HPLC (Agilent Technologies, Santa Clara, CA, USA). A Zorbax Eclipse Plus C18 column was used with an isocratic elution method where the mobile phase was a mixture containing 45% Methanol, 45% Acetonitrile and 10% Water at a flow rate of 1.5 mL/minute and injection volume of 10 μL. The column was maintained at a temperature of 40 °C while the sample holder was kept at 4 °C and the UV detector was set to 214 nm. The samples for drug estimation were prepared in methanol and TAC was eluted at a retention time of 3.3 ± 0.1 min. For samples from dissolution experiments, the samples were directly injected into the column after filtration and analyzed. Calibration was performed in both methanol and dissolution medium between 0 to 100 mg/L [27].

2.7. Microscopy and Imaging

An Olympus polarization microscope BX51 (Olympus Corporation, Tokyo, Japan) was used along with a Sony digital color video camera (Sony Corporation, Tokyo, Japan) to capture images using the analySIS pro software (Soft Imaging Systems, Olympus Corporation, Tokyo, Japan). The extruded strands and milled powders were observed under a microscope under both polarized and ordinary light.

2.8. Powder X-ray Diffraction

The powder X-ray diffraction analysis was done on a Bruker D8 (Bruker AXS GmbH, Karlsruhe, Germany) Advance X-ray diffractometer using Cu Kα radiation (α = 1.5406 Å) with a scanning rate of 1°/min and scanning angles between 4° to 50°.

2.9. Fourier Transform InfraRed (FTIR) Spectrophotometric Analysis

FTIR was performed on a BioRad Spectrophotometer (Bio Rad, Philadelphia, PA, USA). The powder samples were made into KBr pellets and the transmittance in the wave number range of 4000 to 400 cm^{-1} was measured for 64 scans.

2.10. Dissolution Testing

Dissolution studies were done in USP II paddle dissolution apparatus (Agilent 708-DS, Agilent Technologies, Santa Clara, CA, USA). 250 mL of 0.1% sodium lauryl sulfate (SLS) in de-ionized water was used as the medium of dissolution [28]. Crystalline TAC or powdered solid dispersion equivalent to 5 mg TAC was added to the dissolution tank. The temperature of the water bath was set at 37 ± 0.5 °C and the paddle speed was set at 100 rpm. 1 mL of sample was withdrawn at each time point, syringe filtered and analyzed by High Performance Liquid Chromatography (HPLC) as described above.

2.11. Amorphous Stability Testing

The solid dispersion samples were stored in capped glass vials under accelerated conditions in a stability chamber (Climacell EVO, MMM Group, München, Germany) set at 40 °C and 75% RH.

The storage stability testing was done for 3 months. The solid dispersion stability in terms of drug content, amorphous nature and retention of dissolution enhancement was tested.

2.12. Orally-Disintegrating Tablet (ODT) Compression and Characterization

The solid dispersion powders were incorporated into ODTs. The physical mixtures of the excipients were compressed using a hand operated Carver tablet press and a flat faced tablet punch (10 mm diameter). Two hundred and fifty mg of physical mixture containing the excipients and the solid dispersion was weighed into the die and the tablet was compressed by applying a force of 1 ton for 10 s. The Pharmatron Dr. Schleuniger Multi test 50 (SOTAX AG, Aesch, Switzerland) was used for hardness testing and it gave the hardness value in kilopond (kP). The prepared tablets were also evaluated for friability by Agilent Technologies 250 Friabilator and disintegration time by Agilent Technologies 100 Automated Disintegration (Agilent Technologies, Santa Clara, CA, USA).

3. Results

3.1. Hansen Solubility Parameter and Excipient Selection

The solid-solid miscibility of drug and polymers can be predicted by calculating Hansen solubility parameters (δt) from the chemical structure. The solubility parameter of TAC was calculated using molecular dynamic simulation using the method reported by Gupta and coworkers [29]. The difference between the solubility parameters ($\Delta\delta t$) of two materials is known as interaction parameter and is indicative of likely miscibility or immiscibility. Compounds with $\Delta\delta t$ value 7.0 MPa$^{1/2}$ or less are most likely to be miscible whereas compounds with value greater than 10.0 MPa$^{1/2}$ are most likely immiscible [30]. The interaction parameter ($\Delta\delta t$) for TAC and all polymers is less than 1, so it is most likely that drug and polymer melt would be miscible during melt extrusion. The carrier polymers were selected based on their glass transition temperatures and the Hansen solubility parameters (Table 1).

Table 1. Properties of drug and carrier polymers. TAC: Tacrolimus; PVP VA64: Polyvinylpyrrolidone vinyl acetate; HPC: Hydroxypropyl Cellulose.

Drug/Polymer	Aqueous Solubility	Molecular Weight	Glass Transition (°C)	Hansen's Solubility Parameters (MPa$^{1/2}$)	Interaction Parameter ($\Delta\delta t$)	Solid State
TAC	Insoluble (2.6 µg/mL)	804.02 g/mol	78.8 (amorphous form)	19.1 *	-	Crystalline
PVP VA64	Very soluble	45–70 kD	101	19.7 [31]	0.6	Amorphous
Soluplus	Very soluble	118 kD	70	19.4 [31]	0.3	Amorphous
HPC	Soluble	95 kD	105	21.27 [32]	2.17	Semi-crystalline

* Calculated.

3.2. Thermal Stability of Tacrolimus (TAC)

Hot melt extrusion involves the use of temperature and shear for processing physical mixtures into solid dispersions. The thermal stability of materials (both drug and excipients) will play a crucial role in the selection of extrusion parameters.

The TGA of pure crystalline drug shows that it begins decomposing beyond 200 °C. The physical mixtures of TAC with polymers showed a 5–10% weight loss at 100 °C which could be attributed to the evaporation of moisture present in the polymers (Figure 2). The DSC of TAC showed a melting peak at 132.8 °C during the first heating cycle. After cooling at 50 °C/min to −50 °C, and reheating at 10 °C/min, the melting endotherm of the drug disappeared and glass transition temperature (T$_g$) was observed at 78.8 °C confirming conversion of crystalline TAC to amorphous form by melting and rapid cooling in the DSC. These results show that TAC can be converted to its amorphous form by melting and rapid cooling [21,33].

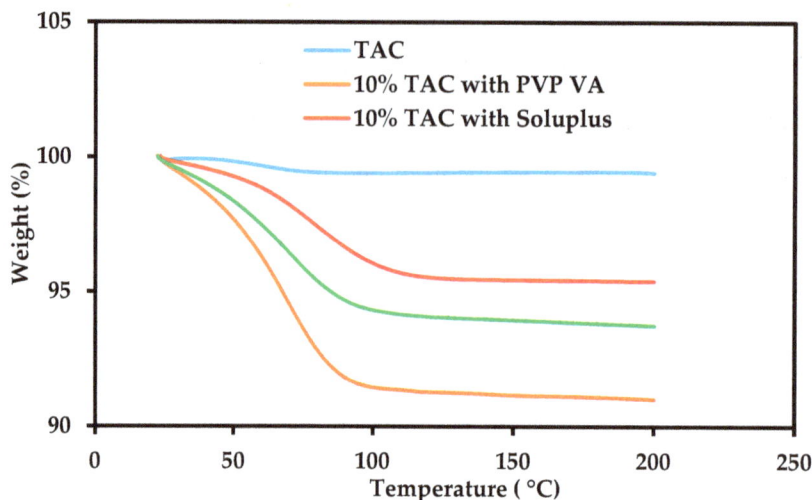

Figure 2. TGA of crystalline TAC and physical mixtures with PVP-VA 64, Soluplus and HPC containing 10% *w/w* TAC.

3.3. Hot Melt Extrusion

The extruded solid dispersions are clear, transparent and brittle strands when observed under a stereo microscope equipped with a digital camera (Leica MZ 16, Leica, Wetzlar, Germany) (Figure 3c,f,i). The milled powder observed under polarized light showed that there were no crystalline particles present in the extruded formulation (Figure 3b,e,h), whereas the corresponding physical mixture showed presence of crystalline TAC (Figure 3a,d,g). TAC content in the extruded and milled solid dispersions was determined by HPLC method. The drug loading efficiency was estimated to be $102 \pm 3\%$, $88 \pm 1\%$ and $79 \pm 8\%$ of the expected drug content (10% *w/w*) in PVP VA 64, Soluplus and HPC solid dispersions respectively. The reduction of TAC content in case of Soluplus and HPC could be due to degradation of TAC during extrusion.

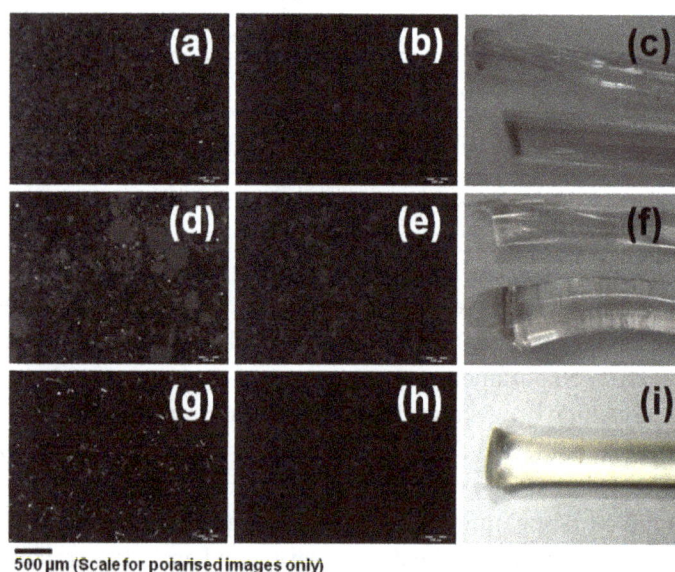

500 μm (Scale for polarised images only)

Figure 3. Polarized light photomicrographs of (**a**) 10% TAC PVP-VA 64 physical mixture, (**b**) 10% TAC PVP-VA 64 extruded and milled powder, (**d**) 10% TAC Soluplus physical mixture (**e**) 10% TAC Soluplus extruded and milled powder (**g**) 10% TAC HPC physical mixture, (**h**) 10% TAC HPC extruded and milled powder, and optical photomicrograph of Extruded strands of (**c**) PVP VA 64 (**f**) Soluplus and (**i**) HPC containing 10% *w/w* TAC.

3.4. Differential Scanning Calorimetry (DSC) Analysis

The DSC thermograms of the physical mixtures of drug and polymer showed a melting peak at 132 °C (see Figure 4A) corresponding to the melting peak of the pure drug while the extruded solid dispersions did not have a melting peak of TAC indicating the absence of crystalline TAC in the solid dispersion. This could be attributed to the conversion of crystalline TAC to amorphous form (Figure 4B).

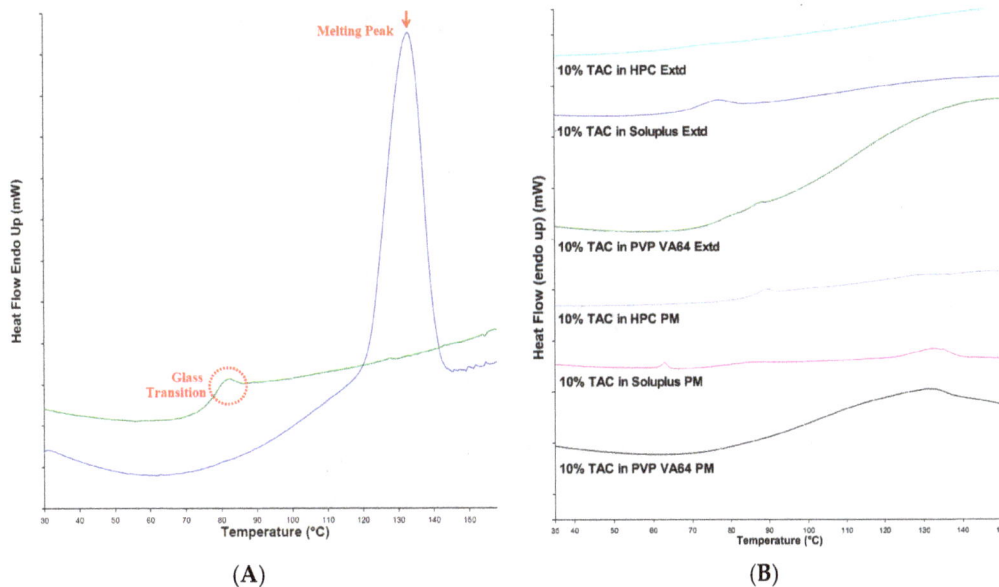

(A)

(B)

Figure 4. (**A**) DSC thermograms of TAC, first heating cycle showing melting peak and second heating cycle showing glass transition; (**B**) DSC of physical mixtures and formulations containing TAC.

3.5. Powder X-ray Diffraction

The diffraction pattern of TAC (Figure 5A) shows characteristic peaks at 2θ values of 8.5, 10.1, 11.2, 19 and 23.5 [4,15]. The powder X-ray diffraction (PXRD) analysis of the physical mixtures shows peaks corresponding to the pure drug while the extruded solid dispersion powders exhibited an amorphous halo (Figure 5B) with all three polymers. These, along with the DSC results confirm that TAC is present in the amorphous form in the extruded samples.

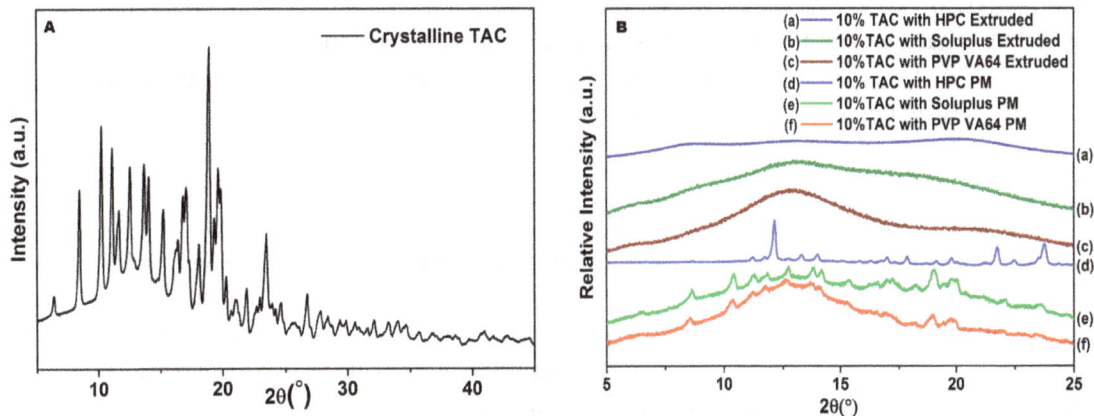

Figure 5. X-ray diffraction patterns of (**A**) TAC and (**B**) physical mixtures and solid dispersion containing 10% TAC.

3.6. FTIR

The FTIR spectra of TAC showed absorption bands of C-O-C (ether) stretching vibrations at 1173 and 1090 cm^{-1}, C-O (ester) stretching vibration at 1194 cm^{-1}, C=O (keto-amide) and C=C stretching vibration at 1640 cm^{-1}, C=O (ester and ketone) stretching vibration peak at 1740, 1724 and 1694 cm^{-1}, and O-H stretching vibration at 3440 cm^{-1} [34].

In the extruded PVP VA64 solid dispersions, the absorption bands attributed to C=O groups at 1724 and 1694 cm^{-1} disappear, and the absorption band at 1640 cm^{-1} was shifted to 1625 cm^{-1}. The peaks at 1173 and 1090 cm^{-1} are found in the physical mixture but the peak at 1090 cm^{-1} disappears and the peak at 1173 cm^{-1} is shifted to 1165 cm^{-1} in the extruded solid dispersion. In the extruded Soluplus solid dispersions, the absorption bands attributed to C=O groups at 1724 and 1694 cm^{-1} are present in the physical mixture but disappear in the extruded solid dispersion, and the absorption band at 1640 cm^{-1} was broadened in the extruded sample. The peak at 1090 cm^{-1} is shifted to 1080 cm^{-1} after extrusion while the peak at 1173 cm^{-1} disappears. The peak at 1194 cm^{-1} is slightly shifted to 1197 cm^{-1} in the extruded solid dispersion of TAC in Soluplus. The drug peaks at 1649, 1724 and 1740 cm^{-1} corresponding to the carbonyl groups are present in the HPC physical mixture while in extruded samples the peaks were shifted (Figure 6).

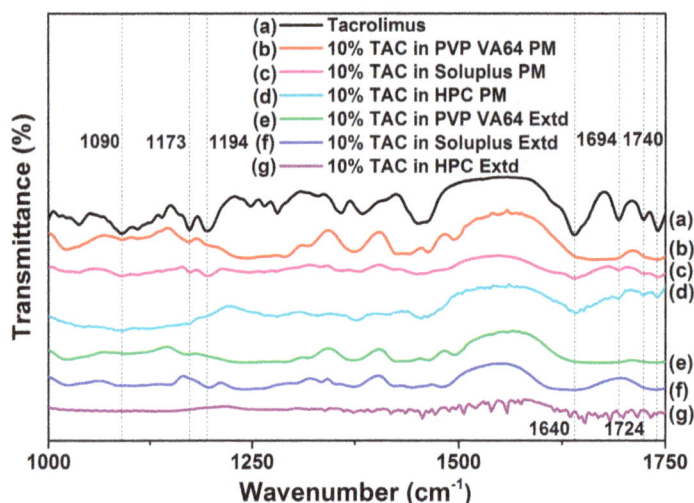

Figure 6. FTIR spectra of TAC and solid dispersion formulations in PVP VA64, Soluplus and HPC.

These observations could be attributed to hydrogen bond formation between PVP VA64, Soluplus and HPC with functional groups of TAC especially carbonyl group and hydroxyl group at molecular level [4]. The reduction in peak intensities could also be attributed to the formation of amorphous TAC in the extruded solid dispersions [34].

3.7. Dissolution Studies

The dissolution profiles of crystalline TAC and extruded formulations are shown in Figure 7. Since TAC is practically insoluble in water, 0.1% SLS was added to the dissolution media. About 5% of crystalline TAC had dissolved in media after 2 h of testing while the solid dispersions showed typical burst release of TAC. PVP-VA64, Soluplus and HPC solid dispersions showed 100%, 90% and 65% drug release in the first 15 min. The Soluplus formulation released 98% of drug in the 2 h of testing while the HPC formulation released 96% in the same time. The amorphous TAC in solid dispersion reaches concentrations of 20 mg/L while the crystalline drug reaches only 2 mg/L after two hours of dissolution testing. The HPC solid dispersion showed slowest release followed by Soluplus and PVP VA64 in first 15 min of dissolution testing. This could be due to the slow solublization behavior of the HPC which first swells and then solubilizes in water.

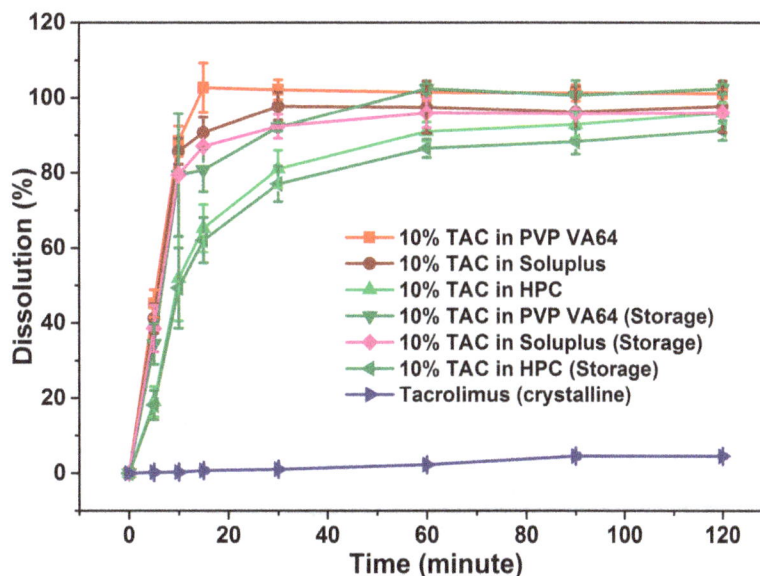

Figure 7. Dissolution profiles of solid dispersions of TAC before and after storage.

3.8. Stability Studies

The TAC solid dispersions were stored in screw capped glass bottles in a stability chamber at 40 °C/75% RH and their physical and chemical stability was studied. The % drug content was found to be at 94%, 86% and 82% for TAC solid dispersions in PVP VA64, Soluplus and HPC respectively after 3 months. The X-ray diffractogram showed an amorphous halo for all three solid dispersions after storage at 40 °C and 75% RH (accelerated conditions) for 3 months (Figure 8). This showed that amorphous TAC in all three formulations has good chemical and physical stability on storage under stressed conditions. The T_g of TAC was found to be 78.8 °C and calculated T_g of PVP-VA 64 solid dispersion was found to be 98.6 °C. As per general convention, storing 50 °C below T_g could significantly reduce the molecular mobility and re-crystallization [35]. The solid dispersions exhibited a typical burst release of TAC similar to the initial dissolution profile with approximately 81%, 87% and 62% of drug release in 15 min for PVP VA64, Soluplus and HPC solid dispersions of TAC respectively (Figure 7).

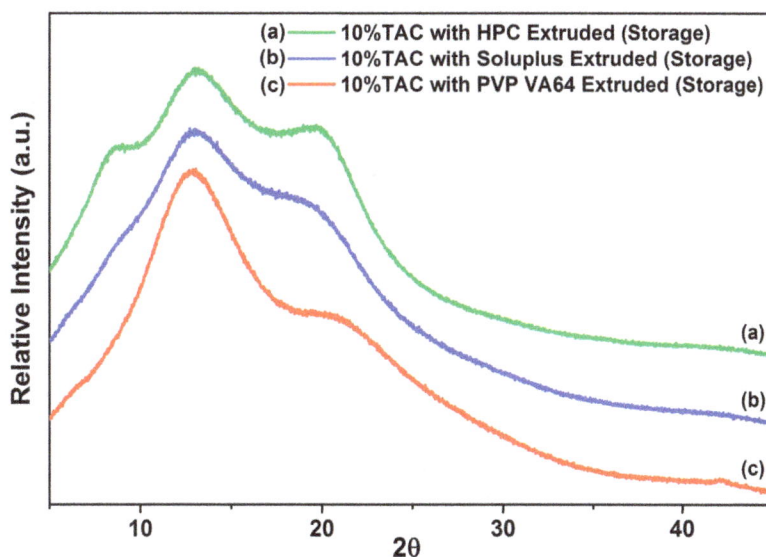

Figure 8. X-ray diffraction patterns of solid dispersion stored at 40 °C and 75% RH for 3 months.

3.9. ODT Formulation and Characterization

Two ODT compositions considered for being compressed into tablets are shown in Table 2. These formulations were punched into 250 mg tablets and the hardness, friability and disintegration were tested (Table 3). The disintegration time in all formulations was influenced by the polymer in the following order.

Soluplus < HPC < PVP VA64

Table 2. Composition of orally-disintegrating tablets (ODT) formulations.

Excipient	Formulation 1	Formulation 2
Microcrystalline cellulose	69.75%	59.5%
Crospovidone	10%	10%
Mannitol	10%	20%
Magnesium Stearate	0.25%	0.5%
Polymer/TAC Solid dispersion	10%	10%

Table 3. Characterization of blank ODTs.

Formulation	Polymer	Hardness (kP)	Friability (%)	Disintegration Time (s)
Formulation 1	PVP VA64	18.6 ± 2.8	0%	83
	Soluplus	11.9 ± 2.5	0.07%	10
	HPC	20.9 ± 2.7	0.06%	50
Formulation 2	PVP VA64	23.0 ± 1.8	0%	60
	Soluplus	17.5 ± 0.8	0.03%	18
	HPC	17.5 ± 1.0	0%	40

It was found that PVP VA64 produced the hardest tablets for each formulation with the least friability and longest disintegration time. It was also observed that increasing the PVP VA64 concentration also contributed to a corresponding increase in the disintegration time (data not shown). The USP stipulates that an ODT should disintegrate within 30 s [36] while the European Pharmacopoeia gives a time limit of 3 min (180 s) [37].

Formulation 2 that showed optimal performance in both hardness and disintegration in all three polymers was chosen and tablets containing solid dispersions of TAC were prepared.

3.10. Dissolution Testing of TAC ODTs

The ODTs were compressed with the polymer component of the blank tablets replaced by the extruded solid dispersion and formulated such that they contained 2.5 mg per 250 mg ODT. All the ODTs showed 100% drug release in the first 30 min of dissolution testing (Figure 9). Slight improvement was observed in rate of TAC release from Soluplus and HPC formulations as compared to powdered solid dispersion where HPC showed 65% release of TAC.

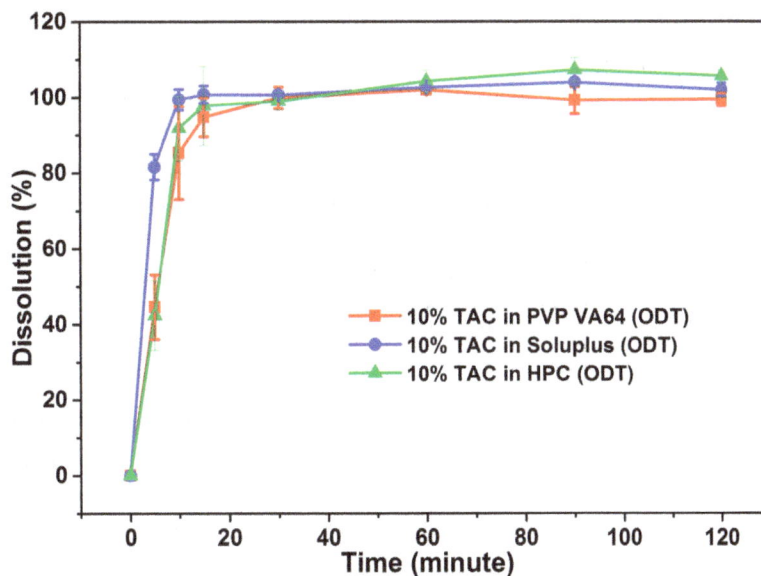

Figure 9. Dissolution profiles of ODTs containing solid dispersions of TAC.

4. Discussion

TAC is an established immunosuppressant that is used to prevent acute rejection of transplanted organ especially in the case of liver and lung transplants [38]. It is chemically classified as a macrolide lactone. The BCS places it in class II implying that the bioavailability of the drug is limited by its solubility at the site of absorption [39].

The DSC results of TAC show that the drug melts above 130 °C and on rapid cooling it solidifies into its amorphous form with a T_g at 78.8 °C. The extrusion was performed at 140 °C with reduced barrel length to decrease the residence time of material in the heated extruder. The material exiting the die was in the form of flexible, transparent, cylindrical rods of melt which cooled quickly on the conveyor belt to form brittle, glassy strands which were later milled to powders before storage. The clear and transparent visual appearance of the strands could mean that the drug is either dispersed as very small particles in the polymeric melt or has dissolved in the polymeric melt after melting in the extruder. This suggests the possibility of formation of a solid solution where the drug is molecularly dispersed in the polymer [40].

The DSC and XRD results confirm that TAC was present in the amorphous form. The melting peak and characteristic XRD peaks of the drug which were seen in the physical mixtures were not found in the extruded solid dispersions.

The molecular structure of TAC shows hydroxy, carbonyl (ester and ketone) and ether moieties in the molecule. The interaction between the drug and the polymers is observed in the region from 1050 to 1200 cm^{-1} in the FTIR. The changes in the spectra of the extruded solid dispersions suggest possibility of hydrogen bond formation between the carbonyl and hydroxyl groups present in TAC and the polymer. The ester and amide functional groups of PVP VA64 could be involved in hydrogen bonding like interactions during extrusion [41]. These interactions could also play a role in maintaining the super saturation of drug in media on dissolution and inhibition of the recrystallization of drug thereby enhancing stability [14].

The extruded solid dispersions exhibit a higher rate and percentage of dissolution of TAC compared to both the physical mixtures and pure crystalline drug. The solid dispersions showed a burst release of the drug in the first 15 min compared to the slow dissolution of pure crystalline TAC. The dissolution results obtained after the storage of solid dispersions in accelerated conditions for 3 months show dissolution profiles similar to those obtained during the initial testing. The increase in drug dissolution could be attributed to the amorphous form being a higher energy state which has been observed to exhibit higher solubility and dissolution rate compared to its crystalline form and the presence of hydrophilic polymer which enhances the rate of dissolution of drug from the extruded solid dispersions. These amorphous solid dispersions of TAC were incorporated into ODTs. PVP VA64 which acts as a binder in the compressed ODT releases the drug faster when it is tested as a solid dispersion powder and there is a marginally faster rate of drug release from the powdered solid dispersions compared to the ODTs. In the case of Soluplus and HPC, the ODT formulation helps disperse the solid dispersion into the media as opposed to the solid dispersion powder which tends to form lumps in the dissolution tub. This explains the slight improvement in the ODT over the solid dispersion powders in the time taken to release the drug.

5. Conclusions

HME was found to be a suitable technique for producing solid dispersions of TAC using PVP VA 64, Soluplus and HPC as carrier polymers at a drug loading of 10% by weight. The solid dispersions were found to be clear, glassy strands of TAC in the carrier polymers where the drug was stabilized in the amorphous form. The extruded solid dispersions which contained TAC in the amorphous form, showed a higher rate of dissolution. These solid dispersions were formulated into ODTs which maintained the dissolution advantage of the solid dispersions and were stable at accelerated conditions for 3 months. This approach can be used to deliver TAC as orally disintegrating tablets with improved dissolution rate.

Acknowledgments: The authors are thankful to GSK-EDB partnership for Green and Sustainable Manufacturing for financial support (ICES/11-322A02).

Author Contributions: Parijat Kanaujia, Wai Kiong Ng and Reginald B. H. Tan conceived and designed the experiments; Poovizhi Ponnammal and Parijat Kanaujia performed the experiments; Poovizhi Ponnammal, Parijat Kanaujia and Wai Kiong Ng analyzed the data; Yin Yani contributed molecular simulation analysis tools.

References

1. Halloran, P.F. Immunosuppressive drugs for kidney transplantation. *N. Engl. J. Med.* **2004**, *351*, 2715–2729. [CrossRef] [PubMed]

2. Kino, T.; Hatanaka, H.; Miyata, S.; Inamura, N.; Nishiyama, M.; Yajima, T.; Goto, T.; Okuhara, M.; Kohsaka, M.; Aoki, H.; et al. Fk-506, a novel immunosuppressant isolated from a streptomyces. Ii. Immunosuppressive effect of fk-506 in vitro. *J. Antibiot.* **1987**, *40*, 1256–1265. [CrossRef] [PubMed]

3. Joe, J.H.; Lee, W.M.; Park, Y.J.; Joe, K.H.; Oh, D.H.; Seo, Y.G.; Woo, J.S.; Yong, C.S.; Choi, H.G. Effect of the solid-dispersion method on the solubility and crystalline property of tacrolimus. *Int. J. Pharm. Investig.* **2010**, *395*, 161–166. [CrossRef] [PubMed]

4. Yamashita, K.; Nakate, T.; Okimoto, K.; Ohike, A.; Tokunaga, Y.; Ibuki, R.; Higaki, K.; Kimura, T. Establishment of new preparation method for solid dispersion formulation of tacrolimus. *Int. J. Pharm.* **2003**, *267*, 79–91. [CrossRef] [PubMed]

5. Tamura, S.; Ohike, A.; Ibuki, R.; Amidon, G.L.; Yamashita, S. Tacrolimus is a class ii low-solubility high-permeability drug: The effect of p-glycoprotein efflux on regional permeability of tacrolimus in rats. *J. Pharm. Sci.* **2002**, *91*, 719–729. [CrossRef] [PubMed]

6. Amidon, G.L.; Lennernas, H.; Shah, V.P.; Crison, J.R. A theoretical basis for a biopharmaceutic drug classification: The correlation of in vitro drug product dissolution and in vivo bioavailability. *Pharm. Res.* **1995**, *12*, 413–420. [CrossRef] [PubMed]

7. Kagayama, A.; Tanimoto, S.; Fujisaki, J.; Kaibara, A.; Ohara, K.; Iwasaki, K.; Hirano, Y.; Hata, T. Oral absorption of fk506 in rats. *Pharm. Res.* **1993**, *10*, 1446–1450. [CrossRef] [PubMed]

8. Grinyo, J.M.; Petruzzelli, S. Once-daily lcp-tacro meltdose tacrolimus for the prophylaxis of organ rejection in kidney and liver transplantations. *Expert Rev. Clin. Immunol.* **2014**, *10*, 1567–1579. [CrossRef] [PubMed]

9. Hashimoto, Y.; Sasa, H.; Shimomura, M.; Inui, K. Effects of intestinal and hepatic metabolism on the bioavailability of tacrolimus in rats. *Pharm. Res.* **1998**, *15*, 1609–1613. [CrossRef] [PubMed]

10. Arima, H.; Yunomae, K.; Hirayama, F.; Uekama, K. Contribution of p-glycoprotein to the enhancing effects of dimethyl-beta-cyclodextrin on oral bioavailability of tacrolimus. *J. Pharmacol. Exp. Ther.* **2001**, *297*, 547–555. [PubMed]

11. Nassar, T.; Rom, A.; Nyska, A.; Benita, S. A novel nanocapsule delivery system to overcome intestinal degradation and drug transport limited absorption of p-glycoprotein substrate drugs. *Pharm. Res.* **2008**, *25*, 2019–2029. [CrossRef] [PubMed]

12. Williams, D.; Haragsim, L. Calcineurin nephrotoxicity. *Adv. Chronic Kidney Dis.* **2006**, *13*, 47–55. [CrossRef] [PubMed]

13. Veroux, P.; Veroux, M.; Puliatti, C.; Valvo, M.; Macarone, M.; Cappello, D. Severe neurotoxicity in tacrolimus-treated living kidney transplantation in two cases. *Urol. Int.* **2003**, *71*, 433–434. [CrossRef] [PubMed]

14. Overhoff, K.A.; McConville, J.T.; Yang, W.; Johnston, K.P.; Peters, J.I.; Williams, R.O., 3rd. Effect of stabilizer on the maximum degree and extent of supersaturation and oral absorption of tacrolimus made by ultra-rapid freezing. *Pharm. Res.* **2008**, *25*, 167–175. [CrossRef] [PubMed]

15. Yoshida, T.; Kurimoto, I.; Yoshihara, K.; Umejima, H.; Ito, N.; Watanabe, S.; Sako, K.; Kikuchi, A. Aminoalkyl methacrylate copolymers for improving the solubility of tacrolimus. I: Evaluation of solid dispersion formulations. *Int. J. Pharm.* **2012**, *428*, 18–24. [CrossRef] [PubMed]

16. Yoshida, T.; Kurimoto, I.; Yoshihara, K.; Umejima, H.; Ito, N.; Watanabe, S.; Sako, K.; Kikuchi, A. Effect of aminoalkyl methacrylate copolymer e/hcl on in vivo absorption of poorly water-soluble drug. *Drug Dev. Ind. Pharm.* **2013**, *39*, 1698–1705. [CrossRef] [PubMed]

17. Arima, H.; Yunomae, K.; Miyake, K.; Irie, T.; Hirayama, F.; Uekama, K. Comparative studies of the enhancing effects of cyclodextrins on the solubility and oral bioavailability of tacrolimus in rats. *J. Pharm. Sci.* **2001**, *90*, 690–701. [CrossRef] [PubMed]

18. Nekkanti, V.; Rueda, J.; Wang, Z.; Betageri, G.V. Design, characterization, and in vivo pharmacokinetics of tacrolimus proliposomes. *AAPS PharmSciTech* **2016**, *17*, 1019–1029. [CrossRef] [PubMed]

19. Wu, X.; Hayes, D., Jr.; Zwischenberger, J.B.; Kuhn, R.J.; Mansour, H.M. Design and physicochemical characterization of advanced spray-dried tacrolimus multifunctional particles for inhalation. *Drug Des. Dev. Ther.* **2013**, *7*, 59–72.

20. Collin, C.; Boussaud, V.; Lefeuvre, S.; Amrein, C.; Glouzman, A.S.; Havard, L.; Billaud, E.M.; Guillemain, R. Sublingual tacrolimus as an alternative to intravenous route in patients with thoracic transplant: A retrospective study. *Transplant. Proc.* **2010**, *42*, 4331–4337. [CrossRef] [PubMed]

21. Srinarong, P.; Pham, B.T.; Holen, M.; van der Plas, A.; Schellekens, R.C.; Hinrichs, W.L.; Frijlink, H.W. Preparation and physicochemical evaluation of a new tacrolimus tablet formulation for sublingual administration. *Drug Dev. Ind. Pharm.* **2012**, *38*, 490–500. [CrossRef] [PubMed]

22. Breitenbach, J. Melt extrusion: From process to drug delivery technology. *Eur. J. Pharm. Biopharm.* **2002**, *54*, 107–117. [CrossRef]

23. *Materials Studio Modeling*; 7.0.100; Accelrys Software Inc.: San Diego, CA, USA, 2013.

24. Sun, H. Compass: An ab initio force-field optimized for condensed-phase applications-overview with details on alkane and benzene compounds. *J. Phys. Chem. B* **1998**, *102*, 7338–7364. [CrossRef]

25. Frenkel, D.; Smit, B. *Understanding Molecular Simulation*, 2nd ed.; Academic Press: San Deigo, CA, USA, 2002.

26. Berendsen, H.J.C.; Postma, J.P.M.; van Gunsteren, W.F.; DiNola, A.; Haak, J.R. Molecular dynamics with coupling to an external bath. *J. Chem. Phys.* **1984**, *81*, 3684–3690. [CrossRef]

27. Akashi, T.; Nefuji, T.; Yoshida, M.; Hosoda, J. Quantitative determination of tautomeric fk506 by reversed-phase liquid chromatography. *J. Pharm. Biomed. Anal.* **1996**, *14*, 339–346. [CrossRef]

28. Azarmi, S.; Roa, W.; Lobenberg, R. Current perspectives in dissolution testing of conventional and novel dosage forms. *Int. J. Pharm.* **2007**, *328*, 12–21. [CrossRef] [PubMed]

29. Gupta, J.; Nunes, C.; Vyas, S.; Jonnalagadda, S. Prediction of solubility parameters and miscibility of pharmaceutical compounds by molecular dynamics simulations. *J. Phys. Chem. B* **2011**, *115*, 2014–2023. [CrossRef] [PubMed]

30. Greenhalgh, D.J.; Williams, A.C.; Timmins, P.; York, P. Solubility parameters as predictors of miscibility in solid dispersions. *J. Pharm. Sci.* **1999**, *88*, 1182–1190. [CrossRef] [PubMed]

31. Kolter, K.; Karl, M.; Gryczke, A. *Hot Melt Extrusion with Basf Pharma Polymers*, 2nd ed.; BASF: Ludwigshafen, Germany, 2012.

32. Mididoddi, P.K.; Repka, M.A. Characterization of hot-melt extruded drug delivery systems for onychomycosis. *Eur. J. Pharm. Biopharm.* **2007**, *66*, 95–105. [CrossRef] [PubMed]

33. Boer, T.M.; Procopio, J.V.; Nascimento, T.G.; Macedo, R.O. Correlation of thermal analysis and pyrolysis coupled to gc-ms in the characterization of tacrolimus. *J. Pharm. Biomed. Anal.* **2013**, *73*, 18–23. [CrossRef] [PubMed]

34. Zidan, A.S.; Rahman, Z.; Sayeed, V.; Raw, A.; Yu, L.; Khan, M.A. Crystallinity evaluation of tacrolimus solid dispersions by chemometric analysis. *Int. J. Pharm.* **2012**, *423*, 341–350. [CrossRef] [PubMed]

35. Hancock, B.C.; Shamblin, S.L.; Zografi, G. Molecular mobility of amorphous pharmaceutical solids below their glass transition temperatures. *Pharm. Res.* **1995**, *12*, 799–806. [CrossRef] [PubMed]

36. *Guidance for Industry Orally Disintegrating Tablets*; U.S. Food and drug administration: Silver Spring, MD, USA, 2008.

37. McLaughlin, R.; Banbury, S.; Crowley, K. Orally disintegrating tablets: The effect of recent fda guidance on odt technologies and applications. *Pharm. Tech.* **2009**. Available online: http://www.pharmtech.com/orally-disintegrating-tablets-effect-recent-fda-guidance-odt-technologies-and-applications (accessed on 9 February 2018).

38. Fitzsimmons, W.E. Tacrolimus. In *Immunotherapy in Transplantation*; Wiley-Blackwell: Hoboken, NJ, USA, 2010; pp. 224–240.

39. Wu, C.-Y.; Benet, L.Z. Predicting drug disposition via application of bcs: Transport/absorption/elimination interplay and development of a biopharmaceutics drug disposition classification system. *Pharm. Res.* **2005**, *22*, 11–23. [CrossRef] [PubMed]

40. Kadajji, V.G.; Betageri, G.V. Water soluble polymers for pharmaceutical applications. *Polymers* **2011**, *3*, 1972–2009. [CrossRef]

41. Jijun, F.; Lishuang, X.; Xiaoguang, T.; Min, S.; Mingming, Z.; Haibing, H.; Xing, T. The inhibition effect of high storage temperature on the recrystallization rate during dissolution of nimodipine-kollidon va64 solid dispersions (nm-sd) prepared by hot-melt extrusion. *J. Pharm. Sci.* **2011**, *100*, 1643–1647. [CrossRef] [PubMed]

4

Sustained Release Drug Delivery Applications of Polyurethanes

Michael B. Lowinger [1,2,*] (iD), Stephanie E. Barrett [2], Feng Zhang [1,*] and Robert O. Williams III [1] (iD)

[1] College of Pharmacy, The University of Texas at Austin, 2409 University Avenue, Austin, TX 78712, USA; bill.williams@austin.utexas.edu
[2] MRL, Merck & Co., Inc., 126 E. Lincoln Ave, Rahway, NJ 07065, USA; stephanie_barrett@merck.com
* Correspondence: michael.lowinger@utexas.edu (M.B.L.); feng.zhang@austin.utexas.edu (F.Z.)

Abstract: Since their introduction over 50 years ago, polyurethanes have been applied to nearly every industry. This review describes applications of polyurethanes to the development of modified release drug delivery. Although drug delivery research leveraging polyurethanes has been ongoing for decades, there has been renewed and substantial interest in the field in recent years. The chemistry of polyurethanes and the mechanisms of drug release from sustained release dosage forms are briefly reviewed. Studies to assess the impact of intrinsic drug properties on release from polyurethane-based formulations are considered. The impact of hydrophilic water swelling polyurethanes on drug diffusivity and release rate is discussed. The role of pore formers in modulating drug release rate is examined. Finally, the value of assessing mechanical properties of the dosage form and approaches taken in the literature are described.

Keywords: polyurethane; isocyanate; long-acting; sustained release; drug delivery

1. Introduction

Polyurethanes are among the most ubiquitous of materials found in society, owing to their versatile properties. They can be found in automobiles, chairs, beds, refrigerators and many other household items [1]. Early research into the chemistry of polyurethanes can be found as early as 1947 [2]. By varying different substituents and their ratios, different polyurethanes with a wide range of physicochemical properties can be synthesized at large scales.

This review presents an overview of recent applications of polyurethanes to sustained release drug delivery. Previous review publications generally focused on the chemistry, synthesis and properties of polyurethanes. Cherng et al. authored an extensive review of polyurethane-based drug delivery systems, however it was published over five years ago [3]. Since that time, there has been significant advancement in the research area of polyurethanes, particularly as applied to parenteral sustained release dosage forms.

Polyurethanes have been applied to drug products in nearly every conceivable configuration. Seo and Na explored modifications to polyurethane membrane porosity from a non-erodible drug eluting stent [4]. Guo et al. developed biodegradable polyurethane stent coatings enabling adjustable drug release [5]. Chen et al. explored the use of polyurethane pressure-sensitive adhesives for transdermal drug delivery [6]. Several studies have explored the controlled release of antibiotics from polyurethane matrices through tissue scaffolds [7], bone grafts [8], microspheres [9] and nanoparticles [10]. Temperature- and pH-responsive polyurethane nanoparticles have been developed to deliver doxorubicin to the tumor microenvironment [11]. Drug loaded polyurethane implants have been studied for the treatment of bacterial infection [12] and inflammation [13]. The polymers have been extensively applied in the development of intravaginal rings [14–25]. Polyurethanes have also been applied to modulate the release characteristics of orally administered tablets [26].

Experimental work exploring monolithic mixtures of a polymer (ethylene vinyl acetate) with model drug compounds has been documented as early as 1964 [27] and the use of polyurethanes in medical devices has been well documented since 1968 [28–34]. Both biodegradable and biostable sub-dermal implant polyurethane formulations have been of more recent interest [3].

2. Chemistry of Polyurethanes

Polyurethanes are a group of condensation polymers that include the urethane (—NHCOO—) group in the chemical structure (Figure 1). They are typically synthesized by a step-growth polymerization reaction between isocyanates and polyols in the presence of a suitable catalyst. Polyurethanes synthesized solely from isocyanates and polyols generally have poor mechanical properties. Therefore, chain extenders are added to the structure in order to induce microphase separation between the two thermodynamically incompatible segments. The two segments are commonly described as hard segments (composed of the isocyanate and chain extender components) and soft segments (composed of the polyol component). The hard segments impart mechanical strength, whereas the soft domains provide flexibility (Figure 1).

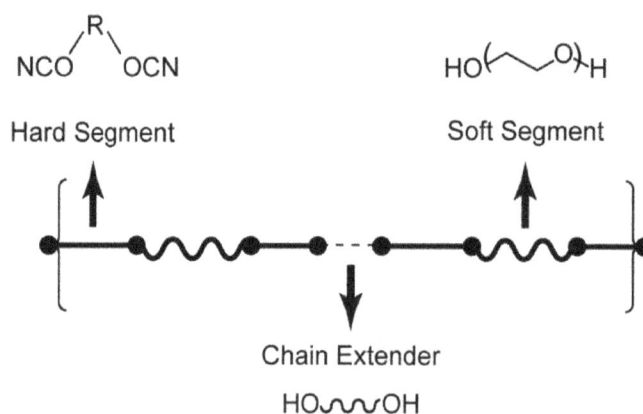

Figure 1. General chemical structure of polyurethanes.

2.1. Isocyanates

Diisocyanates are commonly employed in the synthesis of polyurethanes, which can be divided into aliphatic and aromatic diisocyanates. In general, aromatic diisocyanates are more reactive than aliphatic species. For example, polyurethanes made from aliphatic diisocyanates demonstrated more resistance to ultraviolet radiation, whereas those made from aromatic diisocyanates have been shown to undergo photodegradation [35,36]. Polyurethanes based on aromatic diisocyanates have also been shown to exhibit less biocompatibility than those synthesized from aliphatic diisocyanates, caused by toxic degradation products. Polyurethanes prepared with toluene diisocyanate have been shown to degrade under physiological conditions to yield 2,4-toluene diamine, which has known toxicity [37]. Kääriä et al. conducted an in vivo study using a polyurethane prepared from the aromatic 4,4'-methylenediphenyl diisocyanate and observed cytotoxicity attributed to the aromatic amine 4,4'-methylenedianiline produced as a degradation product of the polymer [38].

2.2. Chain Extenders

Chain extenders are typically low molecular weight (<400 Da) bisamines or diols, such as 1,4-butandiol, 1,3-propanediol and ethylene diamine. The physical and mechanical properties of polyurethanes, including hardness and crystallinity, are dependent on the extent of phase separation between the hard and soft segments. The extent of phase separation is, in part, a function of the type and number of chain extenders used for polymerization. Jabbari and Khakpour investigated the impact of changes to the mole fraction of polyurethane chain extruder to the porosity of prepared microspheres [39]. They observed that the pores in polyurethane microspheres decreased as the content of chain extruder increased from 0 to 50 mol %. When they increased the chain extruder content to 67 mol %, the polymer stiffness increased and formation of pores was inhibited.

2.3. Polyols

Polyols are generally di-hydroxyl terminated macroglycols of polyesters, polyethers and polycarbonates in the molecular weight range of 1000 to 5000 Da. The molecular weight and type of polyol plays a significant role in the physicochemical and mechanical properties of the polyurethane. Polyester-based polyurethanes often have good mechanical strength and thermal stability, however they are susceptible to hydrolysis [40]. Biodegradable poly(ester urethanes) have been prepared from lysine diisocyanate with D,L-lactide, ε-caprolactone and other monomers [41]. Kaur et al. developed a biodegradable intravaginal ring composed of a poly(ester urethane) prepared from bis(4-isocynaatocyclohexyl)methane with poly(tetramethylene ether)glycol and ε-caprolactone, which released the antiretroviral dapivirine at target levels for one month [42]. Yu et al. developed biodegradable polyurethanes based on L-phenylalanine that possess tunable mechanical properties and degradation rates over a wider range than was achievable with poly(lactic acid) [43].

Polyether-based polyurethanes tend to be more hydrolytically stable and exhibit more elasticity at lower temperatures. However, they can be more susceptible to oxidative and thermal lability [44,45]. It was found that poly(ether urethane) used as pacemaker lead insulation suffered from stress cracking due to oxidation after being placed in humans for long periods of time [46]. However, antioxidants have been used to stabilize poly(ether urethanes) to prevent oxidation and prolong the life of the polymer [47]. A polyether-based polyol particularly relevant to pharmaceutical applications is polyethylene oxide (PEO). PEO-based polyurethanes exhibit sensitivity to water due to the hydrophilicity and water-absorbing capacity of the ethylene oxide units [3]. Ikeda et al. demonstrated that the larger the PEO content, the higher the degree of swelling which increased the drug release rate of slowly releasing model compounds [48].

Polycarbonate-based polyurethanes were developed in response to the disadvantages of polyester and polyether based polyurethanes. They exhibit good mechanical properties, heat stability and hydrolytic stability but they have been shown to undergo enzymatic hydrolysis and oxidative degradation by inflammatory cells in long-term in vivo studies [49].

2.4. Synthesis

Polyurethanes are generally synthesized by reacting the isocyanate, polyol and chain extender together at temperatures above 80 °C [50]. The central reaction is the formation of a urethane linkage that occurs when an isocyanate reacts with an alcohol group of the polyol. The exothermic polymerization reaction is generally carried out in one of two ways. The "one-shot method" involves mixing all of the ingredients together, while the "prepolymer method" features the reaction of the polyol with an excess of isocyanate, followed by a subsequent reaction with the chain extender to form a linear block copolymer with alternating blocks of hard segment and soft segment [29]. The prepolymer method has been shown to yield more ordered structure with better control of polymer properties [51].

Two manufacturing methods are typically employed for industrial production: the belt process and the reaction extruder process. During the belt process, all components are mixed using a high efficiency mixing head and the reacting liquid mixture is poured onto a belt, where it solidifies. The solid material is then granulated and may be blended with other components and extruded into pellets. Utilization of a reaction extruder allows for the mixing of prepolymers or all components inside of the extruder, where screw design and temperature can be modified to suit the desired product properties. The urethane reaction is nearly complete by the time the material exits the extruder and uniform pellets may be formed by the use of underwater or strand pelletizers [50].

Since phase separation of polyurethanes is dependent on the temperature and shear conditions during polymerization, the process may have a significant influence on the product properties. Consequently, although two polyurethane batches may start from the same raw materials, their physical properties can be very different [50].

3. Drug Release Mechanisms

Solute diffusion, polymer swelling and polymer erosion or degradation are generally considered to be the main driving forces for drug transport from a polymeric matrix [52]. However, other phenomena may be involved in the control of drug release and are discussed in more detail in other publications [53].

3.1. Solute Diffusion

Fick's law of diffusion is the fundamental basis for the mechanism describing drug transport from a polymer matrix. Fickian diffusion refers to a solute transport process in which the polymer relaxation time is much greater than the solvent diffusion time. When polymer swelling occurs, changes to diffusivity with time result in non-Fickian drug release. Drug release from polyurethane formulations can be categorized into two groups: (i) monolithic systems, where drug is dissolved or dispersed in a polyurethane matrix and (ii) reservoir systems, where a drug depot is surrounded by a rate controlling membrane [53]. Table 1 describes the categories of solute diffusion from polyurethane-based sustained release dosage forms.

Table 1. Categories of Solute Diffusion from Polyurethane-based Sustained Release Dosage Forms.

Dosage Form Type	Drug Concentration in Polymer	Release Kinetics	Examples
Monolithic	$C_{drug} \leq C_{solubility}$	Geometry and drug load dependent	[57,58]
	$C_{drug} > C_{solubility}$	Geometry and drug load dependent	[59]
Reservoir	$C_{drug} \leq C_{solubility}$	First order	[54,55]
	$C_{drug} > C_{solubility}$	Zero order	[56]

In each of those categories, drug release kinetics will be dependent on whether the drug concentration is above or below its solubility in the system. In the case of a reservoir system where the initial drug concentration is below its solubility, those drug molecules that diffuse out of the system will not be replaced by undissolved drug and the drug activity at the rate controlling membrane's surface decreases with time, resulting in first order release kinetics. Models have also been developed which describe first order release kinetics from a cylindrical intravaginal ring [54,55]. However, a reservoir system where the drug concentration exceeds its solubility will feature a saturated solution at the membrane surface, resulting in zero order release kinetics. Over time, drug release kinetics from such a system will approach those of a dosage form with drug concentration below its solubility in the polymer [56].

In the case of monolithic systems, the device geometry and drug loading will significantly affect the drug release kinetics. For a monolithic system where the initial drug concentration is below its solubility in the system, models have been derived to describe the drug release of thin films, spheres and cylinders, many of which assume an exponential function of release rate with time [57,58]. In the case of a monolithic dispersion where the drug is above its solubility in the system, Higuchi described a square root of time relationship between the amount of drug released from a thin film with a large excess of drug [59].

3.2. Polymer Swelling

Depending on the polyol used, polyurethanes may exhibit substantial polymer swelling which can impact drug release kinetics in several ways. When a polymer swells, the length of the diffusion pathways increases. This can result in decreasing drug concentration gradients, which may decrease drug release rates. Guo et al. observed that the swelling of a synthesized polyurethane matrix slowed down the drug release rate, which was attributed to increased diffusion length [5].

Polymer swelling also increases the mobility of the polymer chains, which increases drug mobility and, potentially, increases drug release rates. Once a water content specific to each polymer is reached, the polymer mobility steeply increases in a phenomenon called "polymer chain relaxation" or "glassy-to-rubbery phase transition" [53]. However, polyurethanes commonly employed for pharmaceutical applications exhibit glass transition temperatures below room temperature, so the transition of polyurethanes from the glassy to the rubbery state is generally not of practical significance to drug release [60]. Clark et al. applied similar pseudo-steady state approach as Higuchi's diffusion model to effectively predict the release of tenofovir from an intravaginal ring composed of hydrophilic polyurethane [54]. They argued that polymer swelling had minimal impact on the long-term drug release kinetics since the polymers reach equilibrium swelling at early time points and it was thus unnecessary to account for it in the model.

Beyond polymer chain mobility itself, water swelling increases free volume for diffusion, thereby increasing diffusivity of drugs [61]. Dapivirine, when released from an intravaginal ring composed of a water-swelling polyurethane grade, exhibited faster release than from a ring composed of non-swelling polyurethane (Figure 2) [14]. Given the wide variety of PEO-based polyurethanes available commercially, polymer swelling has the potential to dramatically impact drug release kinetics from dosage forms.

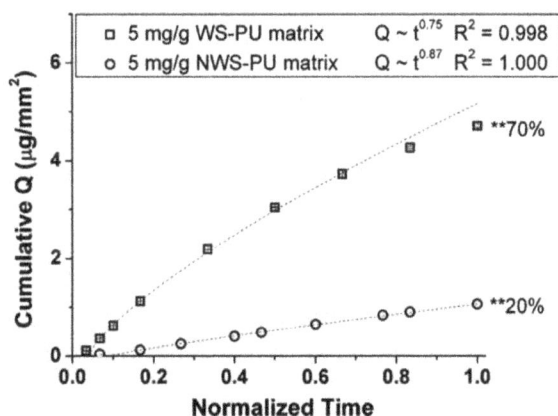

Figure 2. Cumulative flux (Q) of dapivirine as a function of time from a water swelling (WS-PU) and non-water swelling (NWS-PU) polyurethane matrix. ** denotes wt % cumulative release of dapivirine over 30 days. Adapted from [14], Elsevier, 2010 with permission.

3.3. Polymer Erosion and Degradation

The erosion and degradation of polymers to facilitate drug release are often confounded; however, they will be separated for the purpose of this review. Goepferich and Langer differentiated the two processes by defining degradation as involving cleavage of polymer chains into oligomers and monomers, while erosion can be defined as a general loss of weight from the polymer [62]. Consequently, although degradation of water-insoluble polymers is a step in its erosion process, the degradation of the polymer itself is not erosion.

Langer and Peppas defined two extremes of erosion: heterogeneous and homogeneous [63]. Heterogeneous erosion describes a physical situation where water penetration into the polymer is slow relative to polymer degradation rate. Under this scenario, polymer degradation is restricted to the outermost layers and erosion predominantly occurs at the surface of the dosage form. In the case of homogeneous erosion, water penetration occurs rapidly, degradation occurs throughout the device and bulk erosion follows. Although all bioerodible polymers are likely to undergo some combination of the two extremes, surface erosion may be most often observed with hydrophobic polyurethanes and those with highly reactive bonds in their backbone structure, whereas hydrophilic polyurethanes and those with less reactive ester linkages are more likely to undergo bulk erosion [53]. Additionally, the water penetration rate may vary depending on the geometry of the delivery system [64].

Hafeman et al. synthesized hydrophilic polyester-based polyurethanes from ε-caprolactone and observed rapid swelling followed by bulk erosion with approximately 50–80% mass remaining after 36 weeks [65] (Figure 3). In a subsequent study investigating the use of one of these polymers to deliver the antibiotic tobramycin, the authors found that the hydrophilic drug released from the polyurethane scaffold over the course of approximately 30 days. Given the difference in time scales between the drug release and polymer degradation rates, the investigators concluded that tobramycin release was independent of polymer degradation [66]. The study demonstrates the ability to develop biodegradable sustained release dosage forms in which drug release kinetics are not dependent on polymer degradation kinetics.

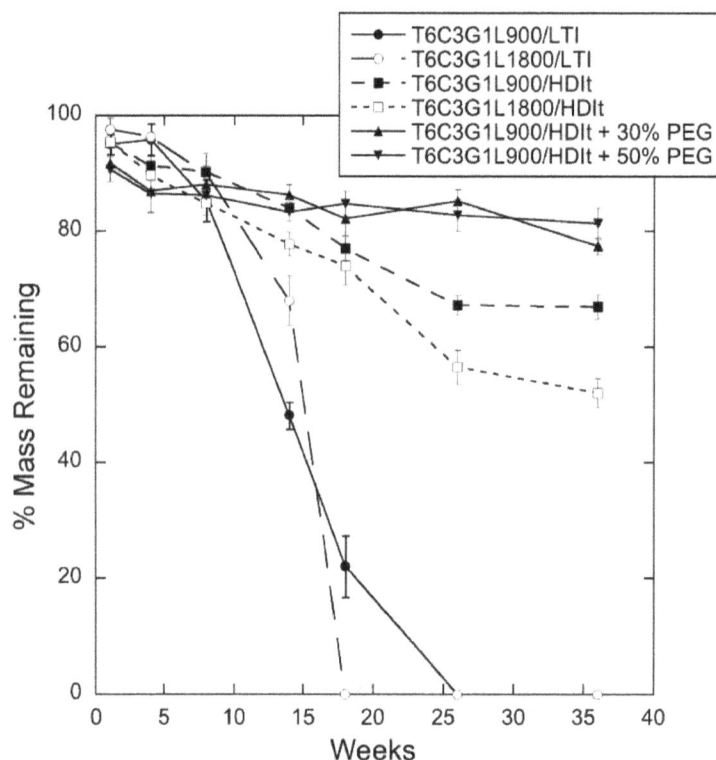

Figure 3. In vitro degradation of polyurethane scaffolds. By 36 weeks, polymers from prepared from lysine triisocyanate (LTI) had completely degraded, while the polyurethanes prepared from hexamethylene diisocyanate trimer remained at 52–81% of their original masses. Adapted from [65], Springer Nature, 2008 with permission.

4. Approaches to Modulate Drug Release Kinetics

Hombreiro-Pérez et al. described the key mass transport phenomena governing drug release through a polymer, including drug dissolution in the polymer; drug diffusion through the polymer matrix and/or through water-filled pores; drug diffusion through the unstirred liquid boundary layer on the surface of the dosage form; and diffusional and convective transport within the release medium [67]. Through deliberate polymer and formulation selection, the release kinetics of a particular drug may be modulated to achieve a target dose. Table 2 summarizes the approaches that may be taken to modulate drug release kinetics from a polyurethane-based reservoir sustained release dosage form.

Table 2. Approaches to Modulate Drug Release Kinetics from a Polyurethane-based Reservoir Sustained Release Dosage Form.

Driver	Approach	Examples
Drug Solubility in Polymer	Polymer selection to increase or reduce drug solubility	[14,17,54,56]
Drug Diffusivity Through Polymer	Polymer selection to increase or reduce polymer crystallinity	[68–70]
	Polymer selection to increase or reduce polymer molecular weight	[71,72]
	Polymer selection to increase or reduce soft segment to hard segment ratio	[73,74]
Drug Diffusion Through Water-filled Channels	Polymer selection to increase or reduce soft segment to hard segment ratio	[73,74]
	Incorporation of additional component as pore former	[75–77]

4.1. Intrinsic Drivers of Drug Release through a Polymer

4.1.1. Drug Solubility in Polymer

In matrix systems where the drug is above its percolation threshold, it is conceivable for drug release to occur by diffusion through drug-rich channels [27,78]. However, for matrix systems where drug load is below its percolation threshold and for all reservoir systems, drug must first dissolve in the polymer in order to diffuse through it. For those formulations, drug solubility in the polymer is an important phenomenon. Johnson et al. found that release of hydrophilic tenofovir with a calculated logP of −2.3 was barely detectable from the hydrophobic polyurethane Tecoflex EG-85A, attributed to poor solubility in the polymer [14]. However, dapivirine with a calculated logP of 6.3 exhibited near zero order release from a similarly hydrophobic polyurethane Tecoflex EG-80A [17]. Van Laarhoven et al. measured the solubility of etonogestrel and ethinyl estradiol in ethylene vinyl acetate copolymers and found that the two hydrophobic drugs were sufficiently soluble in the hydrophobic polymer that they were present in the finished product in a molecularly dissolved state [56]. Clark et al. determined the solubility of tenofovir in a hydrophilic polyurethane and observed that its solubility was 100 to 1000 times lower than the drug loading explored in their studies [54].

4.1.2. Drug Diffusivity through Polymer

The phase state of the polymer has been shown to impact diffusivity of drug through it. Almeida et al. studied the impact of vinyl acetate content on the release rate of metoprolol tartrate from melt extruded ethylene vinyl acetate matrices in the presence of varying levels of polyethylene oxide. Lower vinyl acetate content results in greater crystallinity of the polymer. They found that matrices extruded with lower vinyl acetate content polymers exhibited slower drug release rates than those extruded with higher vinyl acetate content polymers. By fitting the experimental data to an analytical model of Fick's second law of diffusion, they were able to show that release rate differences between polymers could be explained by changes to the apparent diffusion coefficient (Figure 4) [68]. Tallury et al. explored the impact of ethylene vinyl acetate copolymer composition on the release of chlorhexidine and acyclovir from polymer matrices. They observed a strong relationship between vinyl acetate content and drug release for both systems, where higher vinyl acetate content exhibited faster drug release [69]. Although the effect of polymer crystallinity on drug release from nonerodible polyurethane-based dosage forms has not been extensively studied, several investigators correlated the crystallinity of the soft segment to degradation rate of poly(ester urethanes). Reddy et al. proposed that higher crystallinity of the poly(caprolactone) soft segment resulted in reduced polymer degradation rates, which slowed the release of the model drug theophylline [70].

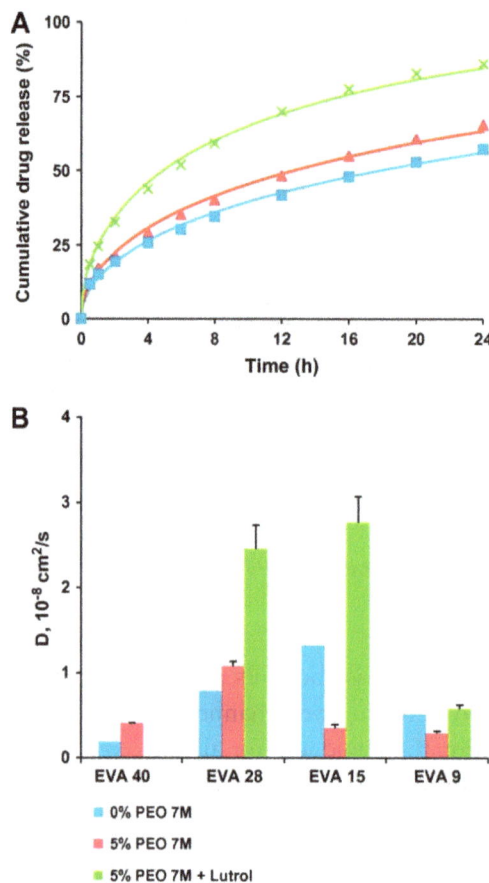

Figure 4. (**A**) Theory (curves) and experiments (symbols): metoprolol tartrate release from EVA 28-based matrices containing 0% PEO 7 M (■), 5% PEO 7 M (▲), or 5% PEG 7 M/Lutrol (9/1, w/w) (×). (**B**) Apparent diffusion coefficients of metoprolol tartrate in EVA-based matrices, containing 0% PEO 7 M, 5% PEO 7 M, or 5% PEO 7 M/Lutrol (9/1, w/w). Adapted from [68], Elsevier, 2012 with permission.

The molecular weight of the polymer may also impact the diffusion of drug through the dosage form. Hsu and Langer investigated the impact of changes to ethylene vinyl acetate molecular weight on the release rate of bovine serum albumin (BSA). They observed a substantial decrease in BSA release rate with relatively small increases in ethylene vinyl acetate molecular weight [71]. Skarja and Woodhouse investigated the effect of molecular weight on the properties of polyurethanes composed of either poly(caprolactone) or poly(ethylene oxide) as the soft segment. They found that phase separation between the hard and soft segments and crystallinity of the soft segment increases with soft segment molecular weight. For polyurethanes based on hydrophobic poly(caprolactone), one might expect reduced drug release rates from a higher molecular weight polymer, however those based on hydrophilic poly(ethylene oxide) might be expected to release drug at faster rates [72].

For polyurethanes, the ratio between soft segment and hard segment has also been shown to affect drug release kinetics. Shoaib et al. explored the effect of soft segment to hard segment ratio on the release of ciprofloxacin. The polyurethane-urea elastomers were synthesized from the aromatic toluene diisocyanate and the hydrophilic polyethylene glycol. As soft segment to hard segment ratio was decreased, the investigators observed a decrease in ciprofloxacin release rate from drug/polymer films. The authors attributed the slower drug release to increased cross-linking of the hard segments in polymers featuring a higher concentration of hard segment. They speculated that increased cross-linking would reduce water penetration into the matrix and drug diffusion out of the matrix [73].

Verstraete et al. investigated the impact of soft segment to hard segment ratio on the release rates of diprophylline, theophylline and acetaminophen for hydrophilic thermoplastic polyurethanes for which the soft segment is composed of polyethylene oxide. As the soft segment to hard segment ratio increased, the fraction of polyethylene oxide in the polymer structure increased. The authors observed an increase in swelling for the polymers Tecophilic SP60D60, SP93A100 and TG2000 ranging from 60% to 900% weight gain. When investigating the drug release kinetics of the three drug compounds from matrices of each polymer, they found that all drugs followed the same trend with the TG2000-based matrix releasing fastest and the SP60D60-based matrix releasing slowest (Figure 5) [74]. Increased water uptake and faster drug release may be due to the formation of a water-filled pore structure or due to higher free volume that increases diffusivity.

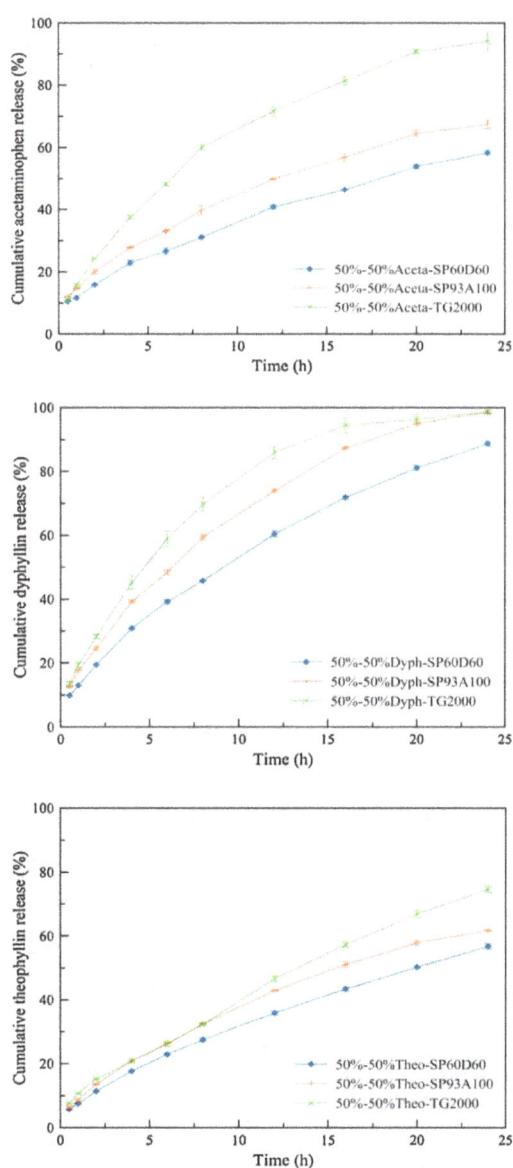

Figure 5. Influence of length of the polyurethane soft segment (polyethylene oxide) on the in vitro release kinetics of drugs with different aqueous solubility (acetaminophen, diprophylline and theophylline) from polyurethane-based matrices (SP60D60, SP93A100 and TG2000). Adapted from reference [74], Elsevier, 2016 with permission.

4.2. The Use of Pore Formers

The incorporation of soluble components to an otherwise poorly soluble barrier has been utilized as an approach to modulate the release of drugs through film coated tablets for decades [79–83]. A similar approach has been applied to the development of drug/polyurethane dosage forms in order to optimize the drug release rate. Kim et al. evaluated the effect of polyethylene glycol, D-mannitol and bovine serum albumin on the release of the antibiotic cefadroxil from a polyurethane matrix [75]. They observed that matrices utilizing bovine serum albumin as the pore former exhibited the fastest drug release. The authors proposed that immiscibility of the pore former with the polyurethane could facilitate channel formation and thus increase drug release rate.

Donelli et al. investigated the utility of incorporating polyethylene glycol and bovine serum albumin into a polyurethane matrix to modify the release rate of the antifungal drug fluconazole [76]. They found that matrices incorporating polyethylene glycol exhibited increased drug release relative to a control without pore former, whereas matrices incorporating bovine serum albumin exhibited sustained drug release relative to the control. Sreenivasan observed an increased release rate of the anti-inflammatory drug hydrocortisone when adding methyl β-cyclodextrin to polyurethane [77]. Claeys et al. explored the impact of polyethylene glycol, polysorbate 80 and the dicarboxylic acids malonic, succinic, maleic and glutaric acid on the release of diprophylline from a polyurethane matrix (Figure 6) [26,60].

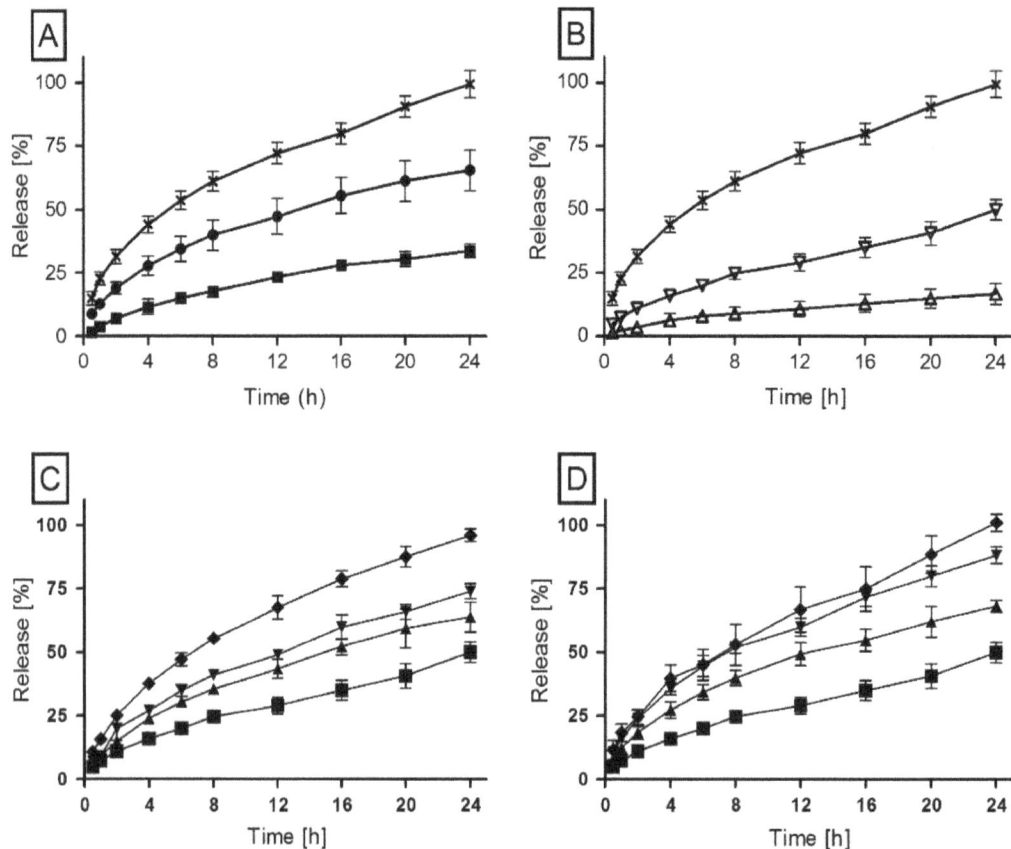

Figure 6. Mean dissolution profiles (±SD) of polyester-based polyurethane (Pearlbond) matrices as a function of (**A**) drug load: 50% (■), 60% (●) and 65% (×) metoprolol tartrate; (**B**) drug solubility: 65 wt % theophylline (△), diprophylline (▽) and metoprolol tartrate (×); pore former (**C**) PEG 4000 or (**D**) Polysorbate 80; 65 wt % diprophylline with 0% (■), 2% (▲), 5% (▼) and 10% (◆) of pore former, respectively. Adapted from [60], Elsevier, 2015 with permission.

5. Mechanical Properties of Polyurethane-Based Dosage Forms

Since many polyurethane-based sustained release dosage forms are intended to remain in vivo for extended periods of time, their mechanical properties are critical to ensure consistent drug release kinetics and good patient adherence. The dosage forms must exhibit enough elasticity to deform seamlessly without causing discomfort to patients during routine daily activities and without causing tissue damage or inflammation [84]. On the other hand, the dosage forms must have sufficient strength to prevent fracture, which would alter geometry and potentially affect drug release rate. For example, intravaginal rings that are too soft may not be effectively retained and could be expelled from the vagina [85].

5.1. Patient Perceptions

Given that many of the mechanical properties are driven by patient perceptions, it can be difficult to determine an appropriate target for a dosage form under development. The target mechanical properties of each dosage form may be dependent on the route of administration and duration of the product. However, patients are likely to have more interaction with intravaginal rings than most other parenteral formulations and therefore investigators have evaluated the mechanical performance of intravaginal rings more extensively than most other presentations.

Morrow Guthrie et al. conducted a clinical study to understand the relationship between user perceptions and mechanical properties of intravaginal rings composed of polyurethane [86]. Users perceived a ring with a matte and textured surface to be easier to manipulate during insertion, whereas they perceived a ring with a glossy and smooth surface to be slicker and more challenging to insert. The study participants also expected rings composed of softer materials to be more comfortable to use. Although the participants preferred a small diameter ring, it conflicted with their general desire for a more pliable dosage form. For a given material at a defined cylinder diameter, a smaller diameter ring will be more difficult to squeeze. Faced with these tradeoffs, users were more comfortable with using softer materials and smaller diameter cylinders, even if the ring diameter were larger.

5.2. Mechanical Testing of Finished Product

Since most investigators lack the clinical data necessary to quantify patient preferences, studies describing the assessment of an investigational dosage form's mechanical properties typically reference their findings back to a marketed product. Baum et al. proposed several techniques to evaluate the mechanical properties of an experimental silicone-based intravaginal ring, comparing it to the commercially available Estring® [87]. The tensile strength, elongation and compression strength were determined using methods adapted from ASTM D2240 and ISO 8009 standards [88,89].

Verstraete et al. built on Baum's efforts by applying those techniques to polyurethane-based intravaginal dosage forms and comparing back to the marketed product Nuvaring® [15]. Shore durometer hardness was measured using an indentation test on the surface of the ring. Elongation and force at maximum extension were measured using an extension testing system. To evaluate elongation, a sample was fixed between two hooks and its axial length was measured after applying a defined force. In order to assess maximum elongation, the sample was stretched at a defined rate until breakage. The researchers sought to evaluate resistance to compression by subjecting a sample to repeated compression cycles at a defined speed and amplitude and assessing changes to the diameter along the axis of compression and orthogonal to it. Table 3 provides a summary of the measured intravaginal ring mechanical properties in comparison to the marketed product. By performing a variety of compression, elongation and indentation tests, the investigators were able to assess the mechanical properties of the dosage form under a variety of circumstances.

Table 3. Overview of intravaginal ring properties (mean $\pm$ SD, n = 3). Devices that featured similar mechanical properties to reference were highlighted in grey. Adapted from [15], Elsevier, 2017 with permission.

Formulation	Hardness [a] (shore A)	Max. Load [a] (N)	Max. Elongation [b] (%)	OD$_1$'/OD$_1$ [c] (%)	OD$_2$'/OD$_2$ [c] (%)
Reference Nuvaring™	75 $\pm$ 4	102.4 $\pm$ 12.7	650.1 $\pm$ 11.8	92.1	107.5
Treatment					
25/75 metronidazole/SP-93-100	72 $\pm$ 3	82.8 $\pm$ 13.7	587.9 $\pm$ 117.4	94.6	104.6
50/50 metronidazole/SP-93-100	91 $\pm$ 2	68.1 $\pm$ 10.2	51.7 $\pm$ 21.4	88.3	110.2
Prophylaxis 20/80 Lactic Acid/EG-80A	51 $\pm$ 1	49.7 $\pm$ 12.4	517.0 $\pm$ 4.9	98.0	101.7
20/80 Lactic Acid/EG-85A	62 $\pm$ 2	68.6 $\pm$ 22.7	389.4 $\pm$ 34.3	98.2	101.3
20/80 Lactic Acid/EG-93A	71 $\pm$ 2	87.7 $\pm$ 8.15	336.7 $\pm$ 24.9	96.0	103.8
20/80 Lactic Acid/EG-100A	80 $\pm$ 2	98.6 $\pm$ 11.6	244.6 $\pm$ 37.4	94.3	105.1
20/80 Lactic Acid/EG-60D	80 $\pm$ 4	105.4 $\pm$ 13.8	173.8 $\pm$ 22.2	93.7	107.2
20/80 Lactic Acid/EG-72D	86.3 $\pm$ 3	129.3 $\pm$ 14.1	125.7 $\pm$ 13.9	89.5	110.0

[a] Hardness and maximum load should be similar to the Nuvaring™ reference values. [b] Mean elongation at break should not be less than 300%. [c] After compression experiments, the diameter along the axis of compression (OD$_1$') and the diameter orthogonal to the axis of compression (OD$_2$') should be at least 90% of their initial values.

Clark et al. performed a destructive extension test on their segmented intravaginal ring samples both before and after 31-day in vitro release testing. Samples were stretched at a defined rate until failure was observed at which point the net extension and net load were recorded [90]. The investigators did not compare measured properties back to a marketed product. Without a benchmark, it can be difficult to interpret the outcome as to whether the failure conditions were beyond what is reasonably expected during normal handling.

Young's modulus measures a material's resistance to being deformed elastically when a stress is applied to it. A stiffer material will have a higher Young's modulus. Ugaonkar et al. leveraged the Young's modulus as a measure of flexibility by subjecting a 25 mm long cylindrical segment to a defined elongation at a specified rate and again compared the measured value for their experimental dosage form to that of the marketed product Nuvaring® [55]. Clark et al. developed a model to predict the force necessary to compress an intravaginal ring material a given distance based on the Young's modulus [54]. Although Young's modulus is an effective measure of stiffness, it does not provide information on elongation and compression properties.

Crnich et al. were interested in understanding the effect of ethanol exposure on the mechanical properties of polyurethane stents. They performed tensile strength testing, including force-at-break, failure stress, elongation at failure, maximum strain and modulus of elasticity in accordance with ISO standard 10555-1 [91]. The investigators concluded that exposure to ethanol had a minimal effect on the mechanical properties of polyurethane catheters.

Johnson et al. performed a tensile strength test on their intravaginal ring samples in a similar fashion to others [14]. Rings were stretched to a defined force at a specific rate and any evidence of failure or changes to diameter were assessed. The investigators also performed compression/retraction force tests in which the rings were compressed at a defined rate to 50% of their initial diameter and force was recorded throughout the experiment (Figure 7). They benchmarked to a marketed product and observed that their hydrophilic polyurethane-based intravaginal ring exhibited similar mechanical properties to the Nuvaring® reference ("EVA-R") when kept dry. However, the hydrated polyurethane-based ring exhibited faster recoil than the reference, which the authors pointed out could improve retention in the vaginal tract.

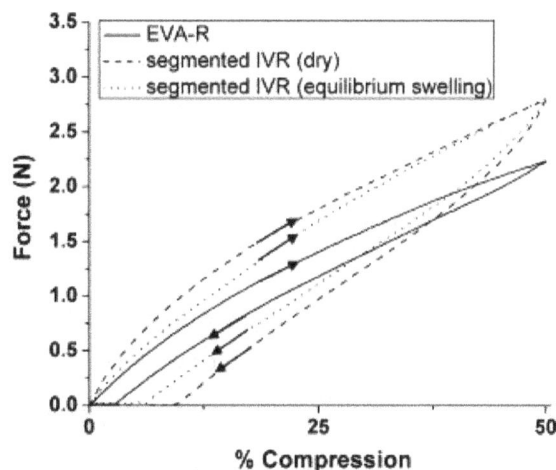

Figure 7. Force versus percent ring compression for experimental (segmented IVR) and Nuvaring® (EVA-R) intravaginal rings. Equilibrium swelling, as determined by mass change, was achieved after 3 days in water. Each ring was brought to 50% compression and subsequently allowed to recover to its original diameter as indicated by the direction of arrows. Adapted from [14], Elsevier, 2010 with permission.

5.3. Gamma Irradiation

Gamma irradiation is an established approach to sterilize materials for biomedical application. However, polymer irradiation may result in crosslinking or chain scission, resulting in physical and mechanical changes to the polymer. It has been generally reported that medical polyurethane products are able to withstand multiple exposures to gamma irradiation without change to physical or mechanical properties [92]. For example, Abraham et al. studied the effect of gamma irradiation on the mechanical properties of an aromatic poly(ether urethane urea) and an aliphatic polycarbonate-based polyurethane [93]. The investigators assessed tensile properties with uniaxial stress-strain data following ASTM D638 methods and elongation properties using a stress hysteresis test. Although they observed a change in molecular weight distribution and soft segment glass transition temperature for both polymers, they found no significant effect of irradiation on the tensile properties and a small increase in hysteresis stress values.

In a separate study, Simmons et al. examined the effect of gamma irradiation on the mechanical properties of an aromatic poly(ether urethane) and an aromatic polyurethane based on both polyether and polysiloxane in the soft segment [94]. They determined the ultimate tensile strength, ultimate elongation and Young's modulus prior to and following sterilization. Gamma irradiation appeared to stiffen the polyether/polysiloxane-based material, with an approximate 20% increase in Young's modulus, while tensile strength and elongation remained largely unchanged. There was no significant effect of irradiation on the measured mechanical properties of the polyether-based polyurethane.

Gorna et al. noted that previous studies had focused on the impact of gamma irradiation on the properties of non-erodible polyurethanes. Therefore, they investigated the effect of gamma irradiation on the mechanical properties of biodegradable polyurethanes based on poly(ethylene oxide) and poly(ε-caprolactone), used for medical implants and scaffolds [95]. They measured the tensile strength, Young's modulus and elongation at break before and after gamma irradiation. The investigators observed a decrease in mechanical strength following gamma irradiation, with the polyurethane based on poly(ethylene oxide) exhibiting a substantial 50% decrease in tensile strength.

However, Ahmed et al. studied the effect of gamma irradiation on the mechanical properties of a non-erodible aromatic poly(carbonate urea) based polyurethane alongside a biodegradable aliphatic polycaprolactone based polyurethane [96]. They observed an approximate 25% decrease in Young's modulus and ultimate tensile strength for both polymers following irradiation. Consequently, no generalized conclusions can be made with regard to the effect of gamma irradiation on the mechanical properties of varying types of polyurethanes, underscoring the importance of verifying mechanical properties of the drug product during development.

6. Conclusions

Owing to their chemical diversity, polyurethanes can be tailored to exhibit a wide variety of physical properties. Crystallinity, hydrophilicity, hydrated porosity, mechanical strength and bioerodibility can be tuned to achieve the desired dosage form characteristics and release rate for a diverse array of treatment duration and route of administration. The diversity of polyurethane chemistry suggests that one may have substantially more degrees of freedom to select a polymer exhibiting good or poor drug solubility than with silicone or poly(ethylene-co-vinyl acetate) elastomers. The ability to tune the extent of water swelling by changing the soft segment to hard segment ratio of polyurethanes presents an exciting route to modulate drug release kinetics independent of drug solubility in polymer. Despite the available opportunities, few commercialized drug products leverage polyurethanes, suggesting that it remains a nascent field with much to be understood before it can be routinely reduced to practice. Polyurethane-based parenteral sustained release dosage forms are well suited toward therapies where high adherence to a consistent dose over a long duration is critical, particularly infectious and neurodegenerative diseases.

Funding: This work was supported by Merck & Co., Inc., Rahway, NJ, USA.

References

1.   Engels, H.-W.; Pirkl, H.-G.; Albers, R.; Albach, R.W.; Krause, J.; Hoffmann, A.; Casselmann, H.; Dormish, J. Polyurethanes: Versatile Materials and Sustainable Problem Solvers for Today's Challenges. *Angew. Chem. Int. Ed.* **2013**, *52*, 9422–9441. [CrossRef] [PubMed]

2.   Bayer, O. Das Di-Isocyanat-Polyadditionsverfahren (Polyurethane). *Angew. Chem.* **1947**, *59*, 257–272. [CrossRef]

3.   Cherng, J.Y.; Hou, T.Y.; Shih, M.F.; Talsma, H.; Hennink, W.E. Polyurethane-based drug delivery systems. *Int. J. Pharm.* **2013**, *450*, 145–162. [CrossRef] [PubMed]

4.   Seo, E.; Na, K. Polyurethane membrane with porous surface for controlled drug release in drug eluting stent. *Biomater. Res.* **2014**, *18*, 15. [CrossRef] [PubMed]

5.   Guo, Q.; Knight, P.T.; Mather, P.T. Tailored drug release from biodegradable stent coatings based on hybrid polyurethanes. *J. Control. Release* **2009**, *137*, 224–233. [CrossRef] [PubMed]

6.   Chen, X.; Liu, W.; Zhao, Y.; Jiang, L.; Xu, H.; Yang, X. Preparation and characterization of PEG-modified polyurethane pressure-sensitive adhesives for transdermal drug delivery. *Drug Dev. Ind. Pharm.* **2009**, *35*, 704–711. [CrossRef] [PubMed]

7.   Li, B.; Brown, K.V.; Wenke, J.C.; Guelcher, S.A. Sustained release of vancomycin from polyurethane scaffolds inhibits infection of bone wounds in a rat femoral segmental defect model. *J. Control. Release* **2010**, *145*, 221–230. [CrossRef] [PubMed]

8.   Gorna, K.; Gogolewski, S. Preparation, degradation, and calcification of biodegradable polyurethane foams for bone graft substitutes. *J. Biomed. Mater. Res.* **2003**, *67A*, 813–827. [CrossRef] [PubMed]

9.   Li, B.; Yoshii, T.; Hafeman, A.E.; Nyman, J.S.; Wenke, J.C.; Guelcher, S.A. The effects of rhBMP-2 released from biodegradable polyurethane/microsphere composite scaffolds on new bone formation in rat femora. *Biomaterials* **2009**, *30*, 6768–6779. [CrossRef] [PubMed]

10.   Martinelli, A.; D'Ilario, L.; Francolini, I.; Piozzi, A. Water state effect on drug release from an antibiotic loaded polyurethane matrix containing albumin nanoparticles. *Int. J. Pharm.* **2011**, *407*, 197–206. [CrossRef] [PubMed]

11. Wang, A.; Gao, H.; Sun, Y.; Sun, Y.; Yang, Y.-W.; Wu, G.; Wang, Y.; Fan, Y.; Ma, J. Temperature- and pH-responsive nanoparticles of biocompatible polyurethanes for doxorubicin delivery. *Int. J. Pharm.* **2013**, *441*, 30–39. [CrossRef] [PubMed]

12. Basak, P.; Adhikari, B.; Banerjee, I.; Maiti, T.K. Sustained release of antibiotic from polyurethane coated implant materials. *J. Mater. Sci. Mater. Med.* **2009**, *20*, 213–221. [CrossRef] [PubMed]

13. Moura, S.A.L.; Lima, L.D.C.; Andrade, S.P.; Silva-Cunha Junior, A. Da; Órefice, R.L.; Ayres, E.; Da Silva, G.R. Local Drug Delivery System: Inhibition of Inflammatory Angiogenesis in a Murine Sponge Model by Dexamethasone-Loaded Polyurethane Implants. *J. Pharm. Sci.* **2011**, *100*, 2886–2895. [CrossRef] [PubMed]

14. Johnson, T.J.; Gupta, K.M.; Fabian, J.; Albright, T.H.; Kiser, P.F. Segmented polyurethane intravaginal rings for the sustained combined delivery of antiretroviral agents dapivirine and tenofovir. *Eur. J. Pharm. Sci.* **2010**, *39*, 203–212. [CrossRef] [PubMed]

15. Verstraete, G.; Vandenbussche, L.; Kasmi, S.; Nuhn, L.; Brouckaert, D.; Van Renterghem, J.; Grymonpré, W.; Vanhoorne, V.; Coenye, T.; De Geest, B.G.; et al. Thermoplastic polyurethane-based intravaginal rings for prophylaxis and treatment of (recurrent) bacterial vaginosis. *Int. J. Pharm.* **2017**, *529*, 218–226. [CrossRef] [PubMed]

16. Mesquita, P.M.M.; Rastogi, R.; Segarra, T.J.; Teller, R.S.; Torres, N.M.; Huber, A.M.; Kiser, P.F.; Herold, B.C. Intravaginal ring delivery of tenofovir disoproxil fumarate for prevention of HIV and herpes simplex virus infection. *J. Antimicrob. Chemother.* **2012**, *67*, 1730–1738. [CrossRef] [PubMed]

17. Gupta, K.M.; Pearce, S.M.; Poursaid, A.E.; Aliyar, H.A.; Tresco, P.A.; Mitchnik, M.A.; Kiser, P.F. Polyurethane Intravaginal Ring for Controlled Delivery of Dapivirine, a Nonnucleoside Reverse Transcriptase Inhibitor of HIV-1. *J. Pharm. Sci.* **2008**, *97*, 4228–4239. [CrossRef] [PubMed]

18. Traore, Y.L.; Chen, Y.; Bernier, A.-M.; Ho, E.A. Impact of Hydroxychloroquine-Loaded Polyurethane Intravaginal Rings on Lactobacilli. *Antimicrob. Agents Chemother.* **2015**, *59*, 7680–7686. [CrossRef] [PubMed]

19. Smith, J.M.; Rastogi, R.; Teller, R.S.; Srinivasan, P.; Mesquita, P.M.M.; Nagaraja, U.; McNicholl, J.M.; Hendry, R.M.; Dinh, C.T.; Martin, A.; et al. Intravaginal ring eluting tenofovir disoproxil fumarate completely protects macaques from multiple vaginal simian-HIV challenges. *Proc. Natl. Acad. Sci. USA* **2013**, *110*, 16145–16150. [CrossRef] [PubMed]

20. Johnson, T.J.; Clark, M.R.; Albright, T.H.; Nebeker, J.S.; Tuitupou, A.L.; Clark, J.T.; Fabian, J.; McCabe, R.T.; Chandra, N.; Doncel, G.F.; et al. A 90-day tenofovir reservoir intravaginal ring for mucosal HIV prophylaxis. *Antimicrob. Agents Chemother.* **2012**, *56*, 6272–6283. [CrossRef] [PubMed]

21. Keller, M.J.; Mesquita, P.M.; Marzinke, M.A.; Teller, R.; Espinoza, L.; Atrio, J.M.; Lo, Y.; Frank, B.; Srinivasan, S.; Fredricks, D.N.; et al. A phase 1 randomized placebo-controlled safety and pharmacokinetic trial of a tenofovir disoproxil fumarate vaginal ring. *AIDS* **2016**, *30*, 743–751. [CrossRef] [PubMed]

22. Teller, R.S.; Malaspina, D.C.; Rastogi, R.; Clark, J.T.; Szleifer, I.; Kiser, P.F. Controlling the hydration rate of a hydrophilic matrix in the core of an intravaginal ring determines antiretroviral release. *J. Control. Release* **2016**, *224*, 176–183. [CrossRef] [PubMed]

23. Smith, J.M.; Srinivasan, P.; Teller, R.S.; Lo, Y.; Dinh, C.T.; Kiser, P.F.; Herold, B.C. Tenofovir disoproxil fumarate intravaginal ring protects high-dose depot medroxyprogesterone acetate-treated macaques from multiple SHIV exposures. *J. Acquir. Immune Defic. Syndr.* **2015**, *68*, 1–5. [CrossRef] [PubMed]

24. Clark, M.R.; Johnson, T.J.; McCabe, R.T.; Clark, J.T.; Tuitupou, A.; Elgendy, H.; Friend, D.R.; Kiser, P.F. A hot-melt extruded intravaginal ring for the sustained delivery of the antiretroviral microbicide UC781. *J. Pharm. Sci.* **2012**, *101*, 576–587. [CrossRef] [PubMed]

25. Friend, D.R.; Clark, J.T.; Kiser, P.F.; Clark, M.R. Multipurpose prevention technologies: Products in development. *Antiviral Res.* **2013**, *100*, S39–S47. [CrossRef] [PubMed]

26. Claeys, B.; Bruyn, S. De; Hansen, L.; Beer, T. De; Remon, J.P.; Vervaet, C. Release characteristics of polyurethane tablets containing dicarboxylic acids as release modifiers—A case study with diprophylline. *Int. J. Pharm.* **2014**, *477*, 244–250. [CrossRef] [PubMed]

27. Lazarus, J.; Pagliery, M.; Lachman, L. Factors Influencing the Release of a Drug from a Prolonged-Action Matrix. *J. Pharm. Sci.* **1964**, *53*, 798–802. [CrossRef] [PubMed]

28. Anderson, J.M.; Hiltner, A.; Wiggins, M.J.; Schubert, M.A.; Collier, T.O.; Kao, W.J.; Mathur, A.B. Recent advances in biomedical polyurethane biostability and biodegradation. *Polym. Int.* **1998**, *46*, 163–171. [CrossRef]

29. Cooper, S.L.; Guan, J. *Advances in Polyurethane Biomaterials*; Woodhead Publishing: Cambridge, MA, USA, 2016; ISBN 9780081006221.

30. Boretos, J.W.; Pierce, W.S. Segmented polyurethane: A polyether polymer. An initial evalution for biomedical applications. *J. Biomed. Mater. Res.* **1968**, *2*, 121–130. [CrossRef] [PubMed]

31. Gogolewski, S. Selected topics in biomedical polyurethanes. A review. *Colloid Polym. Sci.* **1989**, *267*, 757–785. [CrossRef]

32. Gunatillake, P.A.; Martin, D.J.; Meijs, G.F.; McCarthy, S.J.; Adhikari, R. Designing Biostable Polyurethane Elastomers for Biomedical Implants. *Aust. J. Chem.* **2003**, *56*, 545–557. [CrossRef]

33. Lamba, N.M.K.; Woodhouse, K.A.; Cooper, S.L. *Polyurethanes in Biomedical Applications*; CRC Press: Boca Raton, FL, USA, 1997.

34. Vermette, P.; Griesser, H.J.; Laroche, G.; Guidoin, R. (Eds.) *Biomedical Applications of Polyurethanes*; Landes Bioscience: Georgetown, TX, USA, 2001.

35. Irusta, L.; Fernandez-Berridi, M.J. Aromatic poly(ester–urethanes): Effect of the polyol molecular weight on the photochemical behaviour. *Polymer* **2000**, *41*, 3297–3302. [CrossRef]

36. DiBattista, G.; Peerlings, H.W.I.; Kaufhold, W. Aliphatic TPUs for light-stable applications. *Rubber World* **2003**, *227*, 39–42.

37. Szycher, M.; Siciliano, A.A. An Assessment of 2,4 TDA Formation from Surgitek Polyurethane Foam under Simulated Physiological Conditions. *J. Biomater. Appl.* **1991**, *5*, 323–336. [CrossRef] [PubMed]

38. Kääriä, K.; Hirvonen, A.; Norppa, H.; Piirilä, P.; Vainio, H.; Rosenberg, C. Exposure to 4,4′-methylenediphenyl diisocyanate (MDI) during moulding of rigid polyurethane foam: Determination of airborne MDI and urinary 4,4′-methylenedianiline (MDA). *Analyst* **2001**, *126*, 476–479. [CrossRef] [PubMed]

39. Jabbari, E.; Khakpour, M. Morphology of and release behavior from porous polyurethane microspheres. *Biomaterials* **2000**, *21*, 2073–2079. [CrossRef]

40. Thompson, D.G.; Osborn, J.C.; Kober, E.M.; Schoonover, J.R. Effects of hydrolysis-induced molecular weight changes on the phase separation of a polyester polyurethane. *Polym. Degrad. Stab.* **2006**, *91*, 3360–3370. [CrossRef]

41. Saad, B.; Hirt, T.D.; Welti, M.; Uhlschmid, G.K.; Neuenschwander, P.; Suter, U.W. Development of degradable polyesterurethanes for medical applications: In vitro and in vivo evaluations. *J. Biomed. Mater. Res.* **1997**, *36*, 65–74. [CrossRef]

42. Kaur, M.; Gupta, K.M.; Poursaid, A.E.; Karra, P.; Mahalingam, A.; Aliyar, H.A.; Kiser, P.F. Engineering a degradable polyurethane intravaginal ring for sustained delivery of dapivirine. *Drug Deliv. Transl. Res.* **2011**, *1*, 223–237. [CrossRef] [PubMed]

43. Yu, J.; Lin, F.; Lin, P.; Gao, Y.; Becker, M.L. Phenylalanine-Based Poly(ester urea): Synthesis, Characterization, and in vitro Degradation. *Macromolecules* **2014**, *47*, 121–129. [CrossRef]

44. Rychlý, J.; Lattuati-Derieux, A.; Lavédrine, B.; Matisová-Rychlá, L.; Malíková, M.; Csomorová, K.; Janigová, I. Assessing the progress of degradation in polyurethanes by chemiluminescence and thermal analysis. II. Flexible polyether- and polyester-type polyurethane foams. *Polym. Degrad. Stab.* **2011**, *96*, 462–469. [CrossRef]

45. Yilgör, E.; Burgaz, E.; Yurtsever, E.; Yilgör, İ. Comparison of hydrogen bonding in polydimethylsiloxane and polyether based urethane and urea copolymers. *Polymer* **2000**, *41*, 849–857. [CrossRef]

46. Wiggins, M.J.; Wilkoff, B.; Anderson, J.M.; Hiltner, A. Biodegradation of polyether polyurethane inner insulation in bipolar pacemaker leads. *J. Biomed. Mater. Res.* **2001**, *58*, 302–307. [CrossRef]

47. Christenson, E.M.; Dadsetan, M.; Wiggins, M.; Anderson, J.M.; Hiltner, A. Poly(carbonate urethane) and poly(ether urethane) biodegradation: In vivo studies. *J. Biomed. Mater. Res. Part A* **2004**, *69*, 407–416. [CrossRef] [PubMed]

48. Ikeda, Y.; Kohjiya, S.; Takesako, S.; Yamashita, S. Polyurethane elastomer with PEO-PTMO-PEO soft segment for sustained release of drugs. *Biomaterials* **1990**, *11*, 553–560. [CrossRef]

49. Anderson, J.M.; Rodriguez, A.; Chang, D.T. Foreign body reaction to biomaterials. *Semin. Immunol.* **2008**, *20*, 86–100. [CrossRef] [PubMed]

50. Kricheldorf, H.R.; Quirk, R.P.; Holden, G. *Thermoplastic Elastomers*; Hanser Gardner Publications: Munich, Germany, 2004; ISBN 9783446223752.

51. Ahn, T.O.; Choi, I.S.; Jeong, H.M.; Cho, K. Thermal and mechanical properties of thermoplastic polyurethane elastomers from different polymerization methods. *Polym. Int.* **1993**, *31*, 329–333. [CrossRef]

52. Arifin, D.Y.; Lee, L.Y.; Wang, C.-H. Mathematical modeling and simulation of drug release from microspheres: Implications to drug delivery systems. *Adv. Drug Deliv. Rev.* **2006**, *58*, 1274–1325. [CrossRef] [PubMed]

53. Siepmann, J.; Siepmann, F. Mathematical modeling of drug delivery. *Int. J. Pharm.* **2008**, *364*, 328–343. [CrossRef] [PubMed]

54. Clark, J.T.; Johnson, T.J.; Clark, M.R.; Nebeker, J.S.; Fabian, J.; Tuitupou, A.L.; Ponnapalli, S.; Smith, E.M.; Friend, D.R.; Kiser, P.F. Quantitative evaluation of a hydrophilic matrix intravaginal ring for the sustained delivery of tenofovir. *J. Control. Release* **2012**, *163*, 240–248. [CrossRef] [PubMed]

55. Ugaonkar, S.R.; Clark, J.T.; English, L.B.; Johnson, T.J.; Buckheit, K.W.; Bahde, R.J.; Appella, D.H.; Buckheit, R.W.; Kiser, P.F. An Intravaginal Ring for the Simultaneous Delivery of an HIV-1 Maturation Inhibitor and Reverse-Transcriptase Inhibitor for Prophylaxis of HIV Transmission. *J. Pharm. Sci.* **2015**, *104*, 3426–3439. [CrossRef] [PubMed]

56. van Laarhoven, J.A.; Kruft, M.A.; Vromans, H. In vitro release properties of etonogestrel and ethinyl estradiol from a contraceptive vaginal ring. *Int. J. Pharm.* **2002**, *232*, 163–173. [CrossRef]

57. Crank, J. *The Mathematics of Diffusion*, 2nd ed.; Oxford Science Publications; Clarendon Press: Oxford, UK, 1979; ISBN 978-0-19-853411-2.

58. Vergnaud, J.-M. *Controlled Drug Release of Oral Dosage Forms*; CRC Press: Boca Raton, FL, USA, 1993.

59. Higuchi, T. Mechanism of sustained-action medication. Theoretical analysis of rate of release of solid drugs dispersed in solid matrices. *J. Pharm. Sci.* **1963**, *52*, 1145–1149. [CrossRef] [PubMed]

60. Claeys, B.; Vervaeck, A.; Hillewaere, X.K.D.; Possemiers, S.; Hansen, L.; De Beer, T.; Remon, J.P.; Vervaet, C. Thermoplastic polyurethanes for the manufacturing of highly dosed oral sustained release matrices via hot melt extrusion and injection molding. *Eur. J. Pharm. Biopharm.* **2015**, *90*, 44–52. [CrossRef] [PubMed]

61. Yasuda, H.; Lamaze, C.E.; Ikenberry, L.D. Permeability of solutes through hydrated polymer membranes. Part I. Diffusion of sodium chloride. *Die Makromol. Chem.* **1968**, *118*, 19–35. [CrossRef]

62. Go¨pferich, A.; Langer, R. Modeling monomer release from bioerodible polymers. *J. Control. Release* **1995**, *33*, 55–69. [CrossRef]

63. Langer, R.; Peppas, N. Chemical and Physical Structure of Polymers as Carriers for Controlled Release of Bioactive Agents: A Review. *J. Macromol. Sci. Part C* **1983**, *23*, 61–126. [CrossRef]

64. Ritger, P.L.; Peppas, N.A. A simple equation for description of solute release II. Fickian and anomalous release from swellable devices. *J. Control. Release* **1987**, *5*, 37–42. [CrossRef]

65. Hafeman, A.E.; Li, B.; Yoshii, T.; Zienkiewicz, K.; Davidson, J.M.; Guelcher, S.A. Injectable Biodegradable Polyurethane Scaffolds with Release of Platelet-derived Growth Factor for Tissue Repair and Regeneration. *Pharm. Res.* **2008**, *25*, 2387–2399. [CrossRef] [PubMed]

66. Hafeman, A.E.; Zienkiewicz, K.J.; Carney, E.; Litzner, B.; Stratton, C.; Wenke, J.C.; Guelcher, S.A. Local Delivery of Tobramycin from Injectable Biodegradable Polyurethane Scaffolds. *J. Biomater. Sci. Polym. Ed.* **2010**, *21*, 95–112. [CrossRef] [PubMed]

67. Hombreiro-Pérez, M.; Siepmann, J.; Zinutti, C.; Lamprecht, A.; Ubrich, N.; Hoffman, M.; Bodmeier, R.; Maincent, P. Non-degradable microparticles containing a hydrophilic and/or a lipophilic drug: Preparation, characterization and drug release modeling. *J. Control. Release* **2003**, *88*, 413–428. [CrossRef]

68. Almeida, A.; Brabant, L.; Siepmann, F.; De Beer, T.; Bouquet, W.; Van Hoorebeke, L.; Siepmann, J.; Remon, J.P.; Vervaet, C. Sustained release from hot-melt extruded matrices based on ethylene vinyl acetate and polyethylene oxide. *Eur. J. Pharm. Biopharm.* **2012**, *82*, 526–533. [CrossRef] [PubMed]

69. Tallury, P.; Alimohammadi, N.; Kalachandra, S. Poly(ethylene-co-vinyl acetate) copolymer matrix for delivery of chlorhexidine and acyclovir drugs for use in the oral environment: Effect of drug combination, copolymer composition and coating on the drug release rate. *Dent. Mater.* **2007**, *23*, 404–409. [CrossRef] [PubMed]

70. Reddy, T.T.; Hadano, M.; Takahara, A. Controlled Release of Model Drug from Biodegradable Segmented Polyurethane Ureas: Morphological and Structural Features. *Macromol. Symp.* **2006**, *242*, 241–249. [CrossRef]

71. Hsu, T.T.-P.; Langer, R. Polymers for the controlled release of macromolecules: Effect of molecular weight of ethylene-vinyl acetate copolymer. *J. Biomed. Mater. Res.* **1985**, *19*, 445–460. [CrossRef] [PubMed]

72. Zhou, L.; Liang, D.; He, X.; Li, J.; Tan, H.; Li, J.; Fu, Q.; Gu, Q. The degradation and biocompatibility of pH-sensitive biodegradable polyurethanes for intracellular multifunctional antitumor drug delivery. *Biomaterials* **2012**, *33*, 2734–2745. [CrossRef] [PubMed]

73. Shoaib, M.; Bahadur, A.; Iqbal, S.; Rahman, M.S.U.; Ahmed, S.; Shabir, G.; Javaid, M.A. Relationship of hard segment concentration in polyurethane-urea elastomers with mechanical, thermal and drug release properties. *J. Drug Deliv. Sci. Technol.* **2017**, *37*, 88–96. [CrossRef]

74. Verstraete, G.; Van Renterghem, J.; Van Bockstal, P.J.; Kasmi, S.; De Geest, B.G.; De Beer, T.; Remon, J.P.; Vervaet, C. Hydrophilic thermoplastic polyurethanes for the manufacturing of highly dosed oral sustained release matrices via hot melt extrusion and injection molding. *Int. J. Pharm.* **2016**, *506*, 214–221. [CrossRef] [PubMed]

75. Kim, J.-E.; Kim, S.-R.; Lee, S.-H.; Lee, C.-H.; Kim, D.-D. The effect of pore formers on the controlled release of cefadroxil from a polyurethane matrix. *Int. J. Pharm.* **2000**, *201*, 29–36. [CrossRef]

76. Donelli, G.; Francolini, I.; Ruggeri, V.; Guaglianone, E.; D'Ilario, L.; Piozzi, A. Pore formers promoted release of an antifungal drug from functionalized polyurethanes to inhibit Candida colonization. *J. Appl. Microbiol.* **2006**, *100*, 615–622. [CrossRef] [PubMed]

77. Sreenivasan, K. Effect of blending methyl β-cyclodextrin on the release of hydrophobic hydrocortisone into water from polyurethane. *J. Appl. Polym. Sci.* **2001**, *81*, 520–522. [CrossRef]

78. Langer, R.; Folkman, J. Polymers for the sustained release of proteins and other macromolecules. *Nature* **1976**, *263*, 797–800. [CrossRef] [PubMed]

79. Lindholm, T.; Lindholm, B.-Å.; Niskanen, M.; Koskiniemi, J. Polysorbate 20 as a drug release regulator in ethyl cellulose film coatings. *J. Pharm. Pharmacol.* **1986**, *38*, 686–688. [CrossRef] [PubMed]

80. Bodmeier, R.; Paeratakul, O. Theophylline Tablets Coated with Aqueous Latexes Containing Dispersed Pore Formers. *J. Pharm. Sci.* **1990**, *79*, 925–928. [CrossRef] [PubMed]

81. Frohoff-Hülsmann, M.A.; Schmitz, A.; Lippold, B.C. Aqueous ethyl cellulose dispersions containing plasticizers of different water solubility and hydroxypropyl methylcellulose as coating material for diffusion pellets: I. Drug release rates from coated pellets. *Int. J. Pharm.* **1999**, *177*, 69–82. [CrossRef]

82. Sauer, D.; Watts, A.B.; Coots, L.B.; Zheng, W.C.; McGinity, J.W. Influence of polymeric subcoats on the drug release properties of tablets powder-coated with pre-plasticized Eudragit®L 100-55. *Int. J. Pharm.* **2009**, *367*, 20–28. [CrossRef] [PubMed]

83. Irfan, M.; Ahmed, A.R.; Kolter, K.; Bodmeier, R.; Dashevskiy, A. Curing mechanism of flexible aqueous polymeric coatings. *Eur. J. Pharm. Biopharm.* **2017**, *115*, 186–196. [CrossRef] [PubMed]

84. Bounds, W.; Szarewski, A.; Lowe, D.; Guillebaud, J. Preliminary report of unexpected local reactions to a progestogen-releasing contraceptive vaginal ring. *Eur. J. Obstet. Gynecol. Reprod. Biol.* **1993**, *48*, 123–125. [CrossRef]

85. Koetsawang, S.; Gao, J.; Krishna, U.; Cuadros, A.; Dhall, G.I.; Wyss, R.; la Puenta, J.R.; Andrade, A.T.L.; Khan, T.; Kononova, E.S.; et al. Microdose intravaginal levonorgestrel contraception: A multicentre clinical trial. *Contraception* **1990**, *41*, 125–141. [CrossRef]

86. Morrow Guthrie, K.; Vargas, S.; Shaw, J.G.; Rosen, R.K.; van den Berg, J.J.; Kiser, P.F.; Buckheit, K.; Bregman, D.; Thompson, L.; Jensen, K.; et al. The Promise of Intravaginal Rings for Prevention: User Perceptions of Biomechanical Properties and Implications for Prevention Product Development. *PLoS One* **2015**, *10*, e0145642. [CrossRef] [PubMed]

87. Baum, M.M.; Butkyavichene, I.; Gilman, J.; Kennedy, S.; Kopin, E.; Malone, A.M.; Nguyen, C.; Smith, T.J.; Friend, D.R.; Clark, M.R.; et al. An intravaginal ring for the simultaneous delivery of multiple drugs. *J. Pharm. Sci.* **2012**, *101*, 2833–2843. [CrossRef] [PubMed]

88. ASTM International. *ASTM D2240-15e1, Standard Test Method for Rubber Property—Durometer Hardness*; ASTM International: West Conshohocken, PA, USA, 2015.

89. ISO. *ISO 8009 Mechanical Contraceptives—Reusable Natural and Silicone Rubber Contraceptive Diaphragms—Requirements and Tests*; ISO: Geneva, Switzerland, 2014.

90. Clark, J.T.; Clark, M.R.; Shelke, N.B.; Johnson, T.J.; Smith, E.M.; Andreasen, A.K.; Nebeker, J.S.; Fabian, J.; Friend, D.R.; Kiser, P.F. Engineering a Segmented Dual-Reservoir Polyurethane Intravaginal Ring for Simultaneous Prevention of HIV Transmission and Unwanted Pregnancy. *PLoS ONE* **2014**, *9*, e88509. [CrossRef] [PubMed]

91. Crnich, C.J.; Halfmann, J.A.; Crone, W.C.; Maki, D.G. The Effects of Prolonged Ethanol Exposure on the Mechanical Properties of Polyurethane and Silicone Catheters Used for Intravascular Access. *Infect. Control Hosp. Epidemiol.* **2005**, *26*, 708–714. [CrossRef] [PubMed]

92. Massey, L.K. *The Effects of Sterilization Methods on Plastics and Elastomers: The Definitive User's Guide and Databook*; William Andrew Pub: Norwich, NY, USA, 2005; ISBN 0815515057.

93. Abraham, G.A.; Frontini, P.M.; Cuadrado, T.R. Physical and mechanical behavior of sterilized biomedical segmented polyurethanes. *J. Appl. Polym. Sci.* **1997**, *65*, 1193–1203. [CrossRef]

94. Simmons, A.; Hyvarinen, J.; Poole-Warren, L. The effect of sterilisation on a poly(dimethylsiloxane)/poly(hexamethylene oxide) mixed macrodiol-based polyurethane elastomer. *Biomaterials* **2006**, *27*, 4484–4497. [CrossRef] [PubMed]
95. Gorna, K.; Gogolewski, S. The effect of gamma radiation on molecular stability and mechanical properties of biodegradable polyurethanes for medical applications. *Polym. Degrad. Stab.* **2003**, *79*, 465–474. [CrossRef]
96. Ahmed, M.; Punshon, G.; Darbyshire, A.; Seifalian, A.M. Effects of sterilization treatments on bulk and surface properties of nanocomposite biomaterials. *J. Biomed. Mater. Res. Part B Appl. Biomater.* **2013**, *101*, 1182–1190. [CrossRef] [PubMed]

5

Qualification and Application of a Liquid Chromatography-Quadrupole Time-of-Flight Mass Spectrometric Method for the Determination of Adalimumab in Rat Plasma

Yuri Park, Nahye Kim, Jangmi Choi, Min-Ho Park, Byeong ill Lee, Seok-Ho Shin, Jin-Ju Byeon and Young G. Shin * 🆔

College of Pharmacy and Institute of Drug Research and Development, Chungnam National University, Daejeon 34134, Korea; yuri.park.cnu@gmail.com (Y.P.); nahye.kim.cnu@gmail.com (N.K.); jangmi.choi.cnu@gmail.com (J.C.); minho.park.cnu@gmail.com (M.-H.P.); byungill.lee.cnu@gmail.com (B.i.L.); seokho.shin.cnu@gmail.com (S.-H.S.); jinju.byeon.cnu@gmail.com (J.-J.B.)
* Correspondence: yshin@cnu.ac.kr

Abstract: A liquid chromatography–quadrupole time-of-flight (Q-TOF) mass spectrometric method was developed for early-stage research on adalimumab in rats. The method consisted of immunoprecipitation followed by tryptic digestion for sample preparation and LC-QTOF-MS/MS analysis of specific signature peptides of adalimumab in the positive ion mode using electrospray ionization. This specific signature peptide is derived from the complementarity-determining region (CDR) of adalimumab. A quadratic regression (weighted 1/concentration), with an equation $y = ax^2 + bx + c$, was used to fit calibration curves over the concentration range of 1–100 µg/mL for adalimumab. The qualification run met the acceptance criteria of ±25% accuracy and precision values for quality control (QC) samples. This qualified LC-QTOF-MS/MS method was successfully applied to a pharmacokinetic study of adalimumab in rats as a case study. This LC-QTOF-MS/MS approach would be useful as a complementary method for adalimumab or its biosimilars at an early stage of research.

Keywords: adalimumab; immunoprecipitation; liquid chromatography-quadrupole TOF MS; bioanalysis

1. Introduction

Since humanized and fully human monoclonal antibodies (mAbs) were approved as therapeutic pharmaceutical products, the attention for monoclonal antibody products has been growing significantly in the global pharmaceutical market [1,2].

Therapeutic mAbs offer many advantages when compared to small-molecule drugs [3]. In general, mAbs have three main characteristics: (i) target-specific binding ability to increase or decrease an important biological effect, (ii) interaction of the constant domain with cell surface receptors that causes immune-mediated effector functions, including antibody-dependent cell-mediated cytotoxicity (ADCC), complement dependent cytotoxicity (CDC) or antibody-dependent phagocytosis; and (iii) deposition of complement on multimeric immune complexes between the mAb and the target and subsequent activation of complement-dependent cytotoxicity [2,4].

Tumor necrosis factor α (TNF-α) is an inflammatory cytokine produced by activated monocytes or macrophages [5]. Therefore, TNF-α antagonist (anti-TNF) is one of the agents that has the highest affinity for TNF-α molecules and suppresses the biological activity of TNF-α [6]. One of the well-known anti-TNF drugs is adalimumab, which consists of a fully humanized monoclonal antibody and was approved by the FDA in 2002 [7]. Adalimumab is a tetramer composed of two heavy immunoglobulin G1 (IgG1) chains and two light IgG1 chains [7]. It is currently used to treat rheumatoid arthritis, psoriasis, psoriatic arthritis, ankylosing spondylitis and Crohn's disease [8].

Traditionally, pharmacokinetic evaluation of mAbs has been mainly performed by immunoassays such as enzyme-linked immunosorbent assays (ELISA), radioimmunoassay immunofluorescence assay and etc. [9]. Immunoassays have several advantages in terms of high sensitivity, robust performance and high throughput [2,10]. However, these methods also have several disadvantages such as non-specific binding as well as time-consuming and labor-intensive reagent development [8]. Immunoassays also often show cross-reactions with precursors of the target protein or with smaller metabolized fragments that are not suitable for early-stage mAbs bioanalysis [11].

Liquid chromatographic mass spectrometry (LC-MS/MS) is a complementary technique that can quantify not only small molecules or peptides but also proteins [12]. LC-MS/MS is accurate and precise and enables throughput analysis because this combines a robust separation technique with identification and quantification based on the molecular weights of the analytes [10]. In addition, LC-MS/MS is less matrix-dependent than ELISA [13].

The purpose of this paper is to explore an adalimumab quantification method using LC-QTOF-MS/MS and employing adalimumab's specific signature peptides that are involved in variable regions and produced by tryptic digestion.

2. Materials and Methods

2.1. Materials

Adalimumab was purchased from Dongwon Pharmaceutical Wholesale (Deajeon, Korea). Protein A magnetic beads were purchased from Millipore Corp (Billerica, MA, USA). RapiGest surfactant was purchased from Waters Korea (Seoul, Korea). 1,4-Dithiothreitol (DTT) was purchased from Carl Roth (Karlsruhe, Germany). Iodoacetic acid (IAA) was purchased from Wako (Osaka, Japan). The sequencing grade modified trypsin was purchased from Promega (Madison, WI, USA). All other chemicals were commercial products of analytical or reagent grade and were used without further purification.

2.2. Preparation of Stocks, Standard (STD) and Quality Control (QC) Samples

Stock solution of adalimumab was prepared at a concentration of 5000 µg/mL in a phosphate buffer solution (PBS) containing 0.1% tween 20. The stock solution was stored at 4 °C. Stock solution of adalimumab was further diluted at a concentration 500 µg/mL in PBS containing 0.1% tween 20 as sub-stock solution. Calibration working solution was prepared by serial dilution of the sub-stock solution with PBS containing 0.1% tween 20. Then, the working solution was spiked into rat plasma to yield calibration standard concentrations of 1.0, 2.0, 5.0, 10, 20, 40, 80 and 100 µg/mL. The quality control (QC) samples with final concentrations of 2.5, 25 and 50 µg/mL were also prepared in the same manner.

2.3. Preparation of Sample Digests for Quantification

Each 24 µL aliquot of plasma study samples, QCs and standards (STDs) were separately mixed with 370 µL of PBS containing 0.1% tween 20 and 30 µL of magnetic bead suspension. After gentle shaking at room temperature overnight, the magnetic bead was washed using 600 µL PBS containing 0.1% tween 20 and then was washed again using 600 µL PBS. Seventy-five microliters of RapiGest and 10 µL of DTT were added to the mixture, which was incubated for 50 min at 60 °C to denature and reduce the adalimumab bound to the magnetic beads. After a 10-min incubation at room temperature (RT), 25 µL of IAA was added and the sample was incubated in dark conditions for 30 min at RT. Ten microliters of the sequencing grade-modified trypsin were added to the sample to digest the antibody. After 1 min of shaking, the sample was incubated at 37 °C overnight. Fifteen microliters of 2 N HCl were added to the sample for quenching purposes and the sample was incubated for another 30 min at 37 °C to stop the digestion. The resulting sample was centrifuged at 7000 rpm for 5 min at 4 °C and transferred into a HPLC vial.

2.4. Liquid Chromatography–Mass Spectrometry

The liquid chromatography–mass spectrometry system consisted of a Shimadzu CBM-20A HPLC pump controller (Shimadzu Corporation, Columbia, MD, USA), two Shimadzu LC-20AD pumps, a CTC HTS PAL autosampler (CEAP Technologies, Carrboro, NC, USA) and a quadrupole time-of-flight (Q-TOF) TripleTOF™ 5600 mass spectrometer (Sciex, Foster City, CA, USA). The analytical column used for this assay was a Phenomenex Kinetex Phenyl-hexyl column (50 × 2.1 mm, 2.6 μm). The mobile phase consisted of: mobile phase A, distilled and deionized water containing 0.1% formic acid; and mobile phase B, acetonitrile containing 0.1% formic acid. The gradient was as follows: from 0 min to 0.6 min, 5% B; from 0.5 min to 1.6 min by a linear gradient from 5% B to 95% B; 95% B was maintained for 0.2 min; from 1.8 min to 1.9 min by a linear gradient from 95% B to 5% B and then 5% B was maintained for 1.5 min for column re-equilibrium. The gradient was delivered at a flow rate of 0.4 mL/min and the injection volume was 10 μL.

The TOF-MS scan mass spectra and TOF-MS/MS scan mass spectra were recorded in the positive ion mode. For TOF-MS scan, m/z 100~950 with 0.2 s accumulation time was used. For TOF-MS/MS scan, the scan range was m/z 500~1000. For the quantification, doubly charged $[M + 2H]^{2+}$ ion for the specific signature peptide APYTFGQGTK (m/z 535.4) was selected and its product ion at m/z 901.8 was used for the quantitative analysis of adalimumab. High-purity nitrogen gas was used for the nebulizer/Duospray™ and curtain gases. The ESI spray voltage was set at 5500 V. The source temperature was 500 °C. The curtain gas (CUR) was 30 L/min; the auxiliary gas setting (GS1 and GS2) was 50 L/min.

2.5. Method Qualification and Sample Analysis Procedure

2.5.1. Calibration Curve, Accuracy and Precision

Method qualification was carried out with a 'fit-for-purpose' approach. Quality control (QC) samples as well as standards (STDs) were used for batch acceptance. The qualification run contained duplicate calibration curves at eight concentrations and QCs at three concentrations (low, medium and high concentrations). The acceptance criterion for STDs and QCs in the qualification run was within ±25% of precision and accuracy, which is acceptable for early-stage drug discovery. Calibration curve was done by establishing a quadratic regression function, with an equation $y = ax^2 + bx + c$ after 1/concentration weighting. In addition, two blank plasma samples were in the set. QC samples (2.5, 25 and 50 μg/mL) were processed and analyzed three times in the same run (precision). The accuracy was calculated at each QC concentration as the ratio of the measured concentration to the nominal concentration multiplied by 100%.

2.5.2. Species-Dependent Matrix Effect

For species-dependent matrix effect test, three levels of QC samples were prepared in mouse and monkey plasma. Samples were quantitated with a calibration curve prepared in rat plasma. Mean accuracy and precision were also calculated.

2.5.3. Freeze and Thaw Stability

The freeze and thaw stability in rat, mouse and monkey plasma was assessed using low, medium and high QC samples ($n = 3$ at each concentration). For this study, the samples were subjected to three freeze and thaw cycles at −80 °C.

2.6. Software

Analyst® TF Version 1.6 (Sciex, Foster City, CA, USA) operated with Windows® (Microsoft) was used for instrument control and data acquisition. Peak integrations were operated by MultiQuant® Version 2.1.1 (Sciex, Foster City, CA, USA). Calculations including peak area ratios, standard curve regressions, sample concentration values and descriptive statistics were calculated with MultiQuant® Version 2.1.1. Pharmacokinetic calculations were performed using WinNonLin® version 6.4 (Pharsight Corporation, Mountain View, CA, USA).

2.7. Application for a Pharmacokinetic Study in Rat

Four adult male Sprague–Dawley rats (SD, 250–300 g) were purchased from the Samtako Biokorea Co. (Gyeonggi, Korea). The animals were housed in laminar flow cages that were maintained at $22 \pm 2\,°C$ and 50–60% relative humidity. The animals were kept in these facilities for at least a week prior to the experiment and were fasted for at least 24 h before the commencement of the experiments. Rats were cared for and treated in accordance with the Guiding Principles for the Use of Animals in Toxicology adopted by the Society of Toxicology (Reston, VA, USA) and the experimental protocols were approved by the Animal Care Committee of Chungnam National University (protocol No. CNU-00560).

Plasma samples were collected from the Sprague-Dawley rats ($n = 4$) after dosing intravenously with adalimumab at 1 mg/kg. The sampling times were 0.0014, 0.0417, 0.1667, 0.25, 1, 2, 3, 4, 7, 15, 21 and 28 days. The same set of pharmacokinetic study samples was analyzed by LC-QTOF-MS/MS.

3. Results

3.1. Method Development

3.1.1. Sample Preparation Method

In general, biological matrices such as plasma have highly abundant endogenous proteins such as albumin and immunoglobulins [14]. These endogenous proteins often interfere with the analysis of target mAb and decrease the sensitivity of the analyte. Therefore, a sample preparation method with minimal endogenous protein interference was necessary. To solve this problem, several approaches have been considered, such as albumin depletion kit, solid phase Protein A, and specific immunocapture [2,10,15]. In this study, the immunocapture using protein A magnetic beads was considered to be acceptable due to its selectivity as well as specificity. Plasma IgG and mAb were captured by a protein A magnetic bead and then washed out to remove other endogenous interference. After that, plasma IgG and mAb, bound to a protein A magnetic bead, were digested on-bead by the sequencing grade-modified trypsin. Trypsin-cleaved lysine and arginine residues in the amino acid sequence and various digested peptides from plasma IgG and mAbs were released into the supernatants. The supernatants were then analyzed by LC-QTOF-MS/MS for the target-specific signature peptide of adalimumab.

Generally, it would be ideal if trypsin digestion was carried out after acid dissociation and elution. However, one big challenge of this approach would be recovery from the protein A bead after binding. In addition, trypsin digestion efficiency is another challenge to consider due to lower pH after acid dissociation. Other matrix interference from endogenous immunoglobulins and etc. is another factor to carefully evaluate from this conventional trypsin digestion after acid dissociation followed by elution. Our approach, using on-bead digestion with trypsin, could have some disadvantages such as a large excess of tryptic peptide matrices derived from the protein A ligand, which might interfere with our assay. However, this method is very fast and robust and the interference from these endogenous matrix peptides could be minimized by selecting a specific signature peptide as well as its unique parent ion-product ion transition combination in the next section.

3.1.2. Selection of Target-Specific Signature Peptide

A couple of specific signature peptides were sought that would be applicable and specific to adalimumab using freeware software 'Skyline' (MacCoss Lab Software, https://skyline. ms/). As a result, three peptides out of various digested peptides were selected from the complementarity-determining region (CDR) of adalimumab. The three specific peptide sequences are as follows: NYLAWYQQKPGK, APYTFGQGTK and GLEWVSAITWNSGHIDYADSVEGR.

During the LC-QTOF-MS/MS analysis, two out of three peptides were detected (APYTFGQGTK and NYLAWYQQKPGK), while the GLEWVSAITWNSGHIDYADSVEGR peptide was not, possibly due to poor ionization. Although both APYTFGQGTK and NYLAWYQQKPGK peptides looks acceptable, APYTFGQGTK showed better peak intensity and better signal-to-noise ratio than NYLAWYQQKPGK in our experimental conditions (Figure 1). APYTFGQGTK was not detected in rat blank plasma or any other source during sample preparation and therefore was proven to be quite a unique signature peptide representing adalimumab. Therefore, APYTFGQGTK was chosen as the specific signature peptide for the quantitation of adalimumab in our experiment.

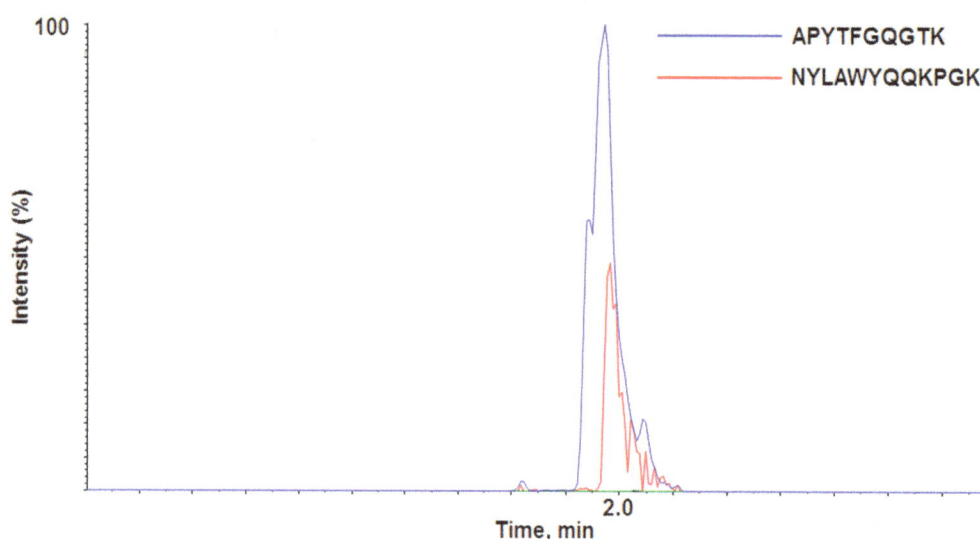

Figure 1. LC-QTOF-MS/MS chromatogram of the two proposed signature peptides.

Figure 2 shows the MS/MS spectrum of the adalimumab-specific signature peptide (APYTFGQGTK). From the doubly charged parent ion observed at m/z 535.27, several product ions were observed and the ion at m/z 901.45 showed the best sensitivity and selectivity.

3.1.3. Liquid Chromatography–Mass Spectrometry Analysis Using Quadrupole Time-of-Flight mass spectrometer

Conventionally, triple quadrupole mass spectrometers (low-resolution instrument) have been used for the quantitative analysis of small molecules. Recently, a Q-TOF mass spectrometer has been introduced to quantify large molecules such as proteins for pharmacokinetic studies [16]. In the past, Q-TOF had drawbacks in terms of sensitivity, linear dynamic range and speed, which meant it was unlikely to fill the need for reliable quantification in bioanalysis when compared to triple quadrupole mass spectrometer. However, the latest Q-TOF is good enough to overcome these shortcomings and shows good sensitivity and selectivity for the analysis of large molecules or peptides in single injection. In this study, the lower limit of quantification (LLOQ), accuracy, precision and linear dynamic range using LC-QTOF-MS/MS were good enough for our discovery non-GLP PK studies in rats.

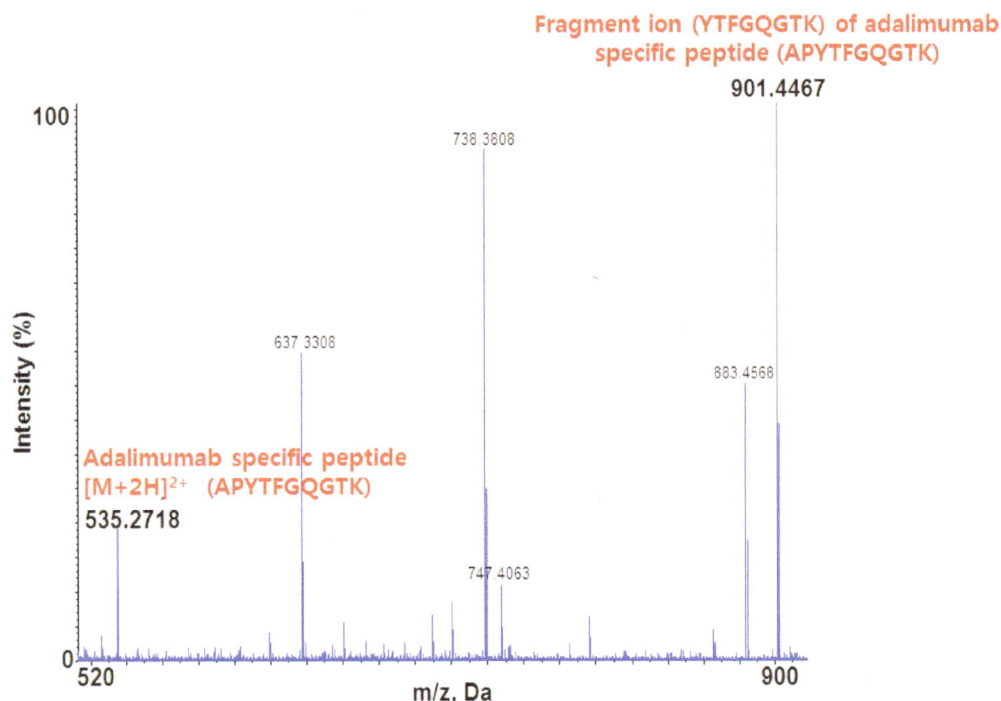

Figure 2. MS/MS spectrum of adalimumab specific peptide [M + 2H]$^{2+}$ and its fragment peptide.

3.2. Method Qualification

3.2.1. Calibration Curve, Linearity and Sensitivity

LC-QTOF-MS/MS analysis using the specific signature peptide in high-resolution mode was used for the quantitation of adalimumab. Calibration curves consisting of eight points in duplicate were prepared fresh for all datasets in rat plasma. The calibration curve range was 1–100 μg/mL. A representative chromatogram at the LLOQ (signal-to-noise ratio: ~9) is shown in Figure 3. This sensitivity was significant enough for most preclinical studies with a dose level ≥1 mg/kg to cover the expected concentration range throughout the PK time course. With a larger volume (~40 μL) of sample (or trypsin), more optimized conditions of LC-QTOF-MS/MS or a more sensitive mass spectrometer, we were also able to improve the LLOQ below 1 μg/mL in the preclinical species plasma, if needed (data not shown). The quadratic regression of the curves using peak area versus concentrations was weighted by 1/concentration. The calculated correlation coefficient value (r) for calibration curve was used to evaluate the linearity of the curve. The correlation coefficient of the calibration curve was ≥0.9931 and the LLOQ of 1 μg/mL was easily achieved in this method.

3.2.2. Accuracy, Precision and Species-Dependent Matrix Effect

Assay performance was determined by assessing inter/intra-day accuracy (%) and precision (%CV) of the QC samples (Table 1). Inter/intra-day accuracy and precision for rat plasma were performed using QC samples ($n = 9$) at low, medium and high QC levels. Accuracy (%) was defined as the calculated concentration, expressed as a percent deviation from nominal concentration. Precision was expressed as the percent coefficient of variation (%CV). The qualification run met the acceptance criteria of ±25% accuracy and precision for all QC samples.

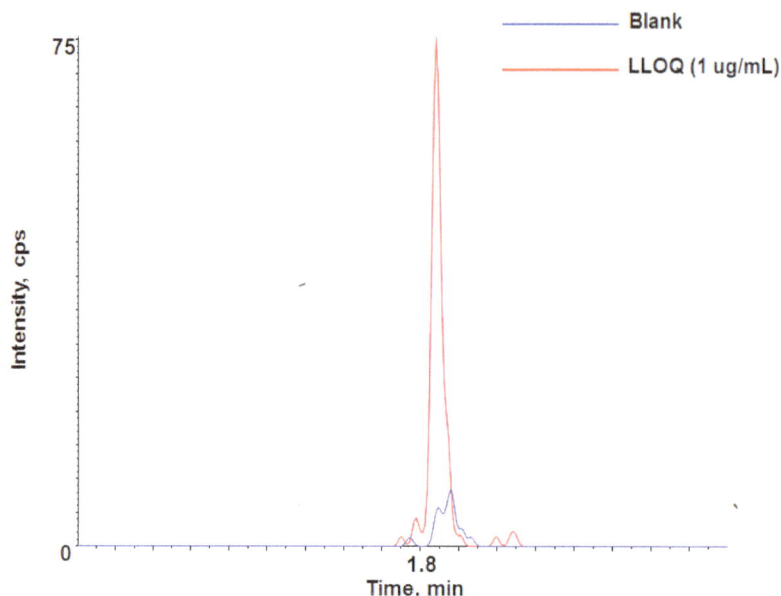

Figure 3. Representative chromatogram of lower limit of quantification (LLOQ, 1 µg/mL) for adalimumab-specific signature peptide in rat plasma.

Table 1. Inter/intra-day accuracy and precision of adalimumab in quality control samples.

Run No.	Statistics	QC Low (2.5 µg/mL)	QC Med (25 µg/mL)	QC High (50 µg/mL)
1	Mean	2.53	25.3	52.3
	Precision (%CV)	13.1	1.76	3.54
	n	3	3	3
	Accuracy (%)	101	101	105
2	Mean	2.73	23.9	56.3
	Precision (%CV)	2.6	11.13	11.55
	n	3	3	3
	Accuracy (%)	109	95	113
3	Mean	2.57	25.1	47.3
	Precision (%CV)	17.3	10.54	4.44
	n	3	3	3
	Accuracy (%)	103	100	95
Inter-day	Mean	2.61	24.77	51.97
	Precision (%CV)	11	7.81	6.51
	n	9	9	9
	Accuracy (%)	104	99	104

This assay developed for rat plasma samples was also evaluated for plasma samples from other species (mouse and monkey). If there are no/few species-dependent matrix effects between species, the rat plasma calibration curve should be able to quantitate adalimumab in other preclinical species as well. Table 2 shows no significant species-dependent matrix effects between rat plasma and other species. Also, Figure 4 shows that the selected signature peptides are unique in the plasma of several preclinical species. Although all three levels of the QC samples were passed, the interference from the blank monkey plasma appeared to be slightly higher than in rat or mouse blank plasma. Therefore, if this method was to be applied to monkey plasma PK samples, a slightly higher LLOQ (e.g., 2 µg/mL) would be helpful for the calibration curve in monkey plasma. Overall, the rat plasma calibration curve should be applicable to analyze adalimumab in mouse and monkey plasma samples if needed.

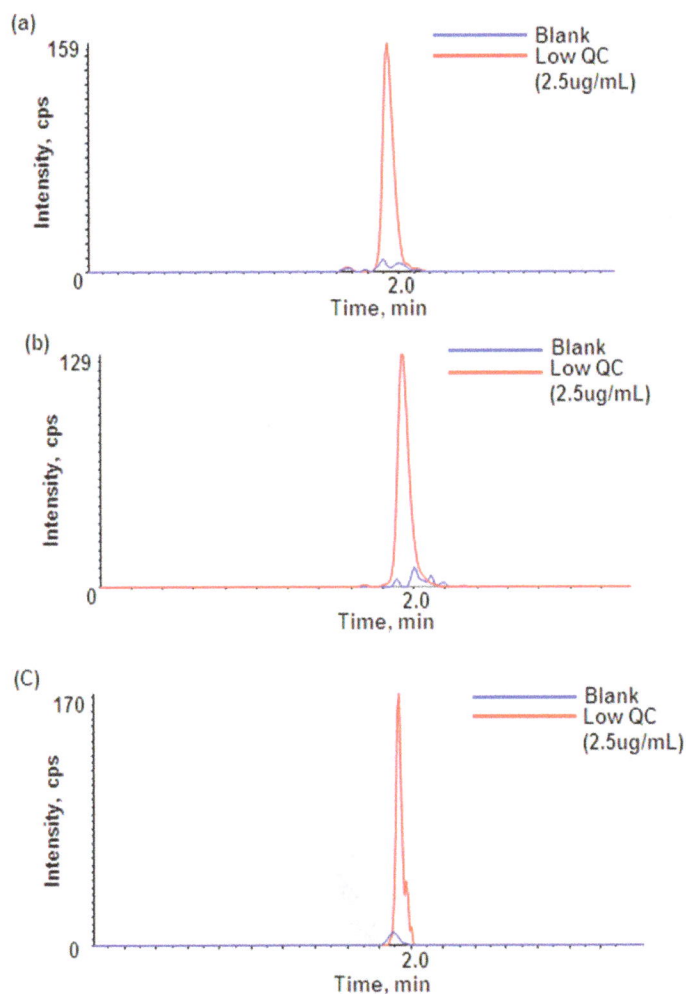

Figure 4. Comparison of peak intensities between blank and QC low in plasma: (**a**) blank and QC low in rat plasma; (**b**) blank and QC low in mouse plasma; (**c**) blank and QC low in monkey plasma.

Table 2. Various species-dependent matrix effects in mouse and monkey plasma. (a) Quality control result in mouse plasma; (b) quality control result in monkey plasma.

(a)					
Mouse	**Theoretical Concentration (μg/mL)**	**Mean Concentration (μg/mL)**	**Precision (%CV)**	***n***	**Accuracy (%)**
QC low	2.5	2.85	13.2	3	114
QC medium	25	29.4	5.74	3	118
QC high	50	57	1.43	3	114
(b)					
Monkey	**Theoretical Concentration (μg/mL)**	**Mean Concentration (μg/mL)**	**Precision (%CV)**	***n***	**Accuracy (%)**
QC low	2.5	2.09	4.9	3	84
QC medium	25	23.4	11.19	3	94
QC high	50	48.1	5.12	3	96

3.2.3. Freeze and Thaw Stability

Freeze and thaw stability assessments were carried out to demonstrate that adalimumab in plasma samples was stable under freeze and thaw conditions. The freeze and thaw stability experiments for rat, mouse and monkey plasma were performed using QC samples (n = 3) at low, medium and high QC levels. The mean values of the freeze and thaw stability QC samples at each level were compared with the nominal concentrations. The results are summarized in Table 3. The acceptance criterion for the freeze and thaw stability samples was within ± 25% precision and accuracy, which is acceptable for early drug discovery studies, and the results all met the acceptance criteria. As a result, adalimumab in rat, mouse and monkey plasma QC samples was stable through three freeze and thaw cycles.

Table 3. Freeze and thaw stability assessment in preclinical species (three cycles) (**a**) Freeze and thaw stability in rat plasma; (**b**) freeze and thaw stability in mouse plasma; (**c**) freeze and thaw stability in monkey plasma.

(a)					
Rat	**Theoretical Concentration (µg/mL)**	**Mean Concentration (µg/mL)**	**Precision (%)**	**n**	**Accuracy (%)**
QC low	2.5	2.58	10.5	3	103
QC medium	25	25.6	13.67	3	102
QC high	50	57.3	8.73	3	115

(b)					
Mouse	**Theoretical Concentration (µg/mL)**	**Mean Concentration (µg/mL)**	**Precision (%)**	**n**	**Accuracy (%)**
QC low	2.5	2.62	16.7	3	105
QC medium	25	28	3.26	3	112
QC high	50	60.2	0.94	3	120

(c)					
Monkey	**Theoretical Concentration (µg/mL)**	**Mean Concentration (µg/mL)**	**Precision (%)**	**n**	**Accuracy (%)**
QC low	2.5	2.26	2.8	3	91
QC medium	25	19.5	12.42	3	78
QC high	50	40.3	8.52	3	81

3.2.4. Application to a Pharmacokinetic Study in Rats

The qualified LC-QTOF-MS/MS method was successfully applied to a pharmacokinetic study of adalimumab in Sprague–Dawley (SD) rats. Plasma samples obtained after intravenous administration of 1 mg/kg were analyzed by LC-QTOF-MS/MS for the quantification of adalimumab concentrations. To assure acceptance of study sample analytical runs, at least two-thirds of the QC samples had to be within ±25% accuracy, with at least half of the QC samples at each concentration meeting these criteria. When 1 mg/kg of adalimumab was administered to the rats, the drug concentrations in rat plasma were all within the calibration curve range. The time–concentration profile is shown in Figure 5. Although no head-to-head comparison for the PK profiles was carried out between this LC-QTOF-MS/MS method and other conventional methods, the PK profile produced by LC-QTOF-MS/MS looked comparable to the reference adalimumab human PK profile published in studies using conventional methods. Unlike the PK profiles of small molecules, most monoclonal antibody drugs typically show bi-phase elimination PK profiles, which consist of a short half-life alpha-phase distribution followed by a beta-phase elimination with a long half-life. Therefore, a two-compartment model was used for the PK parameters of adalimumab in this experiment. (Table 4) [17]. The time-concentration graph of adalimumab in Figure 5 also showed typical two-compartment monoclonal antibody PK characteristics with a short alpha-phase and a long beta-phase half-life (~10 days).

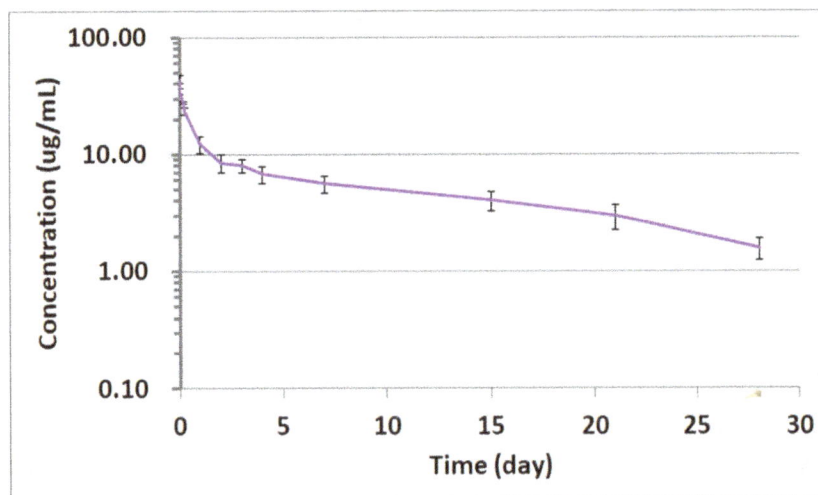

Figure 5. Time-concentration profile of adalimumab in rat plasma from the study subjects receiving 1 mg/kg adalimumab by intravenous administration. The data represent the mean ± standard deviation (SD, $n = 4$).

Table 4. Pharmacokinetic parameters of adalimumab after 1 mg/kg intravenous injection in rats.

Compound	AUC (μg·Day/mL)	Cl (mL/Day/kg)	Alpha Half Life (Day)	Beta Half Life (Day)	C_{max} (μg/mL)	V_1 (mL/kg)	V_{ss} (mL/kg)	Compartment Model
				PK parameters				
Adalimumab	155.29	6.68	0.2	9.82	41.64	24.1	85.83	2

4. Discussion

Immunoassay has been used for over 50 years and has traditionally been used to quantify large molecules. However, this method has some disadvantages [18]. The main disadvantages are that it is time-consuming and requires labor-intensive reagent development [8]. Immunoassays also often show cross-reaction with precursors of the target protein or with smaller metabolized fragments that are not suitable for early-stage mAbs bioanalysis [11]. LC-MS/MS can overcome the disadvantages of immunoassay. Compared to traditional immunoassay, LC-MS/MS technique does not require the preparation of time-consuming and high-cost reagents for specific antibody detection. Combined with LC-MS/MS and immunocapture methods, analytes can be selectively extracted without interferences such as anti-drug antibodies (ADA), which interfere with protein drug targets in the biological matrix [19].

Adalimumab is a recombinant human IgG1 monoclonal antibody [20]. Therefore, human IgG1 is also detected when quantifying adalimumab in the human matrix, making it difficult to distinguish it from the target drug. Therefore, the specific signature peptide of adalimumab was selected because it was distinguishable from human IgG1.

A LC-QTOF-MS/MS method was developed for the determination of adalimumab in rat plasma using a specific signature peptide (APYTFGQGTK) to demonstrate the feasibility of this method for adalimumab or its biosimilars. The calibration curve was acceptable over a concentration range from 1 to 100 μg/mL for adalimumab using quadratic regression with 1/concentration weighting. This LC-QTOF-MS/MS method was sensitive, selective, accurate and reproducible for the determination of adalimumab concentration and has been applied successfully to an adalimumab rat PK study. There was no significant species-dependent matrix effect between rats and other preclinical species, which means this method would be applicable to other preclinical sample analyses without developing new reagents for sample preparation. In conclusion, this method was useful for the analysis of adalimumab and could also be used as a complementary method for adalimumab or its biosimilars in early-stage research and development.

Author Contributions: Y.P., M.-H.P. and Y.G.S. designed the experiment; Y.P., N.K., J.C., M.-H.P., B.i.L., S.-H.S. and J.-J.B. performed the experiments; Y.P., N.K. and J.C. analyzed the data; Y.P. wrote the paper; Y.G.S. reviewed and revised the paper.

Acknowledgments: This research was supported by a research fund of Chungnam National University.

References

1.   Ecker, D.M.; Jones, S.D.; Levine, H.L. The therapeutic monoclonal antibody market. *MAbs* **2015**, *7*, 9–14. [CrossRef] [PubMed]

2.   Park, M.H.; Lee, M.W.; Shin, Y.G. Qualification and application of a liquid chromatography-quadrupole time-of-flight mass spectrometric method for the determination of trastuzumab in rat plasma. *Biomed. Chromatogr.* **2016**, *30*, 625–631. [CrossRef] [PubMed]

3.   Breedveld, F.C. Therapeutic monoclonal antibodies. *Lancet* **2000**, *355*, 735–740. [CrossRef]

4.   Catapano, A.L.; Papadopoulos, N. The safety of therapeutic monoclonal antibodies: Implications for cardiovascular disease and targeting the pcsk9 pathway. *Atherosclerosis* **2013**, *228*, 18–28. [CrossRef] [PubMed]

5.   Voller, A.; Bartlett, A.; Bidwell, D.E. Enzyme immunoassays with special reference to elisa techniques. *J. Clin. Pathol.* **1978**, *31*, 507–520. [CrossRef] [PubMed]

6.   Balkwill, F. Tnf-alpha in promotion and progression of cancer. *Cancer Metastasis Rev.* **2006**, *25*, 409–416. [CrossRef] [PubMed]

7.   Azevedo, V.F.; Troiano, L.D.C.; Galli, N.B.; Kleinfelder, A.; Catolino, N.M.; Martins, P.C.U. Adalimumab: A review of the reference product and biosimilars. *Biosimilars* **2016**, *6*, 29–44. [CrossRef]

8.   Sandborn, W.J.; Hanauer, S.B.; Rutgeerts, P.; Fedorak, R.N.; Lukas, M.; MacIntosh, D.G.; Panaccione, R.; Wolf, D.; Kent, J.D.; Bittle, B.; et al. Adalimumab for maintenance treatment of crohn's disease: Results of the classic ii trial. *Gut* **2007**, *56*, 1232–1239. [CrossRef] [PubMed]

9.   Darwish, I.A. Immunoassay methods and their applications in pharmaceutical analysis: Basic methodology and recent advances. *Int. J. Biomed. Sci.* **2006**, *2*, 217–235. [PubMed]

10.   Liu, H.; Manuilov, A.V.; Chumsae, C.; Babineau, M.L.; Tarcsa, E. Quantitation of a recombinant monoclonal antibody in monkey serum by liquid chromatography-mass spectrometry. *Anal. Biochem.* **2011**, *414*, 147–153. [CrossRef] [PubMed]

11.   Becher, F.; Pruvost, A.; Clement, G.; Tabet, J.C.; Ezan, E. Quantification of small therapeutic proteins in plasma by liquid chromatography-tandem mass spectrometry: Application to an elastase inhibitor epi-hne4. *Anal. Chem.* **2006**, *78*, 2306–2313. [CrossRef] [PubMed]

12.   Domon, B.; Aebersold, R. Mass spectrometry and protein analysis. *Science* **2006**, *312*, 212–217. [CrossRef] [PubMed]

13.   Heudi, O.; Barteau, S.; Zimmer, D.; Schmidt, J.; Bill, K.; Lehmann, N.; Bauer, C.; Kretz, O. Towards absolute quantification of therapeutic monoclonal antibody in serum by lc-ms/ms using isotope-labeled antibody standard and protein cleavage isotope dilution mass spectrometry. *Anal. Chem.* **2008**, *80*, 4200–4207. [CrossRef] [PubMed]

14.   Roopenian, D.C.; Akilesh, S. Fcrn: The neonatal fc receptor comes of age. *Nat. Rev. Immunol.* **2007**, *7*, 715–725. [CrossRef] [PubMed]

15.   Li, H.; Ortiz, R.; Tran, L.; Hall, M.; Spahr, C.; Walker, K.; Laudemann, J.; Miller, S.; Salimi-Moosavi, H.; Lee, J.W. General lc-ms/ms method approach to quantify therapeutic monoclonal antibodies using a common whole antibody internal standard with application to preclinical studies. *Anal. Chem.* **2012**, *84*, 1267–1273. [CrossRef] [PubMed]

16.   Shen, H.W.; Yu, A.M. Conference report: New analytical technologies for biological discovery. *Bioanalysis* **2010**, *2*, 181–184. [CrossRef] [PubMed]

17.   Ferri, N.; Bellosta, S.; Baldessin, L.; Boccia, D.; Racagni, G.; Corsini, A. Pharmacokinetics interactions of monoclonal antibodies. *Pharmacol. Res.* **2016**, *111*, 592–599. [CrossRef] [PubMed]

18.   Cross, T.G.; Hornshaw, M.P. Can lc and lc-ms ever replace immunoassays? *J. Appl. Bioanal.* **2016**, *2*, 108–116. [CrossRef]

19.   Wilffert, D.; Bischoff, R.; van de Merbel, N.C. Antibody-free workflows for protein quantification by lc-ms/ms. *Bioanalysis* **2015**, *7*, 763–779. [CrossRef] [PubMed]

20.   Kaymakcalan, Z.; Sakorafas, P.; Bose, S.; Scesney, S.; Xiong, L.; Hanzatian, D.K.; Salfeld, J.; Sasso, E.H. Comparisons of affinities, avidities, and complement activation of adalimumab, infliximab, and etanercept in binding to soluble and membrane tumor necrosis factor. *Clin. Immunol.* **2009**, *131*, 308–316. [CrossRef] [PubMed]

6

Chitosan Gel to Treat Pressure Ulcers

Virginia Campani [1], Eliana Pagnozzi [2], Ilaria Mataro [2], Laura Mayol [1] (iD), Alessandra Perna [3] (iD), Floriana D'Urso [4], Antonietta Carillo [4], Maria Cammarota [4], Maria Chiara Maiuri [5] and Giuseppe De Rosa [1,* (iD)

[1] Department of Pharmacy, Università degli Studi di Napoli Federico II, Via D. Montesano 49, 80131 Naples, Italy; virginia.campani@unina.it (V.C.); laumayol@unina.it (L.M.)

[2] M.D. Department of Plastic and Reconstructive Surgery and Burn Unit, Hospital Hospital "A. Cardarelli", Via A. Cardarelli 9, 80131 Naples, Italy; elianapagnozzi@virgilio.it (E.P.); ilariamataro@gmail.com (I.M.)

[3] First Division of Nephrology, Department of Cardio-thoracic and Respiratory Sciences, Second University of Naples, School of Medicine, via Pansini 5, Ed. 17, 80131 Naples, Italy; alessandra.perna@unicampania.it

[4] U.O.S.C Farmacia, U.O.S.S. Galenica Clinica e Preparazione Farmaci Antiblastici, Hospital "A. Cardarelli", Via A. Cardarelli 9, 80131 Naples, Italy; florianad-urso@hotmail.it (F.D.); antoniettacarillo1985@gmail.com (A.C.); maresas@tin.it (M.C.)

[5] U.M.R.S. 1138, Centre de Recherche des Cordeliers, 15, rue de l'Ecole de Médecine, 75006 Paris, France; chiara.maiuri@crc.jussieu.fr

* Correspondence: gderosa@unina.it

Abstract: Chitosan is biopolymer with promising properties in wound healing. Chronic wounds represent a significant burden to both the patient and the medical system. Among chronic wounds, pressure ulcers are one of the most common types of complex wound. The efficacy and the tolerability of chitosan gel formulation, prepared into the hospital pharmacy, in the treatment of pressure ulcers of moderate severity were evaluated. The endpoint of this phase II study was the reduction of the area of the lesion by at least 20% after four weeks of treatment. Thus, 20 adult volunteers with pressure ulcers within predetermined parameters were involved in a 30 days study. Dressing change was performed twice a week at outpatient clinic upon chronic wounds management. In the 90% of patients involved in the study, the treatment was effective, with a reduction of the area of the lesion and wound healing progress. The study demonstrated the efficacy of the gel formulation for treatment of pressure ulcers, also providing a strong reduction of patient management costs.

Keywords: chitosan; gel; pressure ulcers; chronic wounds; wound healing; clinical study

1. Introduction

Pressure ulcers are localized areas of injury to the skin and they mainly affect patients that require bed rest. They are caused by external forces, such as pressure, or shear, or a combination of both, and often occur over bony prominence [1]. Wound resolution is often impaired by bacterial proliferation and the production of exudates that causes maceration of healthy skin layers [2–4]. Moreover, many factors like smoking, obesity, old age, and malnutrition can promote the development of chronic skin damage and impair healings processes [3]. Wound care represents a heavy cost on the total health care budget [5]. Pressure ulcers have been shown to increase length of hospital stay and associated hospital costs. Costs are mainly dominated by health professional time and, for more severe ulcers, by the incidence of complications, including hospital admission/length of stay [6]. Advanced wound dressings have prohibitive costs for public health system. The economic care impacts of wound healing represent a serious bottleneck for the correct wound care, especially in public hospitals.

Chitosan (CHI) is a natural polysaccharide that is composed of units of glucasamine linked by a 1–4 glycosid bond to N-acetyl glucosamine units [7]. Due to its characteristics of biodegradability, biocompatibility and safety, CHI has attracted considerable interest for biological applications. The presence of a positive charge at physiological pH makes CHI adhesive, ensuring a longer permanence in the application site [8,9]. Furthermore, the antiseptic activity of CHI was also demonstrated [10]. Finally, its abundance in nature and the low-cost of production make this polymer of commercial interest and suitable to be used for a large-scale production [11]. Many studies have demonstrated the effect of CHI in wound healing due to its microbiological activity, and to the ability to promote homeostasis and angiogenesis processes [12–16]. Moreover, CHI positive charges attract growth factors that enhance cell growth and proliferation [17]. In particular, severe infiltrations of polymorphonuclear cells and thick scab have been reported when treating skin wound with CHI-based dressings in dogs [18]. Recently, our research group reported an experimental protocol to prepare the CHI gel suitable for a hospital pharmacy [19]. These CHI-based gels demonstrated the ability to promote wound healing in vitro and in vivo in an animal model of pressure ulcer [19].

Here, we report a pilot clinical study on 20 patients with pressure ulcers and treated with the CHI gels prepared into the hospital. In this study, the efficacy and the tolerability of the treatment were evaluated. The aim of study was to provide a proof-of-concept to support further study on this device, prepared with low-cost biomaterial and directly into the hospital, to reduce the management cost of hospitalized patients affected by pressure ulcers.

2. Materials and Methods

Chitosan from crab shells, highly viscous (>400 mPa·s 1% acetic acid at 20 °C) was purchased from Farmalabor (Canosa di Puglia, Italy), acetic acid was obtained by Carlo Erba (Milano, Italy), sterile water was purchased from B. Braun (Milan, Italy), regenerated cellulose 0.22 microM membranes were obtained by Corning (Viesbaden, Germany), and the immediate sterile packaging was kindly offered by Alfamed (Naples, Italy).

2.1. Gel Preparation

CHI gels were prepared at the Unità di Manipolazione di Chemioterapici Antiblastici (U.M.A.C.A.) center situated in the Azienda di rilievo nazionale, A.O.R.N. Antonio Cardarelli (Naples, Italy). Gels were prepared, as previously described by Mayol et al. [19] with same modifications. Briefly, CHI powder was sterilized in autoclave at 121 °C for 20 min and 2 atm. Sterilization was checked by microbiological tests carried out on CHI samples at the Laboratorio Chimico Merceologico (Naples, Italy). Samples preparation was made under laminar flow hood and directly in the immediate sterile packaging. The acetic acid aqueous solution was filtered on 0.22 microM membrane filters before use. Then, 0.1 M acetic acid solution was slowly added under continuous stirring to 2% CHI powder until the obtainment of a clear solution. To evaporate the organic solvent, gels were sealed with 0.22 microM filter caps and then placed in oven for 48 h at 37 °C under vacuum (Vuototest, Mazzali, Monza, Italy); finally, filters were removed and the samples were sealed with hermetic caps. Each formulation was prepared in 30 mL sterile container (kindly provided by Alfamed s.r.l., Naples, Italy), intended for a single administration and stored at 4 °C (Figure 1).

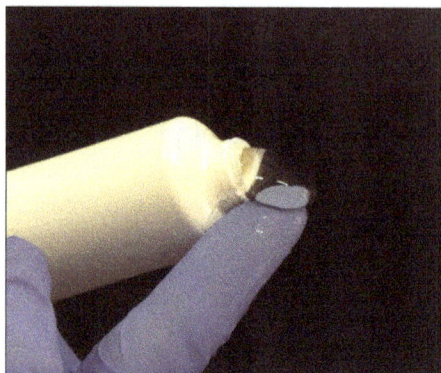

Figure 1. Chitosan gel formulation used in the study.

2.2. Patients Eligibility

Volunteers patients of both sexes, aged between 40 to 80 years with good nutrition conditions, a life expectancy of at least six months with the ability to sign informed consent and affected by pressure ulcers of moderate severity (class II EUPAP/NPUAP 2014) were enrolled. The study excluded subject with: age less than 40 years or older than 80 years, malnutrition state, predisposition to bleeding, or treatment with anticoagulants, infections (including HIV positive), infected injuries, patients not available to follow the procedures envisaged by the study.

A total of 20 adult volunteers with skin ulcers were involved in this 30 days study. Only patients susceptible to outpatient treatment were recruited and hospitalization was not envisaged at any stage of the study. The protocol for the clinical study (identification code: CHITODERM) was examined and approved by ethics committee (No. 558 of 06/24/2016) of "Cardarelli-Santobono" responsible for the experimentation and biomedical research activities carried out at the A.O.R.N. Antonio Cardarelli and A.O.R.N. Santobono-Pausilipon.

2.3. Patients Retirement

Patients had the opportunity to retire from the clinical trial at any time and with no obligation to motivate the interruption. Moreover, treatment discontinuation has been provided in case of adverse events such as erythema, itching, and pain. In this case, motivations were attached to the medical record of the patient and no patient replacement was expected. For these patients a follow-up of 30 days duration was planned.

2.4. Study Design and Treatment

Pressure ulcers were treated according to the EUPAP/NPUAP guidelines. Firstly, the lesion was cleaned with povidone iodine solution and finally washed with physiological solution. The gel preparation was applied on the decubitus ulcer covering the total area of the lesion. Once filled with the CHI gel, the skin lesion was covered with a secondary dressing. Dressing change was performed two times a week at the outpatient clinic for chronic wound treatment. The study lasted 30 days.

2.5. Safety and Efficacy Assessment

The endpoint of the phase II study was the reduction (expressed as a percentage) of the area of the lesion by at least 20% after four weeks of treatment. The secondary endpoint of the study was to establish the tolerability of the gel preparations in the treatment of pressure ulcers. The occurrence of adverse events such as erythema, itching, and pain was evaluated. Patients assessed their degrees of overall satisfaction with the treatment using a 100 mm long horizontal line visual analog scale (VAS).

Patients were treated twice a week. Before each application and at the end of the treatment, the area of the skin lesion was measured. Moreover, any influence of concomitant therapies and the general status of the patient were evaluated.

The area of the lesion was evaluated by digital photography, applying a ruler beside the lesion. Digital images were analyzed using the open source software "Image J" (Java 1.8.0_112) to calculate the area of the wound. At 14 and 30 days visit patient's satisfaction level was assessed by VAS score, ranging from not satisfied (score-0) to fully satisfied (score-100) with the treatment outcomes.

2.6. Statistical Analyses

All of the skin lesion areas were analyzed. The data obtained for each lesion area changes (assessed by image analysis) and presented as area (cm^2) and as percentage (%) of reduction of the area of lesion were then statistically analyzed. A one-sample Student's *t*-test was utilized, and the results were analyzed with the statistics software GraphPad Prism Version 6.0a for Macintosh (GraphPad Software, San Diego, CA, USA).

3. Results and Discussion

The aim of this trial was to test the efficacy of the gel to accelerate the healing of pressure ulcers. CHI is a biocompatible, biodegradable, and low cost natural polymer proposed for several biopharmaceutical applications, among them wound healing [13–16]. Although the clinical use of CHI as a wound healing agent has shown difficulty in taking off, its ability to promote tissue regeneration is well known [13–16]. Different effects, among them inhibition of the microbial growth and increased homeostasis, able to promote healing of injured tissues have been ascribed to CHI. In particular, CHI has been found to be involved in the rapid mobilization of platelets and red blood cells to the injured site and also in vasoconstriction and activation of blood clotting factors responsible for blood clotting [4,12,13]. Thus, CHI accelerates the granulation phase in wound healing and stimulates macrophage activity. Finally, the *N*-acetyl-*D*-glucosamine, which os responsible for fibroblast proliferation, increases collagen and HA synthesis in the wound cavity, and it also allows oxygen permeability at the wound site [12,13]. At the moment, few CHI-based wound dressings (i.e., ChitoFlex®, ChitoGauze®, ChitoSAM™, Celox™ Rapid Gauze) are available on the market, but proposed for their hemostatic properties although than for tissue regeneration. This pilot clinical study is aimed to support the use of a CHI-based device to increase the wound healing rate, independently on the bleeding of the wound.

Here, to carry out the study, the preparation protocol previously developed [19] was reproduced in a sterile manufacturing area at the U.M.A.C.A. center of the A.O.R.N. Antonio Cardarelli. Thus, in the first phase of the work, three batches prepared into the hospital were characterized in terms of viscoelastic behavior, showing no significant differences with gel previously prepared [19]. Gels were prepared and stored in hermetically sealed containers, to avoid following growth of microbiological contamination. Microbiological tests carried out at the Laboratorio Chimico Merceologico of Naples confirmed that all the three pilot batches prepared in this study were sterile and suitable to be administrated on damaged skin (data not shown).

The clinical protocol was designed according to the 2014 EUPAP/NPUAP guidelines. In particular, following the cleansing of the wound, CHI gel was spread on the skin lesions, then covered with a secondary dressing. The primary endpoint to investigate the efficacy of the treatment was the reduction of the area of the lesion at least 20% after 30 days of treatment of the skin lesion. Indeed, a reduction of the area of the lesion of about 20% observed after the first weeks of treatment can be considered a predictive healing factor [20]. In Table 1, the percentages of reduction of the area of the lesion after 30 days of treatment were reported. As shown, a significant reduction of the area of the lesion (higher than 20%) was observed in most patients (about 90%) with a complete wound healing in 20% of the cases after four-week of treatment with CHI gel. Moreover, in 18 patients the treatment was effective, showing a significantly reduction of the area of the lesion and wound healing progression.

Furthermore, in 50% of patients involved in the clinical study, the reduction of the area of the lesion was higher than 50% (patients 1, 2, 5, 6, 7, 9, 10, 14, 16, 17), with a complete wound healing of the ulcers in some cases (patients 2, 5, 9, 16). The results obtained from t test demonstrated that the reduction of the area of the lesions after 30 days of treatment was statistically significant with a two-tailed p value of 0.0002 (t value of 4.16 and a p value of 0.0002).

Table 1. Area of the lesion before and after treatment with chitosan (CHI) formulation and the percentage of reduction of the lesion for each patient.

Patient	Area of the Lesion (before Treatment)	Area of the Lesion (after Treatment)	Reduction of the Area of the Lesion (%)
1	30,238	13,457	55
2	1245	125	90
3	12,580	10,742	15
4	7271	5421	25
5	7356	1031	86
6	7205	3379	53
7	8479	3881	54
8	17,492	9090	48
9	2500	670	73
10	10,832	4329	60
11	2352	1564	34
12	1929	1527	21
13	3687	2901	21
14	2263	146	94
15	33,403	26,336	21
16	33,403	26,336	97
17	1346	460	66
18	14,407	9910	31
19	32,366	20,927	35
20	14,699	13,994	5

In Figure 2, representative images of the wounds in three patients before the treatment (panels A1, B1, C1) and after 30 days of treatment (panels A2, B2, C2) are showed. Interestingly, any patient reported adverse effects of mild, moderate of serious severity after the administration of the gel preparations. Finally, in any case, the discontinuation of the treatment was required.

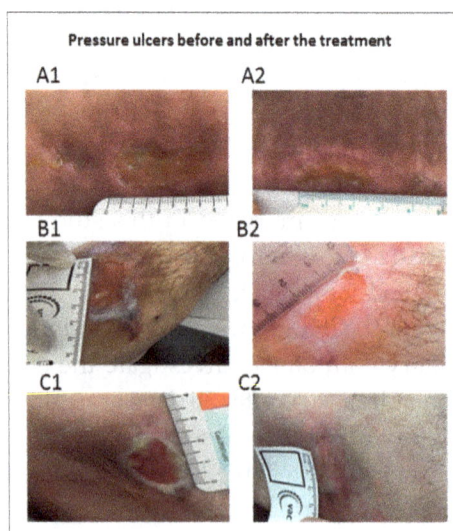

Figure 2. Images of pressure ulcers before (A1, B1, C1) and after 30 days of treatment with chitosan gel (A2, B2, C2).

Furthermore, we evaluated the overall patient satisfaction level on a visual analogue scale (VAS) ranging from not satisfied (score-0) to fully satisfied (score-100). The VAS scale was used due to its advantages in the evaluation of satisfaction outcome; indeed, VAS scale is reported as a very powerful research tool, reliable, sensitive, and easy to use [21]. As expected, the patient who obtained a significant reduction of the area of the lesion gave VAS score higher than those patients who did not obtain a significant result after 30 days of treatment (Table 2).

Table 2. Patient's satisfaction level assessed by visual analogue scale (VAS) score at 14 days and 30 days visit.

Patient	VAS Score 14 Days	VAS Score 30 Days
1	41	75
2	63	94
3	19	25
4	34	36
5	74	91
6	45	82
7	56	68
8	44	70
9	55	88
10	70	86
11	42	59
12	28	43
13	31	59
14	75	100
15	15	40
16	66	95
17	63	84
18	27	49
19	36	45
20	15	21

These results on patients confirm our previous findings in an animal model of pressure ulcers [19], where a significant reduction of the area of the lesion after 3 and 10 days of treatment with CHI gel was found. On the other hand, the healing process should not be observed in chronic wound, such as pressure ulcers, during 12 weeks, from the beginning of the treatment [22]. On the contrary, in this study, significant wound healing progression was observed in the majority of the patients (90%) treated with the CHI gel for four weeks. Interestingly, the 50% of the patients the reduction of the area was superior to the 50% compared to the area before the treatment; finally, 20% of the patients resulted completely healed. These encouraging results confirmed the efficacy of the CHI gel in wound healing, suggesting that this formulation could provide real advantages in term of efficacy and the cost of the treatment. A clinical trial on a larger group of patients (phase III) could provide further information on the use of CHI gels on patients with pressure ulcers and other kind of ulcers. Moreover, in this case, only patients with ulcers at the stage II were enrolled. Other studies should also be organized to investigate the effect of CHI gels also on ulcers of a higher severity.

4. Conclusions

In conclusion, this pivotal study on a restricted group of subjects affected by pressure ulcers demonstrated the tolerability and the efficacy of the CHI-based gel formulation in promoting wound healing. Although on a limited number of volunteers, 90% of the treated patients were responder to treatment, with 20% of the patients completely healed. Furthermore, in this study the gel was prepared directly into the hospital, in the sterile area of the hospital pharmacy. This approach could represent an alternative to the marketed dressing of innovative biomaterials that are generally quite expensive and not always available in public hospital. On the contrary, CHI gel preparation is very easy to perform and the materials that are used in the preparation have negligible costs. Once that the efficacy of this device will be demonstrated on a larger number of patients (Phase III), these findings could represent the basis of new protocols making together increased healing rate with cost-saving for the public health systems.

Acknowledgments: The study was financed by the Italian Minister of Health (Progetto Giovani Ricercatori–bando 2007).

Author Contributions: Virginia Campani: design and characterization of the formulations, analysis of the experimental results, preparation of the manuscript. Eliana Pagnozzi: coordinator of the clinical trial. Ilaria Mataro: analysis and interpretation of clinical results. Laura Mayol: characterization of the formulations. Alessandra Perna: statistical analysis. Floriana D'Urso: preparation of the clinical protocol and dossier for the ethical committee. Antonietta Carillo: preparation of the formulation in the hospital pharmacy. Maria Cammarota: coordination of the HUMACA center in which the formulation has been prepared. Maria Chiara Maiuri: Design of clinical study. Giuseppe De Rosa coordinator together of the study.

References

1.   Westby, M.J.; Dumville, J.C.; Soares, M.O.; Stubbs, N.; Norman, G. Dressings and topical agents for treating pressure ulcers. *Cochrane Database Syst. Rev.* **2017**. [CrossRef] [PubMed]

2.   Mutsaers, S.E.; Bishop, J.E.; McGrouther, G.; Laurent, G.J. Mechanism of tissue repair: From wound healing to fibrosis. *Int. J. Biochem. Cell Biol.* **1997**, *29*, 5–17. [CrossRef]

3.   Pereira, R.F.; Barrias, C.C.; Granja, P.L.; Bartolo, P.J. Advanced biofabrication strategies for skin regeneration and repair. *Nanomedicine* **2013**, *8*, 603–621. [CrossRef] [PubMed]

4.   Agrawal, P.; Soni, S.; Mittal, G.; Bhatnagar, A. Role of polymeric biomaterials as wound healing agents. *Int. J. Low Extrem. Wounds* **2014**, *13*, 180–190. [CrossRef] [PubMed]

5.   Lindholm, C.; Searle, R. Wound management for the 21st century: Combining effectiveness and efficiency. *Int. Wound J.* **2016**, *13*, 5–15. [CrossRef] [PubMed]

6.   Dealey, C.; Posnett, J.; Walker, A. The cost of pressure ulcers in the United Kingdom. *J. Wound Care* **2012**, *6*, 261–264. [CrossRef] [PubMed]

7.   Tomihata, K.; Ikada, Y. In vitro and in vivo degradation of films of chitin and its deacetylated derivatives. *Biomaterials* **1997**, *18*, 567–575. [CrossRef]

8.   He, P.; Davis, S.S.; Illum, L. In vitro evaluation of the mucoadhesive properties of chitosan microspheres. *Int. J. Pharm.* **1998**, *166*, 75–88.

9.   Calvo, P.; Remunan-Lopez, C.; Vila-Jato, J.L.; Alonso, M.J. Novel chitosan derivatives enhance the transport of hydrophilic hydrophilic chitosan-polyethylene oxide nanoparticles as protein carriers. *J. Appl. Polym. Sci.* **1997**, *63*, 125–132. [CrossRef]

10. Burkatovskaya, M.; Castano, A.P.; Demidova-Rice, T.N.; Tegos, G.P.; Hamblin, M.R. Effect of chitosan acetate bandage on wound healing in infected and noninfected wounds in mice. *Wound Repair Regen.* **2008**, *3*, 425–431. [CrossRef] [PubMed]

11. Khor, E.; Lim, L.Y. Implantable applications of chitin and chitosan. *Biomaterials* **2003**, *24*, 2339–2349. [CrossRef]

12. Muzzarelli, R.; Tarsi, R.; Filippini, O.; Giovanetti, E.; Biagini, G.; Varaldo, P.E. Antimicrobial properties of N-carboxybutyl chitosan. *Antimicrob. Agents Chemother.* **1990**, *34*, 2019–2023. [CrossRef] [PubMed]

13. Ueno, H.; Mori, T.; Fujinaga, T. Topical formulations and wound healing applications of chitosan. *Adv. Drug Deliv. Rev.* **2001**, *52*, 105–115. [CrossRef]

14. Wang, W.; Lin, S.; Xiao, Y.; Huang, Y.; Tan, Y.; Cai, L.; Li, X. Acceleration of diabetic wound healing with chitosan-crosslinked collagen sponge containing recombinant human acidic fibroblastgrowth factor in healing-impaired STZ diabetic rats. *Life Sci.* **2008**, *82*, 190–204. [CrossRef] [PubMed]

15. Boateng, J.S.; Matthews, K.H.; Stevens, H.N.; Eccleston, G.M. Wound healing dressings and drug delivery systems: A review. *J. Pharm. Sci.* **2008**, *97*, 2892–2923. [CrossRef] [PubMed]

16. Charernsriwilaiwat, N.; Rojanarata, T.; Ngawhirunpat, T.; Opanasopit, P. Electrospun chitosan/polyvinyl alcohol nanofibre mats for wound healing. *Int. Wound J.* **2014**, *11*, 215–222. [CrossRef] [PubMed]

17. Lee, D.W.; Lim, H.; Chong, H.N.; Shim, W.S. Advances in chitosan material and its hybrid derivatives: A review. *Open Biomater. J.* **2009**, *1*, 10–20. [CrossRef]

18. Ueno, H.; Yamada, H.; Tanaka, I.; Kaba, N.; Matsuura, M.; Okumura, M.; Kadosawa, T.; Fujinaga, T. Accelerating effects of chitosan for healing at early phase of experimental open wound in dogs. *Biomaterials* **1999**, *20*, 1407–1414. [CrossRef]

19. Mayol, L.; De Stefano, D.; Campani, V.; De Falco, F.; Ferrari, E.; Cencetti, C.; Matricardi, P.L.; Maiuri, R.; Carnuccio, A.; Gallo, M.C.; et al. Design and characterization of a chitosan physical gel promoting wound healing in mice. *J. Mater. Sci. Mater. Med.* **2014**, *25*, 1483–1493. [CrossRef] [PubMed]

20. Flanagan, M. Improving accuracy of wound measurement in clinical practice. *Ostomy Wound Manag.* **2003**, *49*, 28–40.

21. Singer, A.J.; Church, A.L.; Forrestal, K.; Werblud, M.; Valentine, S.M.; Hollander, J.E. Comparison of patient satisfaction and practitioner satisfaction with wound appearance after traumatic wound repair. *Acad. Emerg. Med.* **1997**, *4*, 133–137. [CrossRef]

22. Boateng, J.; Catanzano, O. Advanced Therapeutic Dressings for Effective Wound Healing—A Review. *J. Pharm. Sci.* **2015**, *104*, 3653–3680. [CrossRef] [PubMed]

7

Twin Screw Granulation: Effects of Properties of Primary Powders

Sushma V. Lute, Ranjit M. Dhenge ⓘ and Agba D. Salman *

Department of Chemical and Biological Engineering, University of Sheffield, Mappin Street, Sheffield S1 3JD, UK; sushmalute@gmail.com (S.V.L.); ranjitdhenge@gmail.com (R.M.D.)
* Correspondence: a.d.salman@sheffield.ac.uk

Abstract: Lactose and mannitol are some of the most commonly used powders in the pharmaceutical industry. The limited research published so far highlights the effects of process and formulation parameters on the properties of the granules and the tablets produced using these two types of powders separately. However, the comparison of the performance of these two types of powders during twin screw wet granulation has received no attention. The present research is focused on understanding the granulation mechanism of different grades of two pharmaceutical powders with varying properties (i.e., primary particle size, structure, and compressibility). Three grades each of lactose and mannitol were granulated at varying liquid to solid ratios (L/S) and screw speed. It was noticed that primary powder morphology plays an important role in determining the granule size and structure, and tablet tensile strength. It was indicated that the processed powders such as spray-dried and granulated lactose and mannitol can be used in formulation for wet granulation where flowability of active pharmaceutical ingredient (API) is poor.

Keywords: twin screw wet granulation; continuous; excipient; granule; lactose; mannitol; tableting

1. Introduction

In the pharmaceutical industry, granulation of powders to form structured products (i.e., granules) is one of the most important operations in solid oral dosage form manufacturing to improve flow, compaction or homogeneity of powders. It can be carried out using either dry or wet approaches. In wet granulation, liquid binder is added onto a bed of primary powder particles that is being agitated by an impeller (in a high-shear granulator (HSG), screws (in twin screw granulator (TSG), or air (in a fluidized bed granulator (FBG)) to form wet granules.

Amongst various excipient (filler/diluent) powders available for the wet/dry granulation and tableting in the pharmaceutical industry, lactose and mannitol are some of the most common ones. Both lactose and mannitol are commercially available in different grades (e.g., sieved, milled, spray-dried, granulated, etc.) presenting different particle characteristics (i.e., size, size distribution, degrees of fines, shape, surface, flowability, and compressibility) [1,2].

Lactose occurs in α and β forms possessing different melting points, solubility, and hardness [3]. It is known that different grades of lactose have different granulation and compression properties [3,4]. For example, sieved α-lactose monohydrate is used in direct compression, whereas milled α-lactose monohydrate is wet granulated prior to tableting due to its poor compressibility under direct compaction [2]. Spray-dried lactose and anhydrous lactose are recommended for dry granulation and direct compaction owing to their excellent flowability and compressibility [1].

Mannitol is used as a filler/diluent in tablet making with both wet/dry granulation and direct compaction methods in the pharmaceutical industry [5]. Mannitol, due to its non-hygroscopic nature, sweet taste, and negative heat of the solution giving a cooling sensation, is a preferred excipient for formulating the moisture-sensitive drugs [6] and producing chewable tablets or lozenges [7]. Mannitol is known to exist in different polymorphic forms including the α, β, and δ having different compressibility [8]. Like lactose, mannitol is also manufactured in different grades using different approaches for specific application, hence, the different size, shape, and structure. For example, crystalline mannitol is a brittle powder with needle-shaped particles used in wet granulation [9]. Spray-dried mannitol is a crystalline, highly brittle granular powder (high compressibility) with spherical particles used in dry granulation (roller compaction) and direct compaction (tableting) [10]. Granulated mannitol is a crystalline, brittle mannitol powder with high compressibility making it suitable for direct compaction [8].

The particle characteristics of lactose and mannitol powders can play important roles in granulation. For instance, primary powder particle size plays a critical role in determining the size of nuclei during the nucleation step in wet granulation [11], which further influences the final granules' attributes [12,13]. Thus, the effect of particle size and other characteristics of primary powders need to be considered during product development using a wet granulation platform.

In batch high-shear granulation, the effect of primary powder morphology on granulation behavior and properties of granules and tablets have been studied previously [3–6]. Kristensen, et al. [14] investigated the influence of primary particle size of dicalcium phosphate powder on the granules' growth. They found that the granule growth was inversely proportional to the particle size of dicalcium phosphate powder. Badawy, et al. [15] also reported a similar tendency for their powder of interest (code name: DPC 963). They also noticed that the granule size, porosity, and compressibility were inversely proportional to the powder particle size. The smaller powder particles showed reduced tendency for densification than the larger ones. Mackaplow, et al. [16] studied the effect of varying primary particles size of lactose monohydrate powder on granule growth and end point determination during high-shear wet granulation. Unlike Kristensen, et al. [14] and Badawy, et al. [15], Mackaplow, et al. [16] and Badawy and Hussain [17] found that increasing primary particle size of lactose powder results in larger, less porous wet granules. This was attributed to the decrease in both the capillary and viscous interparticle forces with increasing primary particle size making granules more deformable. This difference in the observations in two studies may be attributed to the type of powder used. Keleb, et al. [3] also studied the effect of primary particle size (different grades of milled lactose: Pharmatose 450M, Pharmatose 200M, Pharmatose 100M, and Pharmatose 90M); morphology (anhydrous β-lactose (Pharmatose DCL 21); spray-dried lactose (Pharmatose DCL 11); and milled lactose (Pharmatose 90M)) of lactose powder on properties of tablets (friability, tensile strength, and disintegration time) produced from compression of granules after batch high-shear wet granulation and single-step granulation/tableting (extrusion). In cases of batch high-shear wet granulation, they noticed that the tablet friability and disintegration time decreased and tensile strength increased first with increasing primary particle size (from 450M to 200M), and then the trend was reversed (in cases of 100M and 90M). The morphology of lactose powders also influenced the disintegration time and tensile strength of tablets. The tensile strength of tablets produced from spray-dried and anhydrous lactose powders was similar (stronger than 90 M); however, they differed in terms of disintegration time where spray dried lactose tablets disintegrated slower compared to other powders. The reasons for such trends needed further justifications.

Huang, et al. [1] compared the suitability of four commercial grades of lactose (spray-dried/sieved/milled monohydrate and anhydrous lactose) for a low-dose oral formulation of pentyloxyl paliperidone derivative with drug loading at 1.5% (w/w) and lower using a batch high-shear granulator. The effects on granule size, flowability, and other product attributes were investigated. It was noticed that granule size increases with an increase in the particle size primary powder. It was also found that spray-dried lactose powder produce granules with better flowability, narrow granule, size distribution, and tablets with good hardness and low friability. It can also reduce the degree segregation/agglomeration of granules throughout the manufacturing process.

Compared to batch high-shear wet granulation, the effect of primary powder (i.e., lactose and mannitol) morphology on granulation behavior and properties of granules and tablets has received limited attention in continuous twin screw wet granulation [18,19]. Moreover, the comparison of the performance of different grades of lactose vs. mannitol powders in twin screw wet granulation has not been studied previously. El Hagrasy, et al. [18] granulated three different grades of lactose powder (Pharmatose 200M, Supertab 30GR, and Impalpable) as a major ingredient mixed with three minor ingredients, namely microcrystalline cellulose, hydroxypropylmethyl cellulose, and croscarmellose sodium at different liquid to solid ratios (L/S) in TSG. They concluded that the changes in the lactose grades in the formulation displayed comparable growth behavior at different L/S, while impact of particle size/grade type on granule porosity was inconclusive.

It is only recently that Vanhoorne, et al. [19] investigated the impact of using different polymorphs of mannitol powder (i.e., δ-mannitol (Parteck Delta M), β-mannitol (C*PharmMannidex 16700), and α-mannitol (Pearlitol 200)) on the granules and tablet attributes in twin screw wet granulation. They observed that δ-mannitol changes into β-mannitol during wet granulation leading to a unique granule morphology with a higher specific surface area and better plastic deformability compared to α- and β-mannitol as starting material.

The objective of this study was to compare the performance of different grades of lactose and mannitol powders during twin screw wet granulation. Different types of lactose and mannitol powders having different powder morphology were granulated separately at different L/S and screw speeds and their impact on the properties of the granules (size, shape, and structure) and tablet (tensile strength) was investigated.

2. Materials and Methods

2.1. Materials

2.1.1. Powder

Different grades of lactose and mannitol powders were used in this study for comparing the effects of their physical properties on the granulation behavior and granule properties.

Three types of lactose powders were used in the study: α-lactose monohydrate (Pharmatose 200M), spray-dried lactose (SuperTab11SD), and anhydrous lactose (SuperTab21AN). All powders were supplied by DMV-Fonterra Excipient GmbH and co., Goch, Germany. α-lactose monohydrate powder is manufactured by slow crystallization of a supersaturated lactose solution below 93.5 °C accompanied by roller drying resulting in single crystals of α-lactose monohydrate. The crystals are further milled to produce Pharmatose 200M grade powder (amorphous lactose ~2.6% [20]). Anhydrous lactose is also made from crystallization of a supersaturated solution of lactose, but it is rapidly dried at high temperature (above 93.5 °C) by roller drying. The particles are then milled and sieved to produce SuperTab21AN grade powder. SuperTab21AN particles consist of clusters of micro-crystals of predominantly anhydrous β-lactose together with anhydrous α-lactose [21]. SuperTab21AN contains negligible amounts of amorphous lactose (~0.2%) [20]. Spray-dried lactose consists of particles of α-lactose monohydrate in a matrix of amorphous lactose (~10 to 15%) [20,22]. Finely-milled α-lactose monohydrate is suspended in water and spray dried to make spherical agglomerates to produce SuperTab11SD.

The three types of mannitol powders, used in respective comparison with the three lactose powders, were milled crystalline mannitol (Pearlitol 50C) (β-mannitol [23]), spray-dried mannitol (Pearlitol 200SD) (known to contain both α- and β-mannitol [24] and is crystalline [25]), and granulated mannitol (Pearlitol 300DC) (β-mannitol [8,23]). All mannitol powders were supplied by Roquette (Lestrem cedex, France). Milled crystalline mannitol powder is manufactured by slow crystallization of a supersaturated solution to produce crystals of mannitol which are then crushed to produce Pearlitol 50C. Spray-dried mannitol, as the name suggests, is manufactured by spray drying a suspension of mannitol powder in water to produce spherical agglomerates. The granulated mannitol is produced by pouring a hot slurry of mannitol powder on the cold rotating drum and then crushing into the desired size.

2.1.2. Granulator

A co–rotating twin screw granulator (TSG) (Euro lab 16 TSG (L/D-25/1), Prism, Thermo Scientific (Thermo Electron GmbH), Karlsruhe, Germany) was used for the granulation experiments. A gravimetric, loss-in-weight twin screw powder feeder (K-PH-CL-24-KT20, K-Tron Soder, Niederlenz, Switzerland) having a pair of co-rotating screws was used to feed powder into the granulator. A peristaltic pump (101U, Watson Marlow, Cornwall, UK) was used to inject granulation liquid (distilled water) into the granulator.

2.2. Method

2.2.1. Morphology of Powders

Powder particle size was measured using Camsizer-XT (X-jet module) (Retsch Technology, Haan, Germany). The powder shape and surface were examined using scanning electron microscopy (SEM) (Jeol, Peabody, MA, USA). The lactose and mannitol particles were nonconductive, hence, were coated (for 40 s) with a thin layer (~25 nm) of gold using a coating machine (Leica EM ACE200, Leica Microsystems, Milton Keynes, UK).

2.2.2. Compressibility Factor for Powders

The compressibility of factor K for all six powders was determined from the relationship between the uniaxial stress σ and the resulting powder bed apparent density ρ, as shown in Equation (1) [4]. It is known that the lower the compressibility factor, the more compressible the powder is [4]. This was measured by compressing 405 mg of powders in a die (diameter: 12 mm) using an Instron testing machine (Instron 3367, High Wycombe, Buckinghamshire, UK) under a range of compression forces (1000 to 5000 N) at test speed of 1 mm/min. and determining the apparent density of the tablet (from mass and volume measured out of die (i.e., post tablet ejection, after 24 h)). The compressibility factor K was determined from the slope of a logarithmic plot of the apparent density as a function of stress.

$$\frac{\sigma_1}{\sigma_2} = \left(\frac{\rho_1}{\rho_2}\right)^K \qquad (1)$$

where,

σ_1 = major principal stress
σ_2 = minor principal stress
ρ_1 = powder bulk density at σ_1
ρ_2 = powder bulk density at σ_2

2.2.3. Preparation of Granules

Lactose and mannitol powders were granulated separately using distilled water in the TSG. The granules (60 g in each experiment) were collected after 1 min, when the system reached the equilibrium (based on the stabilization time (~30 s at powder feed rate of 2 kg/h), which was determined by monitoring feed factor variability over time) for a gravimetric, loss-in-weight twin screw powder feeder. The granulation was carried out using the full length of the granulator keeping the screw configuration unchanged (Figure 1).

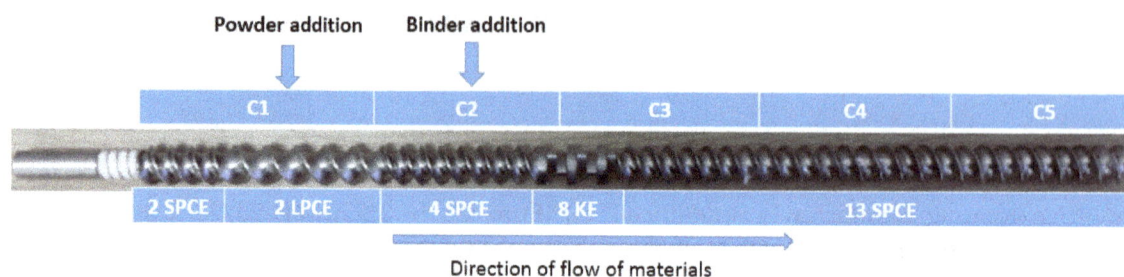

Figure 1. Screw configuration used in the experiments (SPCE, short pitch conveying element; LPCE, long pitch conveying element; KE, kneading element; C1 to C5, compartments/ports along the length of the barrel).

The experimental design is shown in Table 1. In total, 288 experiments (i.e., 16 combinations × 3 repetitions of each combination × 6 powders) were carried out. Each powder was granulated at 4 different L/S and 4 different screw speeds in order to compare its performance under varying process variables, and its effects on the properties of granules (i.e., size, shape, and structure) and tablets (tensile strength).

Table 1. Experimental conditions and variables used in the study. L/S: liquid to solid ratios.

Experiment	Powder Type	Powder Feed Rate (kg/h)	Screw Speed (rpm)	L/S	Liquid Binder
Effect of powder type	Pharmatose 200M SuperTab11SD SuperTab21AN Pearlitol 50C Pearlitol 200SD Pearlitol 300DC	2	200, 450, 700, 950	0.048, 0.07, 0.1, 0.113	Distilled water

2.2.4. Size Analysis of Granules

The granules were air dried at room temperature for 48 h. The median size (d_{50}) of the granules was measured using the particle size analyzer: Camsizer (free-fall module) (Retsch Technology, Haan, Germany). Three repetitions were performed for the size analysis.

2.2.5. Structural Analysis of Granules

The X-ray tomography (XRT) (μCT 35, SCANCO Medical AG, Brüttisellen, Switzerland) of granules was carried out to gain more information on the change in the internal structure of the granules. The granules collected from various processing conditions had varying shapes. For this reason, only the middle area of the granules was scanned to determine the porosity. The stack of 240 images (slices) was threshold to differentiate the void and solid particle using ImageJ Software (National Institutes of Health, Bethesda, MD, USA) [26]. The black area in the X-ray images indicates the air (pores), and the white area indicates the granule or powder particle. The porosity of a granule was determined by dividing the area of air by the total area of the image.

2.2.6. Tableting

The granules produced at two extremes of L/S (i.e., 0.048 and 0.113) at 4 screw speeds were sieved into different size classes (212–600 μm, 600–1000 μm, 1000–1400 μm, and 212–1400 μm) and compressed in a 12 mm die at 10 kN compression force (test speed, 1 mm/min) to produce tablets of about 405 mg using an Instron testing machine. This was done to study the impact of granule size range on the tablet tensile strength [3]. The granules were not pre-lubricated internally or externally;

however, the punch and die of the compression machine were coated with a thin layer of magnesium stearate to minimize sticking and picking.

2.2.7. Analysis of Tablets

The tablets so produced were analyzed for their dimensions (i.e., thickness and diameter) and tensile strength. The thickness and diameter were measured using a digital caliper. The tensile strength of tablets was measured by diametric compression method using Zwick/Roell Z 0.5 (Zwick/Roell, Ulm, Germany) instead of an Instron testing machine. This was done because Zwick/Roell provides more suitable force range compared to the Instron testing machine. The tablets were compressed diametrically (test speed, 1 mm/min) until they fractured. The force-displacement data was recorded. Ten tablets were used for each experimental condition to produce reproducible data. The strength of tablets (σ) was determined by inputting maximum force (F), tablet diameter (D), and thickness (T) in Equation (2) [27,28].

$$\sigma = 2\frac{F}{\pi TD} \tag{2}$$

3. Results

3.1. Morphology of Powder

The morphology of powder (i.e., size and shape) is discussed in this section. The primary particle size of six different powders is shown in Table 2. It can be seen that SuperTab21AN and Pearlitol 300DC had the largest particle size (d_{50}) amongst lactose and mannitol powders, respectively.

Table 2. Primary particle size of powders used in the study.

Powder Grade	Particle Size (μm)		
	d_{10}	d_{50}	d_{90}
Pharmatose 200M	9.3	42.1	110.0
SuperTab11SD	45.0	113.4	191.3
SuperTab21AN	27.5	172.3	330.0
Pearlitol 50C	10.1	33.9	114.9
Pearlitol 200SD	26.0	145.3	200.9
Pearlitol 300DC	58.3	249.9	385.9

The scanning electron microscopy (SEM) images for lactose and mannitol powders are shown in Figures 2 and 3, respectively. The SEM images for lactose and mannitol powders clearly show the difference in their size and shape. Pharmatose 200M is a crystalline milled lactose with tomahawk like shape (Figure 2a,b). SuperTab11SD is spray-dried lactose with porous and relatively spherical particles, and its structure is made from α-lactose monohydrate (Figure 2c,d). SuperTab21AN is crystalline anhydrous lactose, which is an aggregation of lactose microcrystals [29] (Figure 2e,f). Pearlitol 50C powder has elongated particles (Figure 3a,b) with smaller particles sticking on the larger ones. Pearlitol 200SD has more spherical shaped primary particles (Figure 3c,d) having porous shells with elongated thread-like smaller particles embedded in them [30]. Pearlitol 300DC is a granulated mannitol powder with compact and rounded particles (Figure 3e,f).

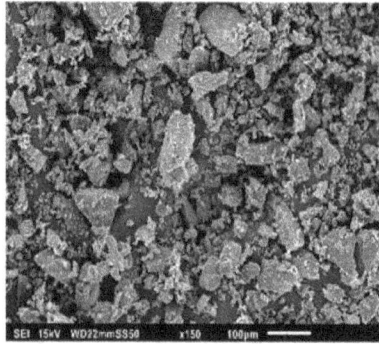

(a) Pharmatose 200M (×150)

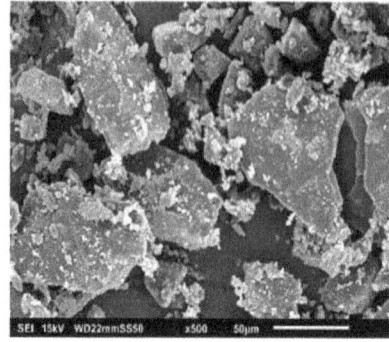

(b) Pharmatose 200M (×500)

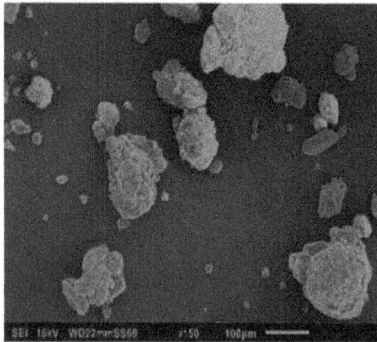

(c) SuperTab11SD (×150)

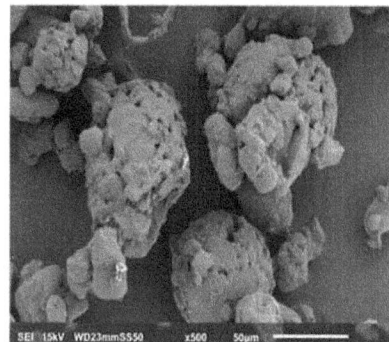

(d) SuperTab11SD (×500)

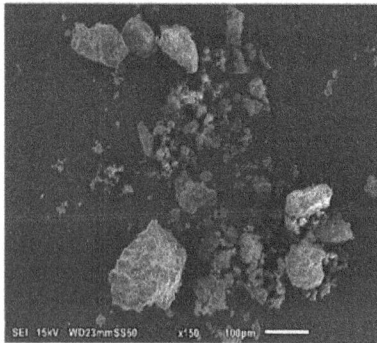

(e) SuperTab21AN (×150)

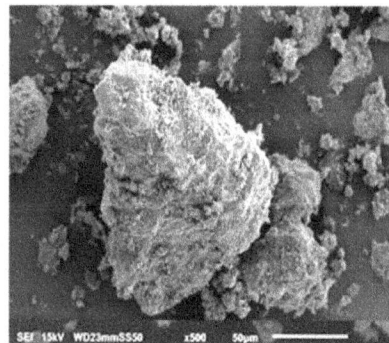

(f) SuperTab21AN (×500)

Figure 2. Scanning Electron Microscope (SEM) images of lactose powder.

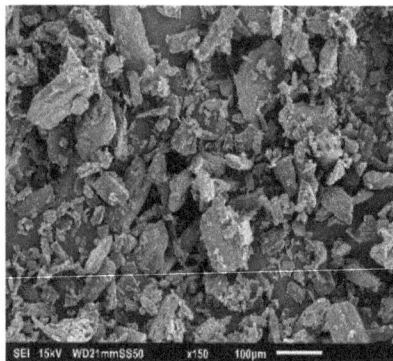

(a) Pearlitol 50C (×150)

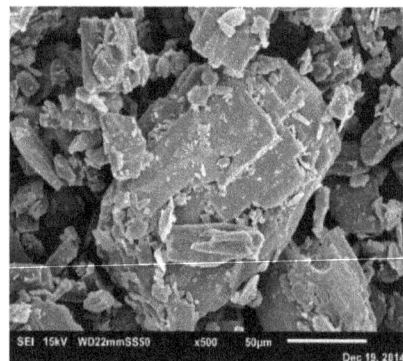

(b) Pearlitol 50C (×500)

Figure 3. *Cont.*

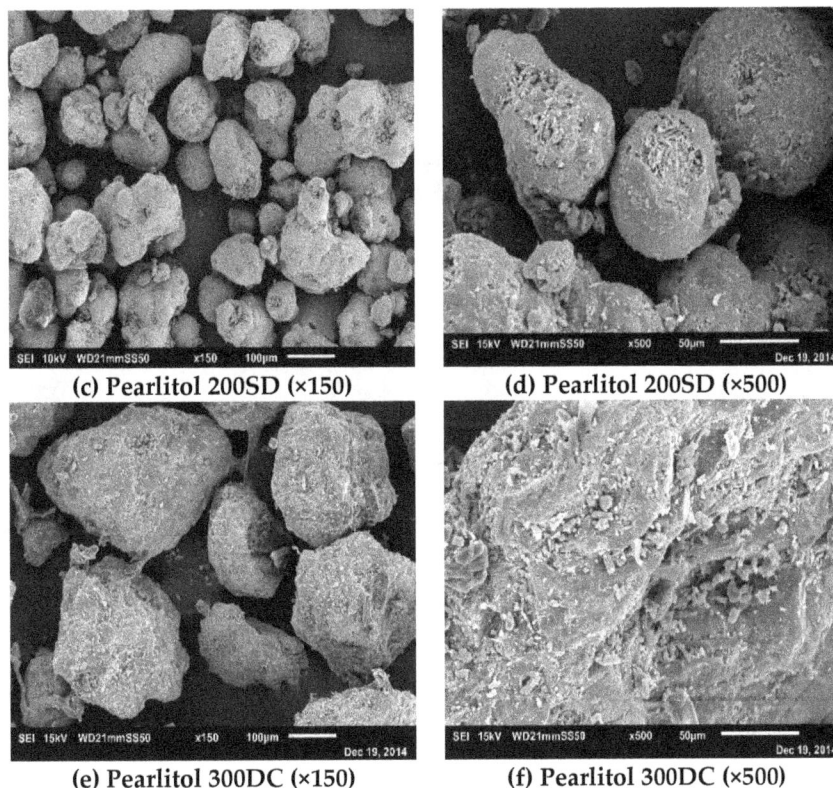

(c) Pearlitol 200SD (×150)

(d) Pearlitol 200SD (×500)

(e) Pearlitol 300DC (×150)

(f) Pearlitol 300DC (×500)

Figure 3. SEM images of mannitol powders.

3.2. Compressibility Factor for Powders

Figure 4 shows compressibility factor (K) for different powders. The compressibility factor results for lactose and mannitol powders were anomalous. Based on the particle size, the expected trend for K value was Pharmatose 200M < SuperTab11SD < SuperTab21AN for lactose and Pearlitol 50C < Pearlitol 200SD < Pearlitol 300DC for mannitol; however, it was not the case. The K value was higher for crystalline Pharmatose 200M and Pearlitol 50C having smaller particle size, while it was lower for spray-dried large sized (meaning higher compressibility) SuperTab11SD and Pearlitol 200SD, respectively. It was also expected that the pre-processed SuperTab21AN and Pearlitol 300DC (which are suitable for direct compression in tableting) to have lower K than SuperTab11SD and Pearlitol 200SD, respectively, but it was not the case. This can be attributed to the structure of the spray-dried lactose and mannitol particles. Scanned electron microscopy images of SuperTab11SD particles (Figure 2c,d) show that they are brittle aggregates of several lactose microcrystals, which during compression or tableting fracture easily into several fine particles, which improve the compressibility (even better than SuperTab21AN). Similar is the case for spray-dried mannitol or Pearlitol 200SD, where the SEM images (Figure 3c,d) clearly show the presence of elongated, smaller particles embedded in the spherical shell. According to Mitra, et al. [31], during compression such Pearlitol 200SD particles may possibly break into smaller fragments and thereby improve compressibility. It can also be noticed from Figure 4 that Pearlitol 200SD has a lower K value (i.e., higher compressibility) compared to Pearlitol 300DC, which is a granular compact.

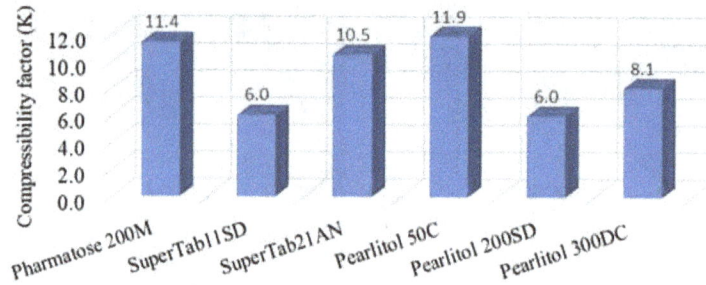

Figure 4. Compressibility factor for different powders.

3.3. *Size of Granules*

3.3.1. Lactose

Figure 5a–d shows the median size of granules produced using different grades of lactose powder at varying L/S and screw speeds. For the ease of understanding the results, they are discussed in two parts viz. the effect of different powder properties on the granule size at varying L/S and the same at varying screw speed.

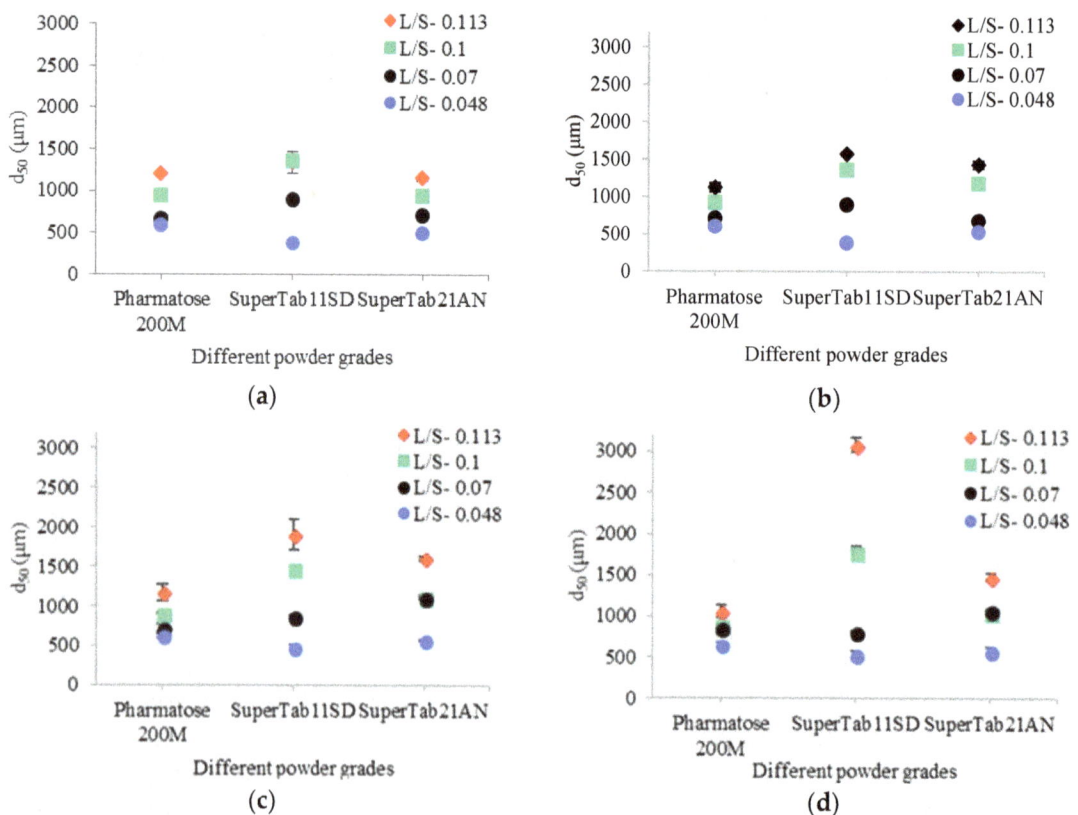

Figure 5. Median size of granules for different grades of lactose powder at varying L/S and screw speeds. (**a**) 200 rpm; (**b**) 450 rpm; (**c**) 700 rpm; (**d**) 950 rpm.

3.3.2. Mannitol

In the case of mannitol (Figure 6a–d), increasing the primary particle size of powder at varying L/S and screw speeds had varying influences on the median granule size. Similar to lactose, for the ease of understanding the results they are discussed in two parts viz. the effect of increasing powder particle size on granule size at varying L/S and the same at varying screw speeds.

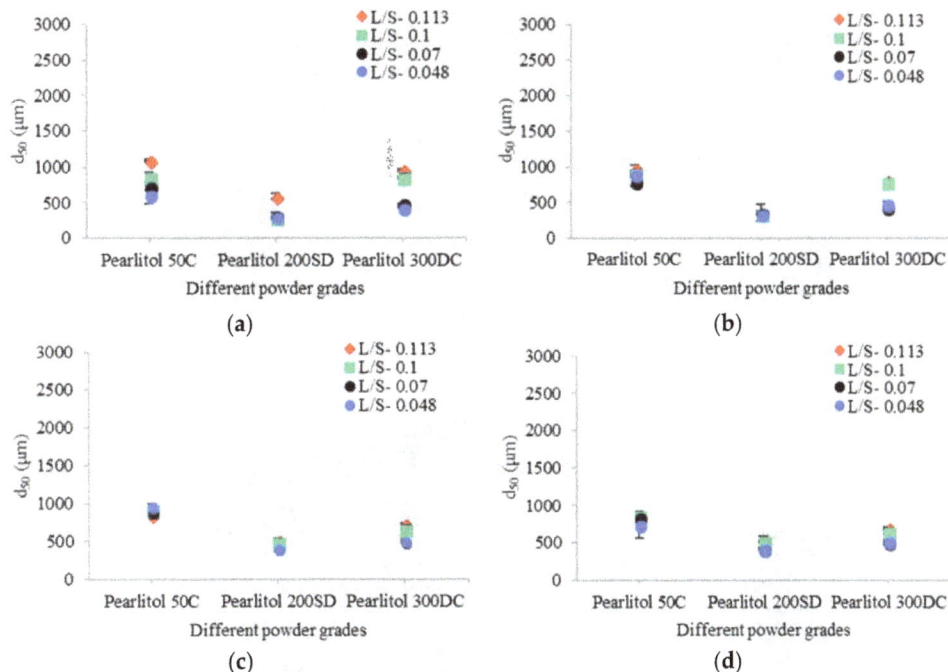

Figure 6. Median size of granules for different grades of mannitol powder at varying L/S and screw speeds. (**a**) 200 rpm; (**b**) 450 rpm; (**c**) 700 rpm; (**d**) 950 rpm.

3.4. Structure of Granules

Figures 7–9 show the XRT images of granules produced using different lactose powders at varying L/S (constant screw speed, 450 rpm). The respective intra-granular porosity within the granules calculated using ImageJ software is presented in Figure 10.

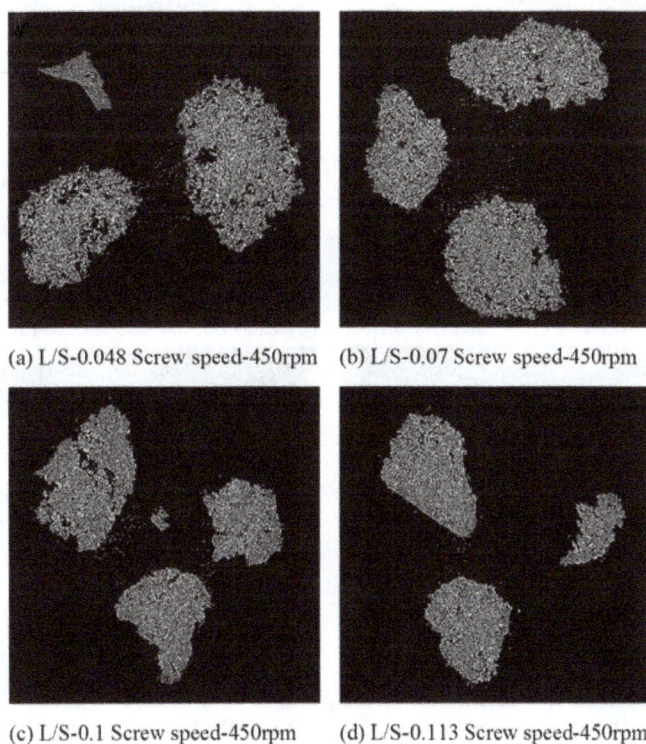

(a) L/S-0.048 Screw speed-450rpm (b) L/S-0.07 Screw speed-450rpm

(c) L/S-0.1 Screw speed-450rpm (d) L/S-0.113 Screw speed-450rpm

Figure 7. X-ray tomographic images of granules produced using Pharmatose 200M at varying L/S (screw speed, 450 rpm).

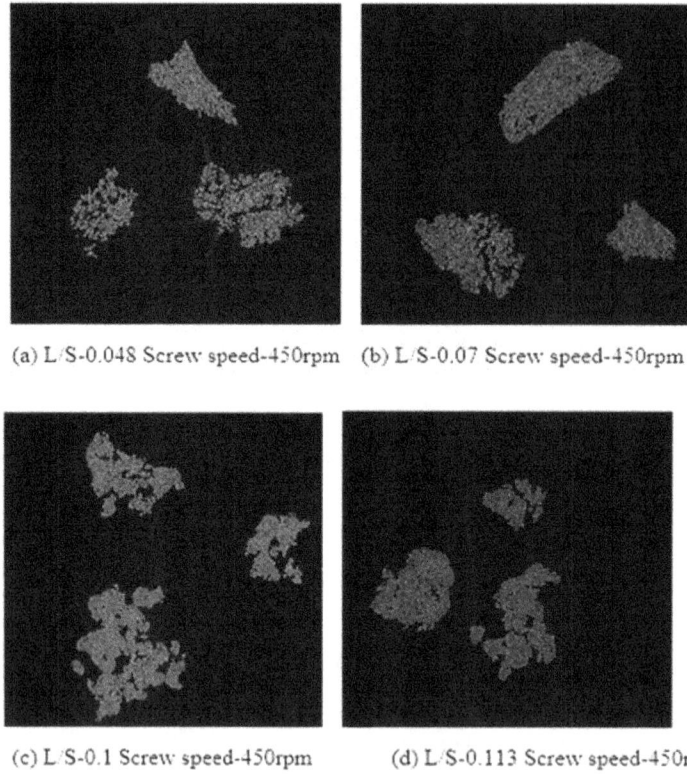

(a) L/S-0.048 Screw speed-450rpm   (b) L/S-0.07 Screw speed-450rpm

(c) L/S-0.1 Screw speed-450rpm   (d) L/S-0.113 Screw speed-450rpm

Figure 8. X-ray tomographic images of granules produced using SuperTab11SD at varying L/S (screw speed, 450 rpm).

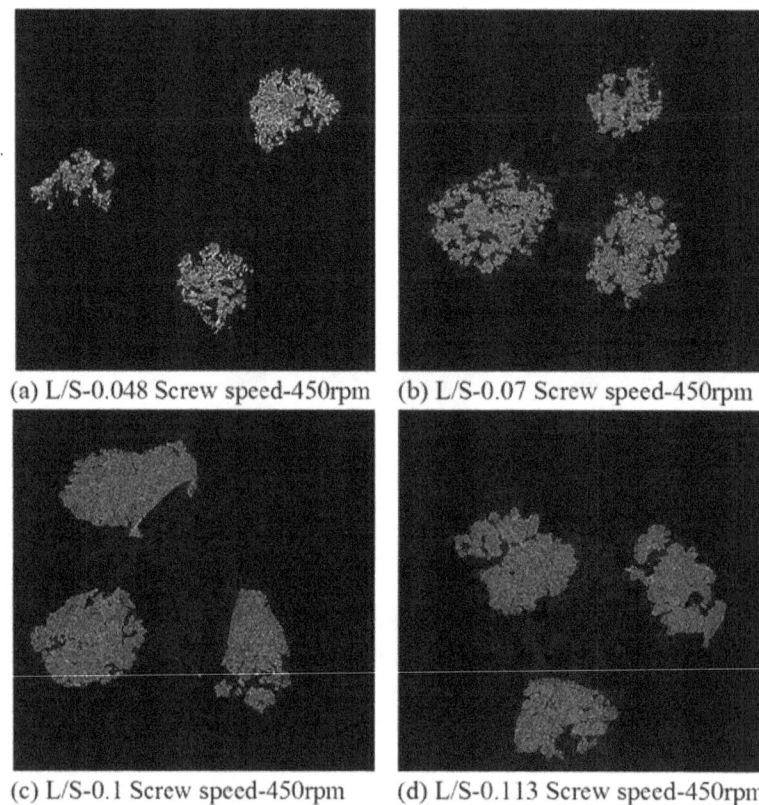

(a) L/S-0.048 Screw speed-450rpm   (b) L/S-0.07 Screw speed-450rpm

(c) L/S-0.1 Screw speed-450rpm   (d) L/S-0.113 Screw speed-450rpm

Figure 9. X-ray tomographic images of granules produced using SuperTab21AN at varying L/S (screw speed, 450 rpm).

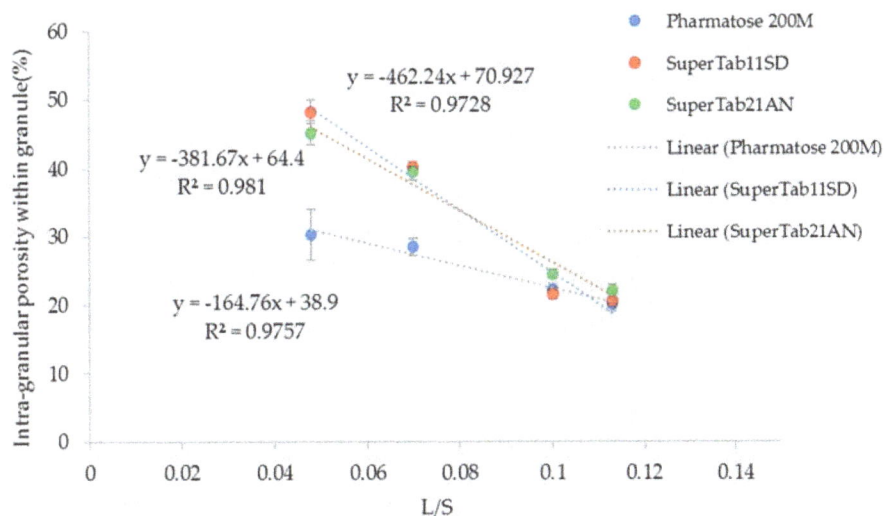

Figure 10. Porosity of granules for different grades of lactose powder at varying L/S (screw speed, 450 rpm).

X-ray tomographic images of granules produced using different grades of mannitol are presented in Figures 11–13. The respective intra-granular porosity within the granules calculated using ImageJ software is presented in Figure 14.

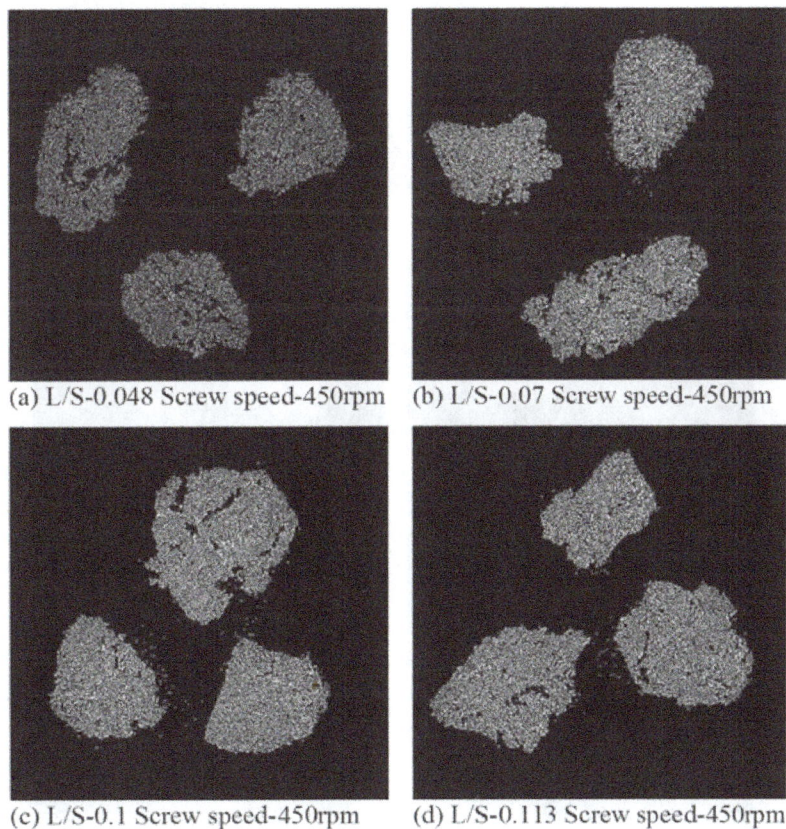

(a) L/S-0.048 Screw speed-450rpm   (b) L/S-0.07 Screw speed-450rpm

(c) L/S-0.1 Screw speed-450rpm   (d) L/S-0.113 Screw speed-450rpm

Figure 11. X-ray tomographic images of granules produced using Pearlitol 50C at varying L/S (screw speed, 450 rpm).

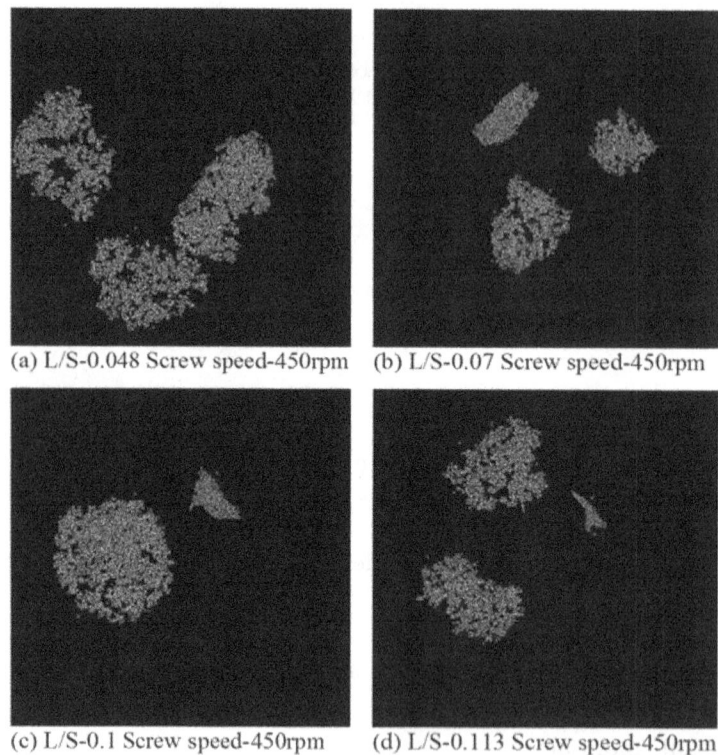

(a) L/S-0.048 Screw speed-450rpm   (b) L/S-0.07 Screw speed-450rpm

(c) L/S-0.1 Screw speed-450rpm   (d) L/S-0.113 Screw speed-450rpm

Figure 12. X-ray tomographic images of granules produced using Pearlitol 200SD at varying L/S (screw speed, 450 rpm).

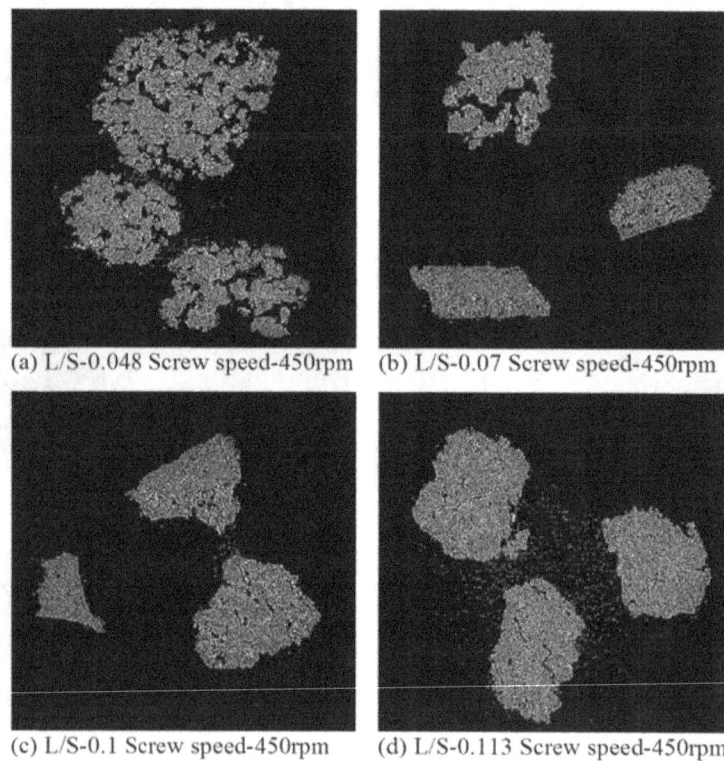

(a) L/S-0.048 Screw speed-450rpm   (b) L/S-0.07 Screw speed-450rpm

(c) L/S-0.1 Screw speed-450rpm   (d) L/S-0.113 Screw speed-450rpm

Figure 13. X-ray tomographic images of granules produced using Pearlitol 300DC at varying L/S (screw speed, 450 rpm).

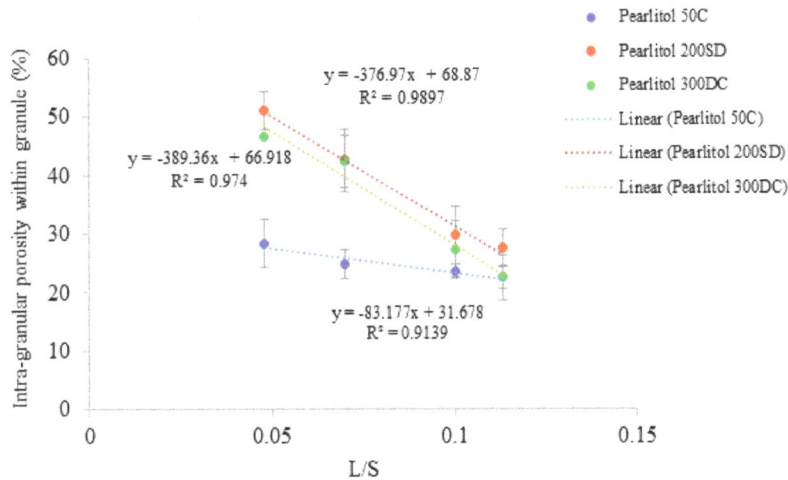

Figure 14. Porosity of granules for different grades of mannitol powder at varying L/S (screw speed, 450 rpm).

3.5. Tensile Strength of Tablets

Granules produced at L/S of 0.048 and 0.113 were sieved in size range of 212–1400 μm and into further subdivisions of 212–600 μm, 600–1000 μm, and 1000–1400 μm. This was done to study the effect of different granule size range on the tableting and tablet tensile strength.

3.5.1. Pharmatose 200M

Figure 15a–d shows the tensile strength of tablets of Pharmatose 200M granules produced at L/S of 0.048 and 0.113 at different screw speeds (200 rpm, 450 rpm, 700 rpm, and 950 rpm) for different granule size ranges (complete range: 212–1400 μm; subdivisions: 212–600 μm, 600–1000 μm, 1000–1400 μm).

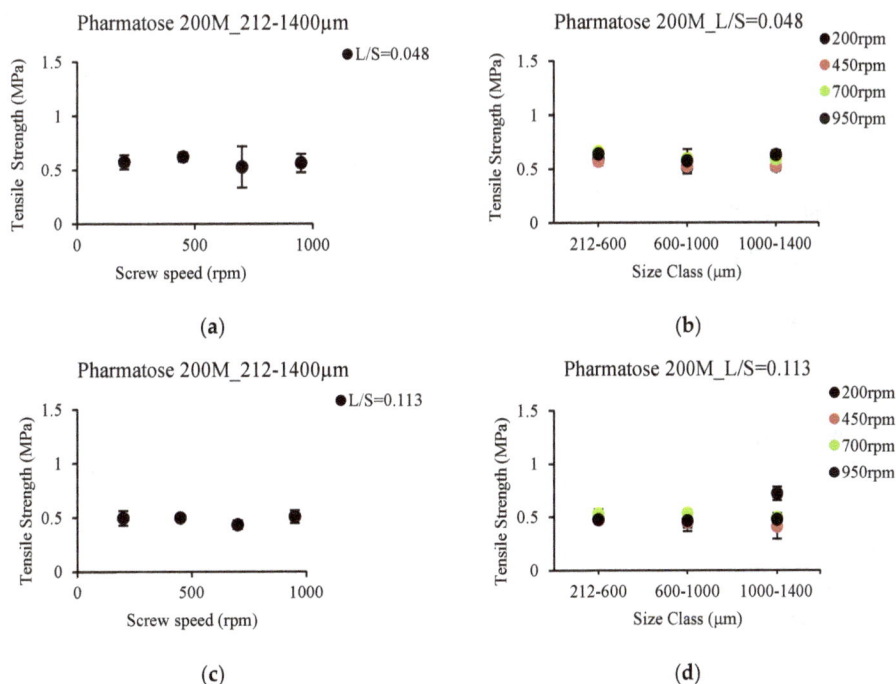

Figure 15. Tensile strength of tablet of granules at different size classes of Pharmatose 200M. (**a**) 212–1400 μm at L/S of 0.048; (**b**) 212–600 μm, 600–1000 μm, and 1000–1400 μm at L/S of 0.048; (**c**) 212–1400 μm at L/S of 0.113; (**d**) 212–600 μm, 600–1000 μm, and 1000–1400 μm at L/S of 0.113.

3.5.2. SuperTab11SD

Figure 16a–d shows the tensile strength of tablets of SuperTab11SD granules produced at L/S of 0.048 and 0.113 (at varying screw speed) for different size classes. Like Pharmatose 200M, tablet strength was similar at all conditions.

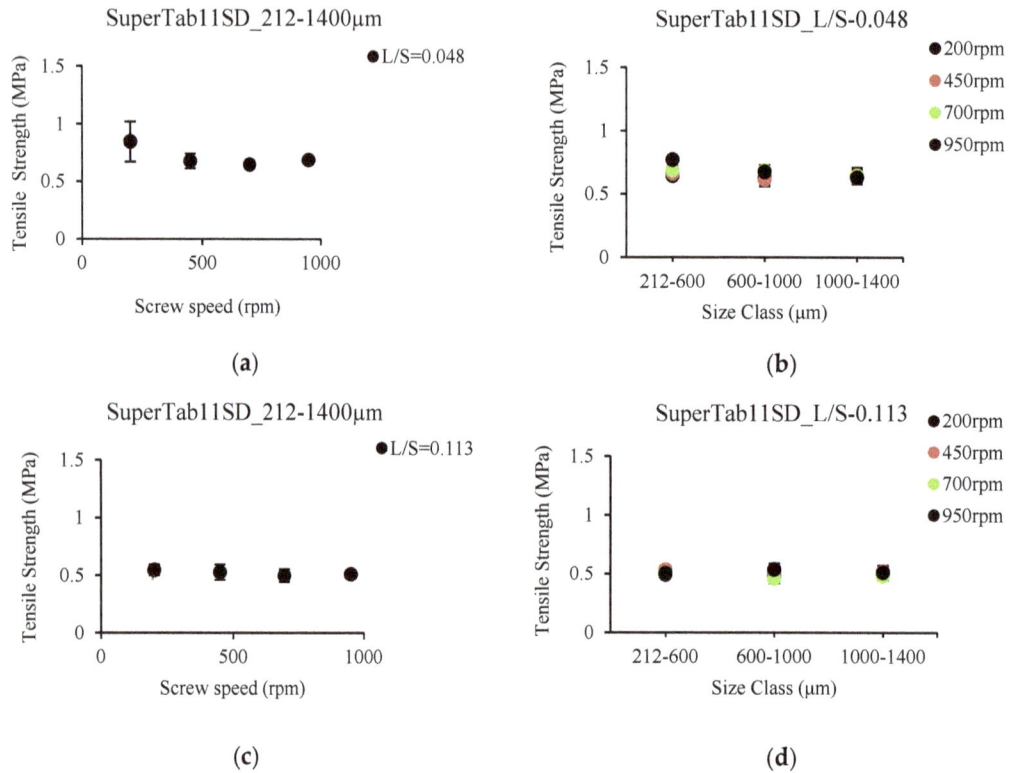

Figure 16. Tensile strength of tablet of granules at different size classes of SuperTab11SD. (a) 212–1400 μm at L/S of 0.048; (b) 212–600 μm, 600–1000 μm, and 1000–1400 μm at L/S of 0.048; (c) 212–1400 μm at L/S of 0.113; (d) 212–600 μm, 600–1000 μm, 1000–1400 μm at L/S of 0.113.

3.5.3. SuperTab21AN

Figure 17a–d shows the tensile strength of tablets of SuperTab21AN granules produced at L/S of 0.048 and 0.113 (at varying screw speed) for different size classes.

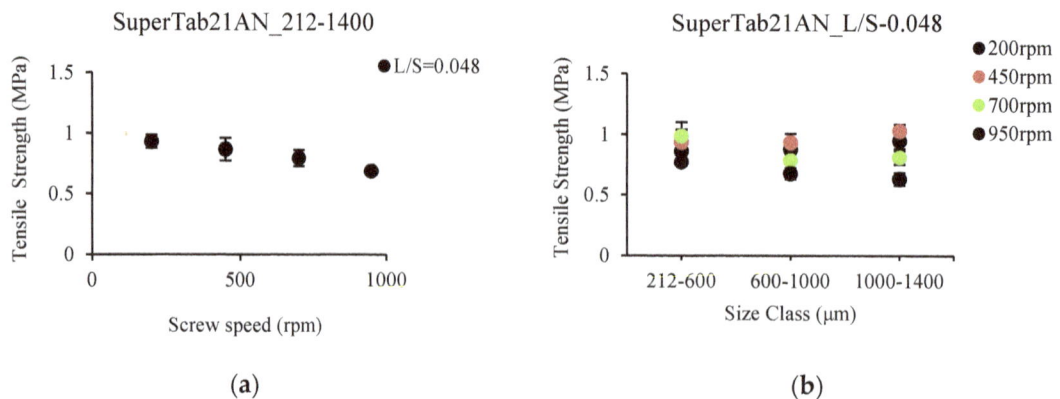

Figure 17. *Cont.*

(c)

(d)

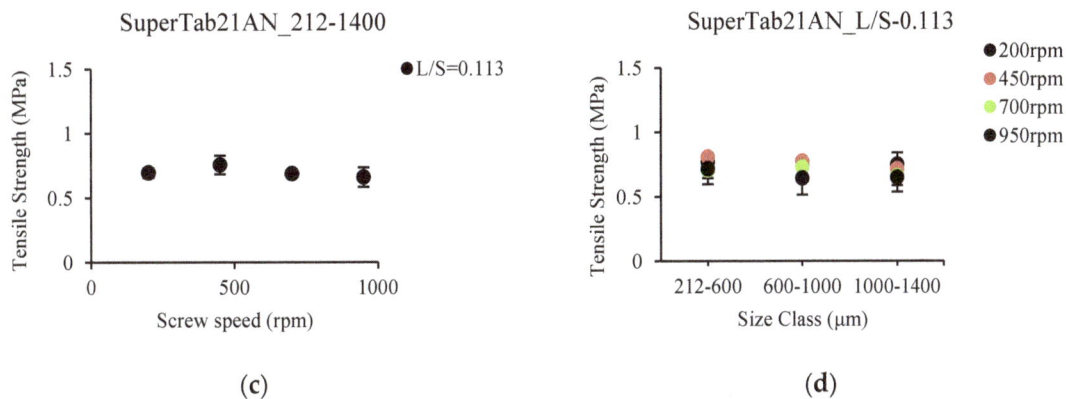

Figure 17. Tensile strength of tablet of granules at different size classes of SuperTab21AN. (**a**) 212–1400 μm at L/S of 0.048 (**b**) 212–600 μm, 600–1000 μm, 1000–1400 μm at L/S of 0.048 (**c**) 212–1400 μm at L/S of 0.113 (**d**) 212–600 μm, 600–1000 μm, 1000–1400 μm at L/S of 0.113.

3.5.4. Pearlitol 50C

Figure 18a–d shows the tensile strength of tablet of Pearlitol 50C granules produced at varying L/S and screw speed for different size ranges.

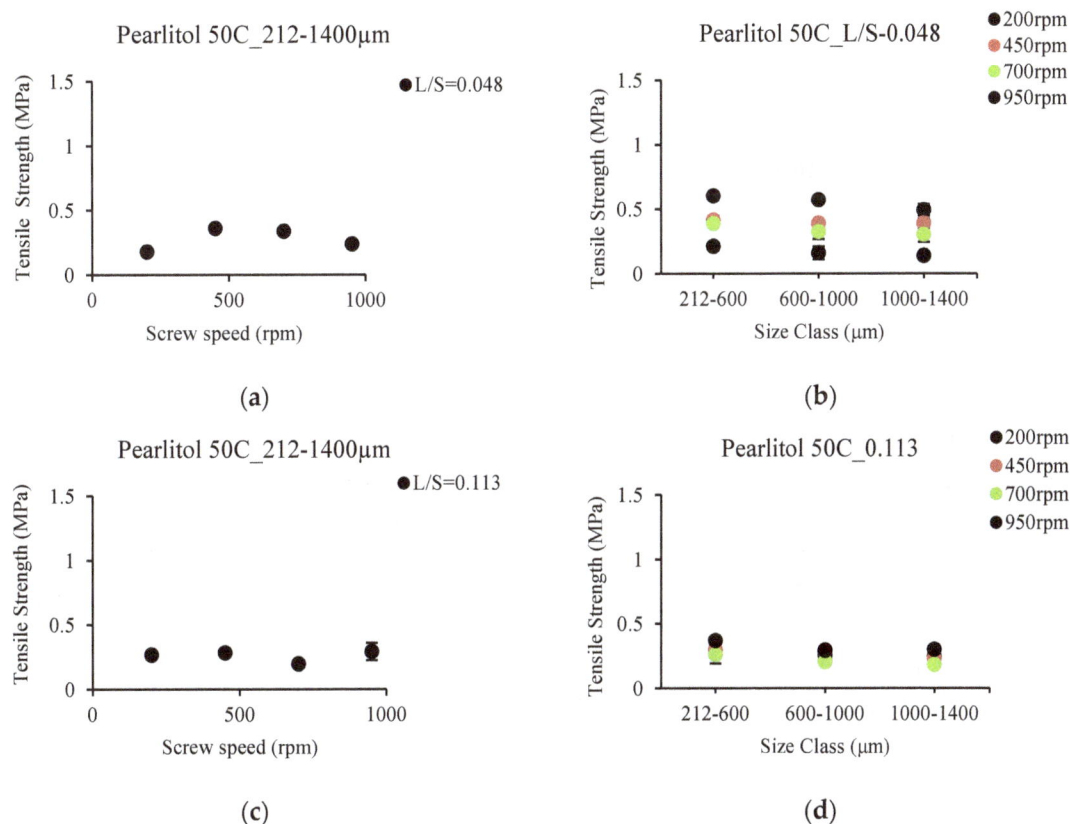

(a)

(b)

(c)

(d)

Figure 18. Tensile strength of tablet of granules at different size classes of Pearlitol 50C. (**a**) 212–1400 μm at L/S of 0.048; (**b**) 212–600 μm, 600–1000 μm, 1000–1400 μm at L/S of 0.048; (**c**) 212–1400 μm at L/S of 0.113; (**d**) 212–600 μm, 600–1000 μm, 1000–1400 μm at L/S of 0.113.

3.5.5. Pearlitol 200SD

Figure 19a–d shows the tensile strength of tablet of Pearlitol 200SD produced at varying L/S and screw speed for different size ranges.

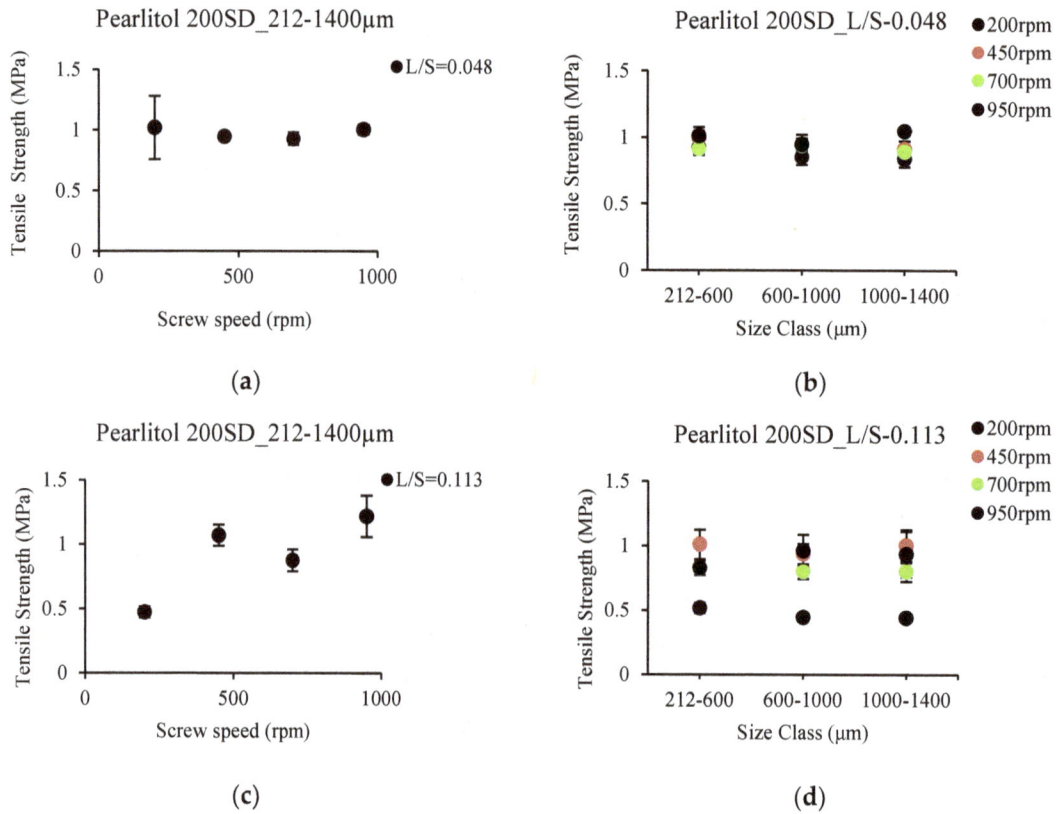

Figure 19. Tensile strength of tablet of granules at different size classes of Pearlitol 200SD. (**a**) 212–1400 μm at L/S of 0.048; (**b**) 212–600 μm, 600–1000 μm, 1000–1400 μm at L/S of 0.048; (**c**) 212–1400 μm at L/S of 0.113; (**d**) 212–600 μm, 600–1000 μm, 1000–1400 μm at L/S of 0.113.

3.5.6. Pearlitol 300DC

Figure 20a–d shows tensile strength of tablets of Pearlitol 300DC produced at varying L/S and screw speed for different size ranges.

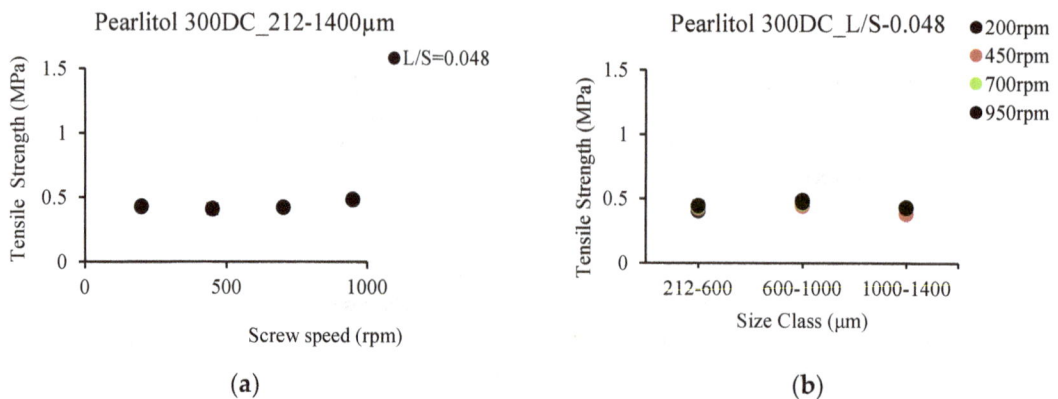

Figure 20. *Cont.*

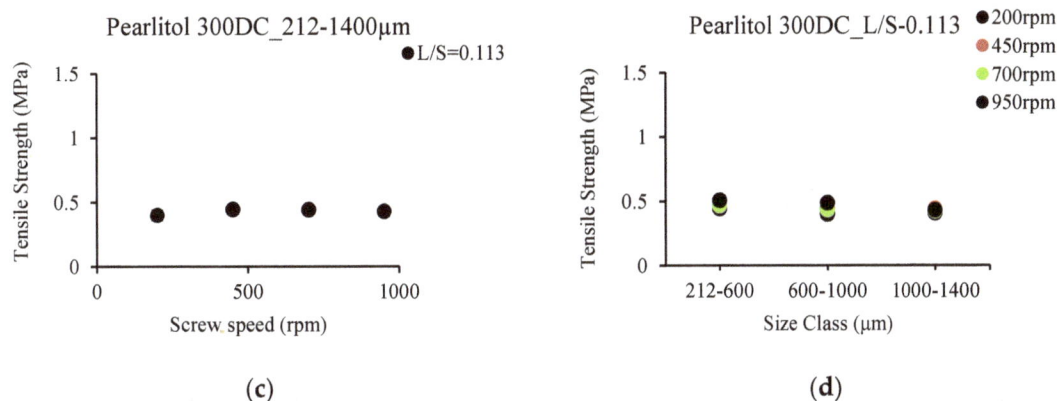

Figure 20.   Tensile strength of tablet of granules at different size classes of Pearlitol 300DC. (**a**) 212–1400 μm at L/S of 0.048; (**b**) 212–600 μm, 600–1000 μm, 1000–1400 μm at L/S of 0.048; (**c**) 212–1400 μm at L/S of 0.113; (**d**) 212–600 μm, 600–1000 μm, 1000–1400 μm at L/S of 0.113.

4. Discussion

4.1. Size of Granules

4.1.1. Lactose

Effect of Varying L/S

From Figure 5a–d, it can be noticed that the granule size increased as the L/S increased for all three lactose powders. At the lowest L/S of 0.048, Pharmatose 200M had the smallest primary particle size (d_{50}) amongst the three lactose powders, but it produced granules comparable to SuperTab21AN, which had larger primary particle size. This indicates that the smaller particles of Pharmatose 200M which promoted the dissolution of particle surface (more than anhydrous lactose [3]), potentially contributed to the formation of stronger liquid bridges between the particles, and thus to the granule growth [1,32,33]. As shown in Table 2, SuperTab21AN powder had larger primary particle size (d_{50}-172.3 μm), and hence, limited dissolution of particle surface [3] and limited granule growth. At same L/S (i.e., 0.048) and screw speeds of 200 rpm and 450 rpm, SuperTab11SD which had larger and more compressible primary particles also produced similar sized granules. This may be because, at such low L/S, larger primary particles remained poorly wetted and were broken into smaller fragments owing to high compressibility, limiting the overall granule growth. No significant change in the granule size was observed at higher screw speeds of 700 rpm and 950 rpm (at the same L/S of 0.048). Although, some differences were observed amongst the three powders at various screw speeds, the overall maximum granule size was limited to ~650 μm due to low availability of liquid at L/S of 0.048.

At L/S of 0.07 and screw speeds of 200 rpm and 450 rpm, SuperTab11SD produced relatively larger granules amongst the three powders. At screw speeds of 700 rpm and 950 rpm, SuperTab21AN had relatively larger median granule size amongst the three powders. This indicated that L/S of 0.07 and a screw speed of 700 rpm may be the parameter settings where SuperTab21AN started exhibiting granule growth. The presence of slightly more granulation liquid (compared to L/S of 0.048) with additional shear/compression force within TSG at higher screw speed resulted in the formation of stronger liquid bridges between SuperTab21AN particles, thus the increase in median granule size.

With further increase in the L/S to 0.1 and 0.113, the solubility of lactose powders increased further resulting in the formation of stronger and higher numbers of liquid bridges between primary particles, meaning formation of bigger and stronger granules. However, apart from the solubility, there are other factors such as compressibility which can also play a key role during wet granulation [1,33,34]. Pharmatose 200M is a crystalline lactose which is smaller in size and less compressible [1]. SuperTab11SD is a more compressible and spherical powder compared to the other two lactose powders. SuperTab21AN is also a crystalline lactose which is more compressible compared to Pharmatose 200M and less compressible compared to SuperTab11SD. At L/S of 0.1 and 0.113 (at all screw speeds except 200 rpm), SuperTab11SD produced the largest granules amongst all three powders. At such higher L/S, shearing action from the kneading elements promoted an even distribution of liquid into the SuperTab11SD powder. This liquid distribution helped to produce the plastic mass of powder, which promoted granules to coalesce and grow further rapidly at all screw speeds [18,35–37].

Effect of Varying Screw Speed

Figure 5a–d also shows that the increase in the screw speed had varying effects on granule size depending on the amount of liquid (L/S). In the case of Pharmatose 200M, the effect of increasing screw speed on the granule size was not prominent. This is in agreement with the observations by Dhenge, et al. [38] and Kumar, et al. [37] where varying screw speed (at lower throughput) resulted in a reduction in oversized granule fraction, and thereby increasing the granulation yield. According to Dhenge, et al. [38] and Kumar, et al. [37], varying screw speed changes the residence time and barrel fill level (surrogate for shear/frictional/compression forces), and thereby impacts the granule size. At lower screw speed, the barrel fill increases and the powder mass experiences a longer residence time. This, based on L/S and powder type, can increase or decrease the granule size. For Pharmatose 200M, all four L/S appeared to be sufficient to promote granule growth. Thus, at lower screw speed, granule growth occurred despite the presence of shear/frictional forces due to a high barrel fill level. As the screw speed increased, both barrel fill level and residence time decreased, but the axial mixing improved and granule–granule and granule–barrel wall impact increased, which resulted in granule growth as well as reduction in oversized granule fraction [37].

In the case of SuperTab11SD, at lower L/S of 0.048 and 0.07 (at all screw speeds), no significant difference was observed due to the porous structure of SuperTab11SD, where liquid was absorbed into the powder particles reducing the availability of liquid on the surface [39]. The absorbed interstitial liquid did not squeeze out sufficiently on the surface of granules due to low granule–granule and granule–barrel wall impact at lower screw speed. As mentioned earlier, at lower screw speed, barrel fill level and residence time also goes up [37] increasing the shear/frictional forces controlling the granule growth [38]. Increasing screw speeds at higher L/S of 0.1 and 0.113, granule size increased noticeably. This may be attributed to improved axial mixing and higher granule–granule and granule–barrel wall impact enhancing granule growth. Furthermore, these results can also be explained using a regime map described by Hapgood, et al. [12], where high liquid amount condition was described as "drop controlled regime", while high shearing condition was indicated by "mechanical agitation controlled regime".

In the case of SuperTab21AN, increasing screw speed at lower L/S of 0.048 did not show a significant effect on the granule growth, because liquid was not sufficient to form an adequate number of liquid bridges between the particles. When increasing screw speed from 200 rpm to 450 rpm at an L/S of 0.07, there was no significant change in granule size, but as the screw speed was increased further to 700 rpm and 950 rpm, the granule size increased noticeably. This is because at lower screw speeds 200 rpm and 450 rpm, the barrel fill level was high and residence time was longer [37,38]. This resulted in more attrition and breakage of formed granules which controlled the granule size. At higher screw speeds of 700 rpm to 950 rpm, the granule size increased because of high impact forces and improved axial mixing [37] which helped granules to squeeze out interstitial liquid on the surface promoting growth. Increasing screw speeds at higher L/S of 0.1 and 0.113 resulted in granule growth due to higher availability and better distribution of granulation liquid [18,35–37].

4.1.2. Mannitol

Effect of Varying L/S

From Figure 6a–d it can be observed that increasing L/S had a powder dependent effect on the granule size. In the case of Pearlitol 50C and Pearlitol 200SD, granule size remained almost similar at L/S of 0.048–0.1 (at a screw speed of 200 rpm). As the L/S increased to 0.113, the granule size increased (Figure 6a) in both Pearlitol 50C and Pearlitol 200SD. Varying L/S at screw speeds of 450 rpm, 700 rpm, and 950 rpm resulted in no change in granule size for Pearlitol 50C and Pearlitol 200SD. In the case of Pearlitol 300DC, the granule size did not vary noticeably at L/S of 0.048 and 0.07, but increased at L/S of 0.1 and 0.113 (at all screw speeds).

Comparing the three powders, Pearlitol 50C, which has the smallest primary particle size (d_{50}) amongst all mannitol powders, generally produced relatively larger granules in almost all cases, while Pearlitol 200SD produced small size granules. This was not the case with similar sized lactose powder (i.e., Pharmatose 200M (similar to Pearlitol 50C)) where granule size was either similar or smaller than the other two lactose powders at various conditions. Pearlitol 300DC, which has the largest primary particles amongst the three mannitol powders, produced granules comparable to Pearlitol 50C. This indicates that there are more dominant variable(s)/properties that controlled the granule size than the primary particle size of the powder. As discussed in the Sections 3.1 and 3.2, the mannitol powders are significantly different in their size, shape, structure, and compressibility. One or more properties of the primary powder can dominate the granulation process outcome. For instance, Pearlitol 50C has the smallest size, elongated shape, and low compressibility. The small particle size of Pearlitol 50C potentially promoted the dissolution of particle surface contributing to the formation of stronger liquid bridges between the particles [1,19], and thus to the granule growth (similar to Pharmatose 200M). Pearlitol 200SD, on the other hand, had larger particles with porous structure and high compressibility. This means that the part of the liquid added may have been absorbed into the particle structure leaving an insufficient amount to promote the formation of sufficient numbers of liquid bridges between the particles, hence, very limited granule growth in the case of Pearlitol 200SD, even at moderately high L/S (0.07–0.113). This suggests that either the binding capacity of Pealrtiol 200SD is poor or it requires further increases in L/S (>0.113) to exhibit an increase in the granule size at increasing shear (i.e., at higher screw speeds). Additionally, the low compressibility factor (Figure 4) also supports the fact that Pearlitol 200SD particles are fragile [40]. Thus, the overall change in growth may be concealed by the volume reduction due to excellent compressibility and/or the breakage of poorly saturated particles. However, spray-dried lactose powder (SuperTab11SD), which has a similar compressibility factor to Pearlitol 200SD, produced larger granules at high L/S (0.1 and 0.113) at all four screw speeds. An attempt was made to understand this contrasting granule growth behavior of these two spray-dried powders (SuperTab11SD and Pearlitol 200SD) by determining differences between their drop penetration time, single particle strength, and dissolution rate (data not shown here). However, none of these additional measurements justified the difference in the granule growth behavior of SuperTab11SD and Pearlitol 200SD. This remains a topic for further investigation in the future.

Compared to Pearlitol 200SD, Pearlitol 300DC had the larger particle size; however, it is relatively low in compressibility (than the porous Pearlitol 200SD). It behaves like Pearlitol 50C at higher L/S. Pearlitol 300DC had large particles, but they are not porous, as in case of Pearlitol 200SD. This means that the liquid was not absorbed in the structure and was available for the inter-particle liquid bridge formation and thereby for granule growth. Additionally, there was less reduction in the volume due to relatively lower compressibility. Hence, it can be concluded that when there is significant difference in the structure and the compressibility, the granule growth is not just controlled by the primary particle size of powder in twin screw wet granulation. The effect on granule size can be a combination of one or more properties of a powder.

Effect of Varying Screw Speed

Figure 6a–d also shows the effect of screw speed on the median size of granules produced using the three mannitol powders. Increasing screw speed at all L/S had limited impact on the granule size.

4.2. Structure of Granules

X-ray tomography images of granules produced using different lactose powders at varying L/S (constant screw speed, 450 rpm) are shown in Figures 7–9. The respective intra-granular porosity within the granules calculated using ImageJ software is presented in Figure 10. The XRT images and the respective calculated intra-granular porosity indicate that the granules generally densify linearly with increase in the L/S at a set screw speed in all three lactose powders. Comparing the XRT images of granules from the three powders, SuperTab11SD and SuperTab21AN granules appeared to be relatively more porous (due to higher inter-granular porosity) [41] due to larger primary particle size. However, they show localized densification (lower intra-granular porosity) within the granule structure owing to their porous primary particles and high compressibility.

Pearlitol 50C (Figure 11a–d) and Pearlitol 200SD (Figure 12a–d) showed less significant change in structure of larger granules at all L/S. However, few densified, elongated granules could be seen at L/S of 0.07–0.113 in the case of Pearlitol 200SD (Figure 12b–d). The intra-particle voids can also be seen in the XRT images. The XRT images support the granule size results for Pearlitol 200SD where the granule size did not change noticeably at increasing L/S and screw speed. The effect of L/S on granule structure was more obvious in the case of Pearlitol 300DC (Figure 13a–d), where granules became denser with increasing L/S. At L/S of 0.048 (Figure 13a), individual large-size particles of Pearlitol 300DC could still be identified in the granule structure. The intra-granular porosity within the granules (Figure 14) supported the observation from XRT images for Pearlitol 300DC. The intra-granular porosity within the granules (Figure 14) also supported the observation from XRT images for Pearlitol 50C where porosity did not vary significantly with increasing L/S. However, in the case of Pearlitol 200SD, the intra-granular porosity decreased with increasing L/S. This is due to the localized densification within the granules.

4.3. Tensile Strength of Tablets

4.3.1. Pharmatose 200M

It was found that the tensile strength of tablets was similar at both L/S of 0.048 and 0.113 (and at all screw speeds of 200 rpm, 450 rpm, 700 rpm, and 950 rpm) (Figure 15a–d). The granule size also had very limited impact on the tablet strength. It appears that compression force applied during tableting overcame the granule strength (at low or high L/S or screw speeds), thus a minimum effect on the tablet strength.

4.3.2. SuperTab11SD

The tensile strength of tablets of SuperTab11SD granules was similar at L/S of 0.048 and 0.113 (at varying screw speed) for different size classes (Figure 16a–d).

4.3.3. SuperTab21AN

From Figure 17a–d it can be observed that the tensile strength of tablets of SuperTab21AN granules was similar to Pharmatose 200M and SuperTab11SD where it did not change (for broader granule size class of 212–1400 μm) with an increase in the L/S and screw speed (Figure 17a,c). The results agree with findings by Keleb, et al. [3], where tensile strength of tablets produced from milled lactose (Pharmatose 200M), spray-dried lactose (Pharmatose DCL 11), and anhydrous lactose (Pharmatose DCL 21) remained almost similar when wet granulated using batch high-shear granulator.

Subdividing the granules into narrower size classes showed a screw speed dependent effect on the tablet strength to some extent (Figure 17b). The tablet strength increased at lower screw speeds of 200 rpm and 450 rpm, while it decreased at higher screw speeds of 700 rpm and 950 rpm, with increasing granule size class from 212–600 μm to 600–1000 μm, and then to 1000–1400 μm. It may be interpreted that the granules in the size of 600–1000 μm and 1000–1400 μm, which are bigger (which are generally stronger according to Dhenge, et al. [42]), dictated the trend of decrease in the tablet strength with increasing screw speed in the broader granule size range (212–1400 μm). At higher L/S of 0.113, the effect of screw speed was concealed by the liquid amount available for the granulation.

4.3.4. Pearlitol 50C

From Figure 18a–d, it can be seen that the tablets produced using broader granule size range (212–1400 μm) does not vary significantly upon increasing screw speed at both L/S (Figure 18a,c). But subdividing the granules from 212–1400 μm into 212–600 μm, 600–1000 μm and 1000–1400 μm showed effect of granule size on the tablet tensile strength at different screw speed (Figure 18b). Increasing the granule size range from 212–600 μm to 600–1000 μm and to 1000–1400 μm, decreased the tensile strength of the tablet [43,44]. The smaller granule size range (212–600 μm) produced stronger tablets [36,45]. This is because the small particles helped to make higher numbers of inter-particle bonds and pack better, making stronger tablets [45]. As granule size range increased to 600–1000 μm and to 1000–1400 μm, the number of bonds between the particles decreased resulting in weaker tablets. As the L/S increased to 0.113, the availability of sufficient liquid promoted the formation of stronger granules that masked the effect of screw speed.

4.3.5. Pearlitol 200SD

In Pearlitol 200SD, varying screw speed at lower L/S of 0.048 showed no significant change in tablet tensile strength for broader (212–1400 μm) and subdivided granule size ranges (212–600 μm, 600–1000 μm and 1000–1400 μm) (Figure 19a,b). The outcome was similar at L/S of 0.113 except at condition at 200 rpm where tablet tensile strength was lower for both broader and subdivided granule size ranges (Figure 19c,d). This indicate that in presence of sufficient availability of granulation liquid (at L/S of 0.113), lower screw speed (meaning longer residence time and higher barrel fill) resulted in stronger granules, thus weaker tablets.

4.3.6. Pearlitol 300DC

Figure 20a–d shows that the tensile strength of Pearlitol 300DC tablets was similar but very low at both lower and higher L/S at all screw speeds.

It is clear that the tensile strength of tablets was low for all three mannitol powders at both lower and higher L/S at all screw speeds. It is likely that the differences in the granule strength or compressibility may have been concealed by the compression force used in the study [3].

5. Conclusions

Powders differ in their size and structure due to the way they are manufactured for their intended application (suitability for dry or wet granulation or direct compaction). In this study, the effects of the properties of powder on twin screw wet granulation behavior and properties of so-produced granules and tablets were studied. It was found that the granulation behavior of powder is controlled by size, structure, and compressibility of primary powder, which agrees with findings in previous research works [1,18,19,46]. The porous structure of a particle may enhance the compressibility in dry granulation or direct compaction, but in wet granulation it can limit the binding between the particles due to absorption of water in the structure of the particles. In general, increasing L/S resulted in an increase in the granule size and weaker tablets in all powders. The effect of screw speed on granule properties was dependent on the amount of liquid added and type of powder. Considering the granule size data, this work suggests that spray-dried lactose and anhydrous lactose can be used in twin screw wet granulation while operating at lower settings of L/S and screw speed. In case of mannitol, Pearlitol 200SD and 300DC are suitable for twin screw wet granulation at all L/S and screw speeds tested in this study. In general, processed powders such as spray-dried and granulated lactose and mannitol can also be used in formulation for wet granulation where flowability of active pharmaceutical ingredient (API) is poor. They may even be preferred over crystalline milled excipient powders (i.e., Pharmatose 200M and Pearlitol 50C, which have relatively poor flowability) while improving granule properties. In the future, the impact of twin wet granulation on the physicochemical characteristics of the granules and tablets of lactose and mannitol powders may be investigated to understand if they undergo form change due to wetting.

Author Contributions: Conceptualization, S.V.L., R.M.D. and A.D.S.; Methodology, S.V.L.; Formal Analysis, S.V.L.; Investigation, S.V.L., R.M.D. and A.D.S.; Data Curation, S.V.L. and R.M.D.; Writing-Original Draft Preparation, S.V.L.; Writing-Review & Editing, R.M.D. and A.D.S.; Supervision, A.D.S.

Acknowledgments: The authors would like to thank Dr. Chalak Omar at The University of Sheffield, for the help on powder compressibility testing experiments.

References

1. Huang, W.; Shi, Y.; Wang, C.; Yu, K.; Sun, F.; Li, Y. Using spray-dried lactose monohydrate in wet granulation method for a low-dose oral formulation of a paliperidone derivative. *Powder Technol.* **2013**, *246*, 379–394. [CrossRef]

2. Jivraj, M.; Martini, L.G.; Thomson, C.M. An overview of the different excipients useful for the direct compression of tablets. *Pharm. Sci. Technol. Today* **2000**, *3*, 58–63. [CrossRef]

3. Keleb, E.I.; Vermeire, A.; Vervaet, C.; Remon, J.P. Single-step granulation/tabletting of different grades of lactose: A comparison with high shear granulation and compression. *Eur. J. Pharm. Biopharm.* **2004**, *58*, 77–82. [CrossRef] [PubMed]

4. Lerk, C.F. Consolidation and Compaction of Lactose. *Drug Dev. Ind. Pharm.* **1993**, *19*, 2359–2398. [CrossRef]

5. Kibbe, A.H. *Handbook of Pharmaceutical Excipients*; American Pharmaceutical Association: Washington, DC, USA, 2000.

6. Westermarck, S.; Juppo, A.M.; Kervinen, L.; Yliruusi, J. Pore structure and surface area of mannitol powder, granules and tablets determined with mercury porosimetry and nitrogen adsorption. *Eur. J. Pharm. Biopharm.* **1998**, *46*, 61–68. [CrossRef]

7. Wade, A.; Weller, P.J. *Handbook of Pharmaceutical Excipients*; American Pharmaceutical association: Washington, DC, USA; Pharmaceutical Press: London, UK, 1994.

8. Debord, B.; Lefebvre, C.; Guyot-Hermann, A.M.; Hubert, J.; Bouché, R.; Cuyot, J.C. Study of Different Crystalline forms of Mannitol: Comparative Behaviour under Compression. *Drug Dev. Ind. Pharm.* **1987**, *13*, 1533–1546. [CrossRef]

9. Gabbott, I.P.; Al Husban, F.; Reynolds, G.K. The combined effect of wet granulation process parameters and dried granule moisture content on tablet quality attributes. *Eur. J. Pharm. Biopharm.* **2016**, *106*, 70–78. [CrossRef] [PubMed]

10. Chang, C.K.; Alvarez–Nunez, F.A.; Rinella, J.V., Jr.; Magnusson, L.-E.; Sueda, K. Roller Compaction, Granulation and Capsule Product Dissolution of Drug Formulations Containing a Lactose or Mannitol Filler, Starch, and Talc. *AAPS PharmSciTech* **2008**, *9*, 597–604. [CrossRef] [PubMed]

11. Schæfer, T.; Mathiesen, C. Melt pelletization in a high shear mixer. *IX. Effects of binder particle size. Int. J. Pharm.* **1996**, *139*, 139–148.

12. Hapgood, K.P.; Litster, J.D.; Smith, R. Nucleation regime map for liquid bound granules. *AIChE J.* **2003**, *49*, 350–361. [CrossRef]

13. Kayrak-Talay, D.; Litster, J.D. A priori performance prediction in pharmaceutical wet granulation: Testing the applicability of the nucleation regime map to a formulation with a broad size distribution and dry binder addition. *Int. J. Pharm.* **2011**, *418*, 254–264. [CrossRef] [PubMed]

14. Kristensen, H.G.; Holm, P.; Schaefer, T. Mechanical properties of moist agglomerates in relation to granulation mechanisms part II. Effects of particle size distribution. *Powder Technol.* **1985**, *44*, 239–247. [CrossRef]

15. Badawy, S.I.F.; Lee, T.J.; Menning, M.M. Effect of drug substance particle size on the characteristics of granulation manufactured in a high-shear mixer. *AAPS PharmSciTech* **2000**, *1*, 55–61. [CrossRef] [PubMed]

16. Mackaplow, M.B.; Rosen, L.A.; Michaels, J.N. Effect of primary particle size on granule growth and endpoint determination in high-shear wet granulation. *Powder Technol.* **2000**, *108*, 32–45. [CrossRef]

17. Badawy, S.I.F.; Hussain, M.A. Effect of starting material particle size on its agglomeration behavior in high shear wet granulation. *AAPS PharmSciTech* **2004**, *5*, 16–22. [CrossRef] [PubMed]

18. El Hagrasy, A.S.; Hennenkamp, J.R.; Burke, M.D.; Cartwright, J.J.; Litster, J.D. Twin screw wet granulation: Influence of formulation parameters on granule properties and growth behavior. *Powder Technol.* **2013**, *238*, 108–115. [CrossRef]

19. Vanhoorne, V.; Bekaert, B.; Peeters, E.; de Beer, T.; Remon, J.P.; Vervaet, C. Improved tabletability after a polymorphic transition of delta-mannitol during twin screw granulation. *Int. J. Pharm.* **2016**, *506*, 13–24. [CrossRef] [PubMed]

20. Omar, C.S.; Dhenge, R.M.; Palzer, S.; Hounslow, M.J.; Salman, A.D. Roller compaction: Effect of relative humidity of lactose powder. *Eur. J. Pharm. Biopharm.* **2016**, *106*, 26–37. [CrossRef] [PubMed]

21. DFE Pharma: Application notes–Anhydrous lactose. Available online: https://www.dfepharma.com/en/excipients/lactose/application-notes/ (accessed on 28 May 2018).

22. DFE Pharma: Application notes—Spray-dried lactose. Available online: https://www.dfepharma.com/en/excipients/lactose/application-notes/ (accessed on 28 May 2018).

23. Paul, S.; Chang, S.-Y.; Dun, J.; Sun, W.-J.; Wang, K.; Tajarobi, P.; Boissier, C.; Sun, C.C. Comparative analyses of flow and compaction properties of diverse mannitol and lactose grades. *Int. J. Pharm.* **2018**, *546*, 39–49. [CrossRef] [PubMed]

24. Littringer, E.M.; Noisternig, M.F.; Mescher, A.; Schroettner, H.; Walzel, P.; Griesser, U.J.; Urbanetz, N.A. The morphology and various densities of spray dried mannitol. *Powder Technol.* **2013**, *246*, 193–200. [CrossRef]

25. Hulse, W.L.; Forbes, R.T.; Bonner, M.C.; Getrost, M. The characterization and comparison of spray-dried mannitol samples. *Drug Dev. Ind. Pharm.* **2009**, *35*, 712–718. [CrossRef] [PubMed]

26. Silva, A.F.; Sarraguça, M.C.; Fonteyne, M.; Vercruysse, J.; de Leersnyder, F.; Vanhoorne, V.; Bostijn, N.; Verstraeten, M.; Vervaet, C.; Remon, J.P.; et al. Multivariate statistical process control of a continuous pharmaceutical twin-screw granulation and fluid bed drying process. *Int. J. Pharm.* **2017**, *528*, 242–252. [CrossRef] [PubMed]

27. Fell, J.T.; Newton, J.M. Determination of Tablet Strength by the Diametral-Compression Test. *J. Pharm. Sci.* **1970**, *59*, 688–691. [CrossRef] [PubMed]

28. Mangwandi, C.; JiangTao, L.; Albadarin, A.B.; Dhenge, R.M.; Walker, G.M. High shear granulation of binary mixtures: Effect of powder composition on granule properties. *Powder Technol.* **2015**, *270*, 424–434. [CrossRef]

29. Omar, C.S.; Dhenge, R.M.; Osborne, J.D.; Althaus, T.O.; Palzer, S.; Hounslow, M.J.; Salman, A.D. Roller compaction: Effect of morphology and amorphous content of lactose powder on product quality. *Int. J. Pharm.* **2015**, *496*, 63–74. [CrossRef] [PubMed]

30. Littringer, E.M.; Paus, R.; Mescher, A.; Schroettner, H.; Walzel, P.; Urbanetz, N.A. The morphology of spray dried mannitol particles—The vital importance of droplet size. *Powder Technol.* **2013**, *239*, 162–174. [CrossRef]

31. Mitra, B.; Hilden, J.; Litster, J.D. Effects of the granule composition on the compaction behavior of deformable dry granules. *Powder Technol.* **2016**, *291*, 487–498. [CrossRef]

32. Lute, S.V.; Dhenge, R.M.; Hounslow, M.J.; Salman, A.D. Twin screw granulation: Understanding the mechanism of granule formation along the barrel length. *Chem. Eng. Res. Design* **2016**, *110*, 43–53. [CrossRef]

33. Iveson, S.M.; Litster, J.D.; Hapgood, K.; Ennis, B.J. Nucleation, growth and breakage phenomena in agitated wet granulation processes: A review. *Powder Technol.* **2001**, *117*, 3–39. [CrossRef]

34. Vanhoorne, V.; Vanbillemont, B.; Vercruysse, J.; de Leersnyder, F.; Gomes, P.; Beer, T.D.; Remon, J.P.; Vervaet, C. Development of a controlled release formulation by continuous twin screw granulation: Influence of process and formulation parameters. *Int. J. Pharm.* **2016**, *505*, 61–68. [CrossRef] [PubMed]

35. Saleh, M.F.; Dhenge, R.M.; Cartwright, J.J.; Hounslow, M.J.; Salman, A.D. Twin screw wet granulation: Binder delivery. *Int. J. Pharm.* **2015**, *487*, 124–134. [CrossRef] [PubMed]

36. Vercruysse, J.; Burggraeve, A.; Fonteyne, M.; Cappuyns, P.; Delaet, U.; van Assche, I.; de Beer, T.; Remon, J.P.; Vervaet, C. Impact of screw configuration on the particle size distribution of granules produced by twin screw granulation. *Int. J. Pharm.* **2015**, *479*, 171–180. [CrossRef] [PubMed]

37. Kumar, A.; Alakarjula, M.; Vanhoorne, V.; Toiviainen, M.; de Leersnyder, F.; Vercruysse, J.; Juuti, M.; Ketolainen, J.; Vervaet, C.; Remon, J.P.; et al. Linking granulation performance with residence time and granulation liquid distributions in twin-screw granulation: An experimental investigation. *Eur. J. Pharm. Sci.* **2016**, *90*, 25–37. [CrossRef] [PubMed]

38. Dhenge, R.M.; Fyles, R.S.; Cartwright, J.J.; Doughty, D.G.; Hounslow, M.J.; Salman, A.D. Twin screw wet granulation: Granule properties. *Chem. Eng. J.* **2010**, *164*, 322–329. [CrossRef]

39. Bouffard, J.; Kaster, M.; Dumont, H. Influence of Process Variable and Physicochemical Properties on the Granulation Mechanism of Mannitol in a Fluid Bed Top Spray Granulator. *Drug Dev. Ind. Pharm.* **2005**, *31*, 923–933. [CrossRef] [PubMed]

40. Souihi, N.; Dumarey, M.; Wikström, H.; Tajarobi, P.; Fransson, M.; Svensson, O.; Josefson, M.; Trygg, J. A quality by design approach to investigate the effect of mannitol and dicalcium phosphate qualities on roll compaction. *Int. J. Pharm.* **2013**, *447*, 47–61. [CrossRef] [PubMed]

41. Dhenge, R.M.; Cartwright, J.J.; Doughty, D.G.; Hounslow, M.J.; Salman, A.D. Twin screw wet granulation: Effect of powder feed rate. *Adv. Powder Technol.* **2011**, *22*, 162–166. [CrossRef]

42. Dhenge, R.M.; Cartwright, J.J.; Hounslow, M.J.; Salman, A.D. Twin screw wet granulation: Effects of properties of granulation liquid. *Powder Technol.* **2012**, *229*, 126–136. [CrossRef]

43. Vercruysse, J.; Díaz, D.C.; Peeters, E.; Fonteyne, M.; Delaet, U.; van Assche, I.; de Beer, T.; Remon, J.P.; Vervaet, C. Continuous twin screw granulation: Influence of process variables on granule and tablet quality. *Eur. J. Pharm. Biopharm.* **2012**, *82*, 205–211. [CrossRef] [PubMed]

44. Meier, R.; Moll, K.-P.; Krumme, M.; Kleinebudde, P. Impact of fill-level in twin-screw granulation on critical quality attributes of granules and tablets. *Eur. J. Pharm. Biopharm.* **2017**, *115*, 102–112. [CrossRef] [PubMed]

45. Djuric, D.; Kleinebudde, P. Impact of screw elements on continuous granulation with a twin-screw extruder. *J. Pharm. Sci.* **2008**, *97*, 4934–4942. [CrossRef] [PubMed]

46. Fonteyne, M.; Correia, A.; de Plecker, S.; Vercruysse, J.; Ilić, I.; Zhou, Q.; Vervaet, C.; Remon, J.P.; Onofre, F.; Bulone, V.; et al. Impact of microcrystalline cellulose material attributes: A case study on continuous twin screw granulation. *Int. J. Pharm.* **2015**, *478*, 705–717. [CrossRef] [PubMed]

8

Impact of Particle Size and Polydispersity Index on the Clinical Applications of Lipidic Nanocarrier Systems

M. Danaei, M. Dehghankhold, S. Ataei, F. Hasanzadeh Davarani, R. Javanmard, A. Dokhani, S. Khorasani and M. R. Mozafari * ⓘ

Australasian Nanoscience and Nanotechnology Initiative, 8054 Monash University LPO, Clayton, Victoria 3168, Australia; danagenepk@gmail.com (M.Da.); m_dehghan.kh@yahoo.com (M.De.); s.ataei@umsha.ac.ir (S.A.); Hasanzadeh.fatemeh1662@gmail.com (F.H.D.); r.javanmard@gmail.com (R.J.); info@anni.com.au (A.D.); dr.sepideh.khorasani@gmail.com (S.K.)
* Correspondence: dr.m.r.mozafari@gmail.com

Abstract: Lipid-based drug delivery systems, or lipidic carriers, are being extensively employed to enhance the bioavailability of poorly-soluble drugs. They have the ability to incorporate both lipophilic and hydrophilic molecules and protecting them against degradation in vitro and in vivo. There is a number of physical attributes of lipid-based nanocarriers that determine their safety, stability, efficacy, as well as their in vitro and in vivo behaviour. These include average particle size/diameter and the polydispersity index (PDI), which is an indication of their quality with respect to the size distribution. The suitability of nanocarrier formulations for a particular route of drug administration depends on their average diameter, PDI and size stability, among other parameters. Controlling and validating these parameters are of key importance for the effective clinical applications of nanocarrier formulations. This review highlights the significance of size and PDI in the successful design, formulation and development of nanosystems for pharmaceutical, nutraceutical and other applications. Liposomes, nanoliposomes, vesicular phospholipid gels, solid lipid nanoparticles, transfersomes and tocosomes are presented as frequently-used lipidic drug carriers. The advantages and limitations of a range of available analytical techniques used to characterize lipidic nanocarrier formulations are also covered.

Keywords: drug delivery; encapsulation; lipidic nanovesicles; nanocarriers; particle size; toxicity

1. Introduction

The number of products on the market manufactured using lipidic nanocarriers is increasing in parallel with increasing public awareness of the health benefits of such products. These products are mainly in the field of cosmetics, food/nutrition, nutraceuticals and pharmaceuticals. Lipid-based encapsulation systems are among the most promising technologies employed in drug delivery and sustained release of bioactive compounds. They include liposomes, nanoliposomes, archaeosomes, solid lipid nanoparticles (SLN), tocosomes and some other drug carrier systems. Figure 1 lists a number of currently available lipidic carrier systems and a brief description of each. One of the first and most applied drug delivery technologies is the liposome, which is also known as a bilayer lipid and/or a phospholipid vesicle. The word liposome has been adopted generally to refer to mesomorphic structures composed of lipid, phospholipid and water molecules. The main chemical components of liposomes are amphiphilic lipid/phospholipid molecules [1]. They improve the efficacy of pharmaceutical, nutraceutical and other bioactive compounds by entrapment and release of water-soluble, lipid-soluble and amphiphilic materials, as well as targeting the encapsulated compounds to particular cells or tissues [2]. Liposomes can be made on a small scale (e.g., for laboratory research) or industrial scales using natural ingredients such as soy or egg lecithin. However, it is also possible to include other molecules such as sterols (mainly cholesterol), polypeptides (e.g., antigens), polymers (such as poly-ethylene-glycol or chitosan), as well as antioxidants (e.g., α-tocopherol) in the structure of the lipid vesicles. These additives assist in targeting the lipidic vesicles (and their encapsulated molecules) where their effect is needed, or improving the stability and shelf life of the product. Nanoliposomes (lipidic nanovesicles or nanometric versions of liposomes), on the other hand, can be briefly defined as colloidal nanostructures composed of lipid/phospholipid bilayers [3]. In general, liposomes and nanoliposomes have the same physical, chemical and thermodynamic properties that are mainly determined by their ingredients and the media in which they are suspended. This is while the smaller the particle size, the larger the surface-to-volume ratio they will possess. Consequently, in comparison with liposomes, nanoliposomes provide more surface area and have more potential to increase solubility, enhance bioavailability, improve controlled release and enable accurate targeting of the encapsulated material. The manufacture of both liposomes and nanoliposomes requires the input of energy to a dispersion of lipid and phospholipid molecules in an aqueous medium [1–5]. Although lipid vesicles are initially prepared as a liquid suspension, they can be subsequently incorporated in a cream, lotion, aerosol, soft-gel, powder (upon freeze drying or spray drying for instance) or other formulations and dosage forms. Vesicular phospholipid gel (VPG) is an example of a highly concentrated phospholipid dispersion of semisolid consistency and vesicular morphology. VPG can be prepared by high-pressure homogenization using high concentrations of phospholipid molecules. Upon dilution with an aqueous solution, VPG constitutes a liquid liposome dispersion [6,7]. Solid lipid nanoparticles (SLN), on the other hand, are a recently-developed nanocarrier utilized as an alternative to the existing drug delivery technologies including polymeric nanocarriers, emulsions and liposomes. They are a new generation of submicron-sized lipidic carriers in which the liquid lipid (oil) has been substituted by a solid lipid, i.e., the lipid particle matrix being solid at room temperature, as well as body temperature [5]. Some of the solid lipids used in the preparation of SLN include triglycerides, emulsifying wax, cetyl alcohol, carnauba wax, beeswax, cholesterol and cholesterol butyrate. The underlying mechanism for the formation of the lipid vesicles is the hydrophilic–hydrophobic interactions and van der Waals forces between phospholipids and water molecules. There are a number of review articles describing the preparation methods of lipid-based vesicles, which readers are referred to for a broader coverage [1,2,5,8].

In addition to their application in the fields of encapsulation of bioactive compounds and drug delivery and targeting, lipid vesicles are being used as simplified models of cells and biological membranes. Their similarity to biomembranes makes them an ideal structure, not only for the study of existing biosystems, but also in the investigation of the emergence, functioning and evolution of original cells [9,10]. Applications of phospholipid vesicles in the area of food fortification are also rapidly growing. Food fortification is the process of adding micronutrients, including vitamins, minerals and essential fatty acids, to food products. These molecules and compounds may change the sensory qualities of food and adversely affect its smell, taste or colour. One of the main advantages of employing nanovesicles in the food industry is their ability to evade our sensory perception, enabling fortification of food and beverages with bioactive materials (such as omega fatty acids) without adversely affecting the sensory attributes of the original product [11–13]. If nanovesicles are kept below a size of around 80 nm in diameter (and not at very high concentrations, or particle refractive index not very different from that of the suspension medium), they hardly scatter any visible light and hence maintain transparency. Such invisible vesicles are very useful, for instance, for the fortification of clear beverages with hydrophobic molecules or those with undesirable odours or flavours [14]. The particle size distribution and polydispersity index (PDI) of lipid-based nanocarriers are highly important physical characteristics to be considered when creating food-grade or pharmaceutical-grade products. These attributes of the lipidic nanocarriers can affect the bulk properties, product performance, processability, stability and appearance of the end product. When formulating lipid-based bioactive carrier systems, a reliable and reproducible analysis of their mean diameter, heterogeneity and charge is important. Determination of the average diameter and determination of the size distribution of lipidic nanocarriers are fundamental quality control assays for such products [15]. In this review, the consideration of size and PDI parameters in the formulation and clinical utilization of lipidic nanocarriers are explained. The advantages and restrictions of a number of currently available analytical techniques used to characterize lipid-based nanocarrier formulations are also presented.

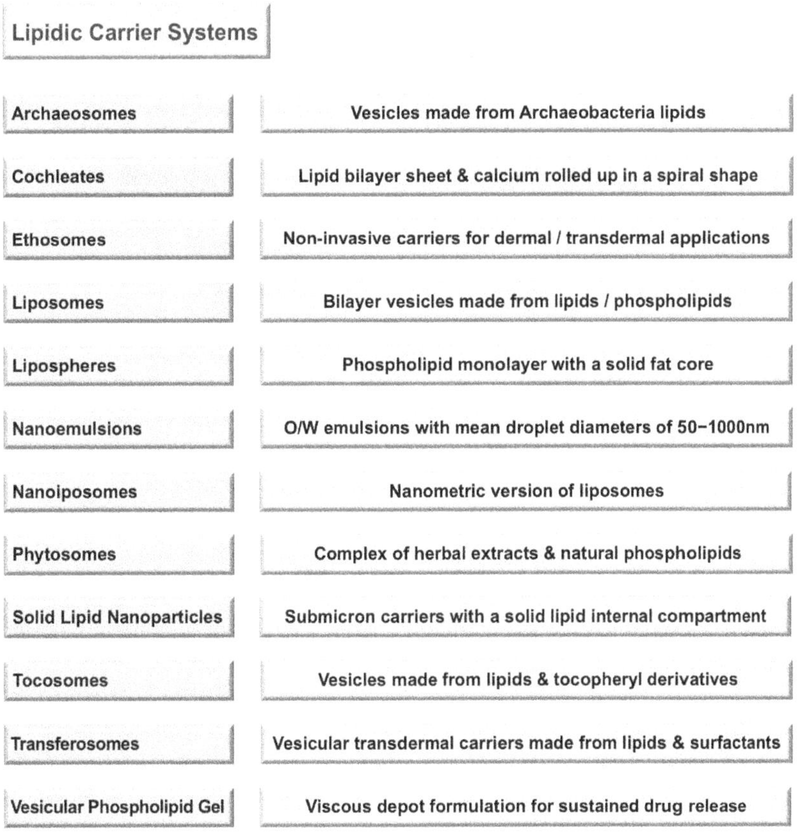

Lipidic Carrier Systems	
Archaeosomes	Vesicles made from Archaeobacteria lipids
Cochleates	Lipid bilayer sheet & calcium rolled up in a spiral shape
Ethosomes	Non-invasive carriers for dermal / transdermal applications
Liposomes	Bilayer vesicles made from lipids / phospholipids
Lipospheres	Phospholipid monolayer with a solid fat core
Nanoemulsions	O/W emulsions with mean droplet diameters of 50–1000nm
Nanoiposomes	Nanometric version of liposomes
Phytosomes	Complex of herbal extracts & natural phospholipids
Solid Lipid Nanoparticles	Submicron carriers with a solid lipid internal compartment
Tocosomes	Vesicles made from lipids & tocopheryl derivatives
Transferosomes	Vesicular transdermal carriers made from lipids & surfactants
Vesicular Phospholipid Gel	Viscous depot formulation for sustained drug release

Figure 1. Main lipidic nanocarrier systems and a concise definition of each.

2. Impact of Particle Size

Different types of lipidic nanocarriers have been applied as drug delivery systems for diagnostic and targeted nanotherapy (employing active or passive targeting mechanisms) to achieve the maximum cellular uptake and therapeutic index [2,16,17]. Nanocarriers can be formulated and processed to differ in terms of composition, size, charge and lamellarity. Techniques such as extrusion, sonication, homogenization and/or freeze-thawing are being employed to control the size and size distribution of different drug carrier systems [1–3]. Continuous physicochemical improvements in the development of the lipid-based nanocarriers may have substantial implications in the cellular uptake and internalization, as well as the bioavailability of the encapsulated therapeutic compound. Particle size is a very critical attribute of lipidic nanocarriers, which affects stability, encapsulation efficiency, drug release profile, bio-distribution, mucoadhesion and cellular uptake [18].

Cellular uptake or internalization is one of the most important physicochemical criteria to be considered prior to in vivo applications. Uptake of small molecules and particles by any cell depends mainly on endocytosis among all other mechanisms (Figure 2). Endocytosis is the process of actively transporting materials into the cell by engulfing them with its phospholipid bilayer using energy in the form of ATP. The two main endocytosis mechanisms are reported to be pinocytosis and phagocytosis [19]. Cellular internalization by phagocytic cells such as macrophages, neutrophils and dendritic cells is mostly achieved by engulfing particles larger than 1 µm [20]. On the other hand, pinocytosis is another mechanism of endocytosis and involves taking extracellular fluids into the cells. Through pinocytosis, the cell can internalize fluids (including dissolved solutes) using a small amount of energy (in the form of ATP). It is mainly associated with particle uptake by the cells via different pathways such as macro-pinocytosis, clathrin-mediated, caveolin-dependent and caveolin-independent pinocytosis, as depicted in Figure 2. The particle size and PDI of nanocarrier systems are the main physicochemical attributes that influence the endocytosis-dependent cellular uptake.

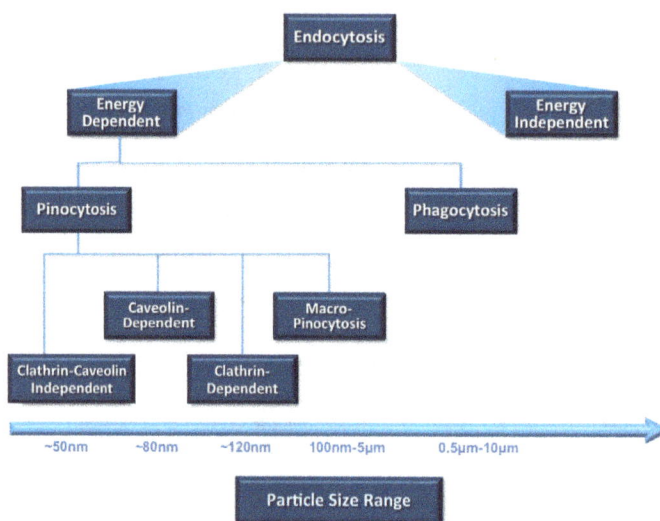

Figure 2. Relative sizes of particles and nanocarriers favourable for cellular uptake and ingestion through different endocytotic pathways. Vesicle size is one of the main parameters that determines clearance by the reticuloendothelial system (RES). The rate of uptake by the immune system cells increases by the increase in the size of the lipidic carriers.

2.1. Impact of Particle Size on Systemic Drug Delivery

It is well documented that the size of drug delivery systems influences pharmacokinetics, tissue distribution and clearance. Certain physiological processes such as hepatic uptake and accumulation, tissue diffusion, tissue extravasation and kidney excretion significantly depend on particle size. Only nanocarriers, including SLN, of a certain size (≤150 nm) are able to enter or exit fenestrated capillaries in the tumour microenvironment or liver endothelium [21,22]. Nanocarriers circulating in normal blood vessels do not easily leave the capillaries that perfuse tissues such as the kidney, lung and heart if they have a diameter range of 100–150 nm [18,22]. However, smaller particles in the size range of 20–100 nm may distribute to bone marrow, spleen and liver sinusoids and may leave the bloodstream via the leaky capillaries of these organs to some extent. It is known that lung alveoli may trap particles of several micrometres in diameter, and the pore size of the pulmonary capillary barrier is estimated to be approximately 35 nm [23]. This pore size is two- to three-times lower than that of the pores within the endothelial lining of kidney capillaries. Glomerulus in the kidneys and islet tissues in the pancreas have smaller pores with diameters around 10–15 nm [24]. Particles with diameters less than 10 nm experience renal filtration via the wall of the glomerular capillary and are not reabsorbed. These tissue and capillary pore size ranges are the reason why most nanocarriers of 50–200 nm in size in their intact form are not able to escape from continuous blood capillaries. Nevertheless, when extravasated from blood vessels (typically via discontinuous capillaries in the bone marrow, liver, spleen and to some extent in the lungs), liposomes and lipidic nanocarriers larger than 100–150 nm can be taken up by phagocytes or remain in these tissues for an extended time [25]. The majority of these phagocytes accumulate in the liver and spleen for subsequent elimination. Once in a tissue, lipidic nanocarriers could be retained because of the capillary pore size or dimensions of the interstitial space of the tissue [26,27].

2.2. Impact of Particle Size on Pulmonary Drug Delivery

Drug administration to human lungs is advantageous for local treatments of diseases such as cystic fibrosis, lung cancer, asthma or other related respiratory distress syndromes. This route can also be applied for systemic delivery of bioactive materials such as peptides and nucleic acids, which are unstable in the gastrointestinal tract, for instance. The advantage of topical drug administration to the lung is the potential of delivering an adequate drug dose to the target site with reduced undesirable extrapulmonary side effects. There are many distinct advantages of lipidic carriers, which make them particularly attractive for drug administration to the lung. These favourable attributes include biocompatibility, ideal specific gravity, targetability and the possibility of producing them in diverse size ranges [28]. The attractiveness of using phospholipid-based carriers (e.g., liposomes and nanoliposomes) as a pulmonary drug delivery system also stems from the fact that phospholipids are naturally-occurring components of lung surfactant and, therefore, should not pose a toxicological risk to this organ [28,29].

When drug carrier systems are intended for inhalation, their size distribution is of primary consideration, since it influences the in vivo fate of the carrier system and the encapsulated therapeutic molecules. It is known that lung deposition of an aerosol depends on its mean aerodynamic particle size, which can also impact the clinical effectiveness of the therapeutic agent [29–32]. It has been postulated that aerosol particle size characteristics can play an important role in avoiding the physiological barriers of the lung, as well as targeting therapeutic compounds to the appropriate pulmonary region [29]. However, it is difficult to predict the actual site of drug deposition, due to the fact that airway calibre and anatomy differ among people. In general, aerosols with a mass median aerodynamic diameter (MMAD) of 5–10 μm are mainly deposited in the large conducting airways and oropharyngeal region [30]. Particles with a 1–5 μm MMAD range are deposited in the small pulmonary airways and alveoli, whereas more than 50% of the particles with 3 μm MMAD are deposited in the alveolar region. In the case of employing the pulmonary route for systemic drug delivery, aerosols with a small average particle size are required to ensure peripheral penetration of the drug [31,32]. Particles smaller than 3 μm have an approximately 80% probability of reaching the lower airways, while around 50–60% of these particles will be deposited in the alveoli [20,29]. On the other hand, nanosized carrier systems have recently gained increasing attention for pulmonary drug delivery. This is due to their advantages for targeted deposition, bioadhesion, sustained release and reduced dosing frequency to improve patient convenience [33,34]. While the most effective particle size for the treatment of systemic diseases has not been determined yet, particles smaller than 150 nm are reported to have delayed lung clearance, increased protein interactions and more transepithelial transport compared to larger particles [33,35].

2.3. Impact of Particle Size on Drug Delivery to Tumours

Particle size is one of the main parameters employed to passively target therapeutic agents to tumours [36]. The tumour vasculature is very different from that of the normal tissues. They are larger in size, more heterogeneous in distribution, have high vascular density and are more permeable and leaky [37]. Consequently, there will be accumulation of vascular mediators at the tumour sites along with the impaired lymphatic drainage of macromolecules. The leaky vasculature of tumours allows accumulation of high molecular weight therapeutics in the tumours. This phenomena is known as the enhanced permeability and retention (EPR) effect, which eventually enables the circulating nanocarriers smaller than around 150 nm to extravasate from circulation through the tumour vasculature and increase the concentration of the chemotherapeutic agents within the tumour [36–38]. However, some literature mentions a size of below 200 nm for passive targeting tumour tissues via EPR [39,40].

It has been reported that decreasing the nanoliposome size to 50 nm in diameter or below greatly reduced mononuclear phagocyte system (MPS)-mediated clearance in mice models and achieved a plasma half-life comparable to that achieved by long-circulating (PEGylated) vesicles with 100–150 nm diameters [41,42]. MPS uptake can be prevented or reduced by saturating the blood circulation with high doses of nanoliposomes containing the encapsulated active compound or by predosing with large quantities of control (empty) nanoliposomes to inhibit phagocytic activity. These strategies may not be effective for clinical applications due to the adverse effects resulting from the destruction of phagocytic functions of the MPS (a natural mechanism to protect the body from pathogenic invasions). Consequently, to avoid MPS uptake and to prolong blood circulation time, most therapeutic nanoliposomes are designed to possess 50–100 nm diameters. For instance, DaunoXome (a nanoliposomal anticancer formulation) consists of 50–80 nm diameter particles intended to reduce MPS uptake [43,44]. Serum protein binding and associated complement-dependent activation are reported to be dependent on nanoliposome size [45]. These two mechanisms together increase the rate of particle clearance in vivo [46]. Nanoliposomes with diameters less than 50–80 nm are subject to significantly lower MPS-dependent clearance in humans. Once PEGylated, vesicles with diameters less than 100–150 nm exhibit reduced plasma protein binding, as well as decreased hepatic and MPS uptake. The presence of PEG polymer coating on the surface of the lipidic carriers has been shown to reduce their uptake by phagocytic cells. As a result, these long-circulating carriers (also known as stealth vesicles) attain longer blood circulation times [45,46].

For the treatment of lung cancer, inhalable nanocarriers have gained more attention in recent years. This is due to their ability to highly associate with therapeutic agents and sustain their release. Moreover, they can be targeted to cancer tissues in the lungs and have the ability to be efficiently transferred into aerosols and highly endure nebulization forces [47]. Lipidic nanocarriers can avoid mucociliary clearance and lung phagocytic mechanisms, thus prolonging the residence of the therapeutic agent within the pulmonary system [48]. The particle size of the aerosol plays a crucial role in specific targeting to different lung regions based on the position of diseased cells within the lung. Larger aerosol particles with diameters of 5–10 µm are principally deposited in oropharynx and large airways, while smaller particles with diameters of 1–5 µm are located in the small airways and alveoli [49]. Nanocarriers in the size range of 100–150 nm display 8–9-times more internalization into lung tumour cells compared to microparticles with a size range of 3–5 µm [50]. Consequently, precise tailoring of aerosol particle size is required to achieve deep lung deposition and the best internalization into the tumour cells.

2.4. Impact of Particle Size on Transdermal Drug Delivery

Transdermal delivery of therapeutic agents involves the application of the formulation to the intact skin and delivery of the drug at a controlled rate locally or to the systemic circulation. As a convenient route of drug administration, transdermal drug delivery has made an important contribution to medical practice. However, it has yet to achieve its full potential as an alternative to oral delivery and hypodermic injections [51]. The mechanisms involved in transdermal drug delivery applications depend on the formulation of nanocarriers; in particular, factors such as chemical composition, surface charge, number of lamella and particle size must be carefully considered. The first studies on exploring the potential use of lipid vesicles in topical applications for the skin were reported in the 1980s [52–54]. Phospholipid vesicles have proven to be useful in the treatment of skin diseases such as psoriasis and skin cancer [55]. Through the utilization of transdermal dosage forms, bioactive compounds can be targeted to the site of the infection or disease and side effects can be kept to a minimum by the prevention of systemic absorption of the drug [56]. The particle size of lipidic vesicles has been shown to have a significant influence on bioactive delivery into the skin [57,58]. Generally, vesicles with a diameter of 600 nm or above are not able to deliver the encapsulated material into deeper layers of the skin. These vesicles are inclined to stay in or on the stratum corneum and may form a lipid layer on the skin after drying [57–59].

Nanovesicles with a diameter of 300 nm or below are able to deliver their contents to some extent into the deeper skin layers. However, nanovesicles with a diameter of 70 nm or below have shown maximum deposition of contents in both viable dermal and epidermal layers [57,59]. Nanoparticles below 6–7 nm in size can be absorbed through the lipidic transepidermal routes, while those with a particle size of below 36 nm can be absorbed through the aqueous pores. Particles in the size range of 10–210 nm, however, may preferentially penetrate through the transfollicular route [60,61]. There are specialized lipid-based encapsulation systems for topical and transdermal drug delivery based on skin penetration enhancement mechanisms and/or certain molecules referred to as "edge activators" [61,62]. They include transfersomes [63], ethosomes [64], solid lipid nanoparticles [65] and the more recently introduced tocosomes [66], a brief definition of which is given in Figure 1 (for a detailed description of these specialized drug delivery systems, see [61–67]).

2.5. Impact of Particle Size on Drug Delivery to Brain

The impermeable characteristic of the blood brain barrier (BBB) has been considered to be the main reason for the failure to achieve therapeutic drug concentrations in the brain tissue. There are fundamental differences between brain capillaries and peripheral capillaries. While peripheral capillaries are fenestrated with gaps up to 50 nm wide, brain capillary endothelial cells are closely connected to each other by tight intercellular junctions and zonulae occludentes [68,69]. The BBB prevents many therapeutic agents, including peptides and medicinal macromolecules, from entering the brain and the rest of the central nervous system (CNS). Consequently, many researchers have tried to overcome the BBB for therapeutic purposes in several different CNS disorders [70,71]. However, these trials have been hampered by limited information on the molecular basis of BBB. A number of therapeutic compounds has proven to be ineffective in the treatment of cerebral diseases due to difficulties to deliver and sustain these drugs within the brain efficiently. As a result, any method that can enhance drug delivery to the brain is of great interest.

In a study aimed at overcoming BBB and targeting brain tumour, Zong et al. [72] prepared doxorubicin-loaded liposomes containing two peptides (TAT and T7) as targeting moieties. The formulation exhibited an improvement in the therapeutic efficacy in the treatment of glioma in animal models as compared to vesicles containing a single targeting moiety and free doxorubicin [72]. Recently, Zhang et al. [73] reported the formulation of PEGylated nanoliposomes within the size range of ca. 93–96 nm, encapsulating two anticancer agents (vincristine and doxorubicin), for the treatment of brain glioma. The nanoliposomes were composed of distearoyl- phosphoethanolamine (DSPE) conjugated with polyethylene glycol (PEG) and two targeting ligands (i.e., T7 and DA7R peptides). The dual targeting strategy resulted in higher therapeutic efficacy as a result of improved drug delivery to the brain of glioma-bearing mice [73]. Another study similarly reported successful drug targeting to brain tumour and overcoming BBB in mice using nanovesicles with a ca. 100-nm average diameter [74]. The approximate particle size range for drug deposition in the brain and some other body organs depending on the dosage form and route of administration are presented in Table 1.

Table 1. Approximate particle size range for drug deposition in various body organs via different dosage forms and routes of administration.

Route of Administration/Dosage Form	Particle Size Range
Lymphatic (RES) *	10–50 nm
Long-circulating carriers (brain, tumour)	50–200 nm
Transdermal	10–600 nm
Intravenous/intramuscular	200–2000 nm
Ocular	100–3000 nm
Aerosol	1–10 μm
Nasal	8–20 μm

* Reticuloendothelial system.

3. Polydispersity Index

The safety and efficacy of therapeutic compounds are limited by inadequate drug delivery to the target tissue or undesired side effects such as severe toxicities in healthy tissues and organs.

Both of these concerns can be addressed by encapsulating the drug inside lipidic nanocarriers with defined and predictable characteristics, which provide maximum bioavailability and minimal side effects. The tendency of lipidic nanocarriers to accumulate in the target tissue depends on their physicochemical characteristics including particle size distribution. Successful formulation of safe, stable and efficient nanocarriers, therefore, requires the preparation of homogenous (monodisperse) populations of nanocarriers of a certain size. However, it is difficult to control the particle size distribution without considering the composition of the nanocarriers and the nature of the solvents and co-solvents used during their preparation [8,75,76]. Following preparation, nanocarriers must be characterized to assure their suitability for in vitro and in vivo applications. With respect to particle size distribution characterization, a parameter used to define the size range of the lipidic nanocarrier systems is called the "polydispersity index" (PDI). The term "polydispersity" (or "dispersity" as recommended by IUPAC) is used to describe the degree of non-uniformity of a size distribution of particles [77,78]. Also known as the heterogeneity index, PDI is a number calculated from a two-parameter fit to the correlation data (the cumulants analysis). This index is dimensionless and scaled such that values smaller than 0.05 are mainly seen with highly monodisperse standards. PDI values bigger than 0.7 indicate that the sample has a very broad particle size distribution and is probably not suitable to be analysed by the dynamic light scattering (DLS) technique (explained more in the next section). Different size distribution algorithms work with data that fall between these two extreme values of PDI (i.e., 0.05–0.7). The calculations used for the determination of size and PDI parameters are defined in the ISO standard documents 13321:1996 E and ISO 22412:2008 [79].

In the field of polymer science, PDI is employed to measure the breadth of the molecular weight distribution (MWD) of the polymer. PDI can be defined as Mw/Mn, where Mw is the weight average and Mn is the number average molecular weight [80,81]. In the fields of molecular science (using chromatography techniques), nanotechnology and nanoparticle research (using light scattering), there are in principle two different aspects of polydispersity, depending on the property of interest. In size exclusion chromatography and gel permeation chromatography, the property of interest is the molecular weight of the sample. The distribution obtained from these techniques is typically a molecular weight distribution describing how much material there is in each of the different molecular weight "segments". When employing the DLS technique, however, the property of interest is the size distribution of molecules, particles or nanovesicles. The distribution describes how many vesicles there are in each of the various size "segments" [77,78].

PDI is basically a representation of the distribution of size populations within a given sample. The numerical value of PDI ranges from 0.0 (for a perfectly uniform sample with respect to the particle size) to 1.0 (for a highly polydisperse sample with multiple particle size populations). Values of 0.2 and below are most commonly deemed acceptable in practice for polymer-based nanoparticle materials [82]. In drug delivery applications using lipid-based carriers, such as liposome and nanoliposome formulations, a PDI of 0.3 and below is considered to be acceptable and indicates a homogenous population of phospholipid vesicles [83–85]. Although the last edition of the FDA's "Guidance for Industry" concerning liposome drug products [86] emphasizes the importance of size and size distribution as "critical quality attributes (CQAs)", as well as essential components of stability studies of these products, it does not mention the criteria for an acceptable PDI. More specific standards and guidelines for the acceptability of product PDI range for different applications (e.g., food, cosmetic, pharmaceutical, etc.) and different routes of bioactive administration need to be set by the regulatory authorities. Figure 3 schematically represents the relationship between the particle size distribution and PDI values.

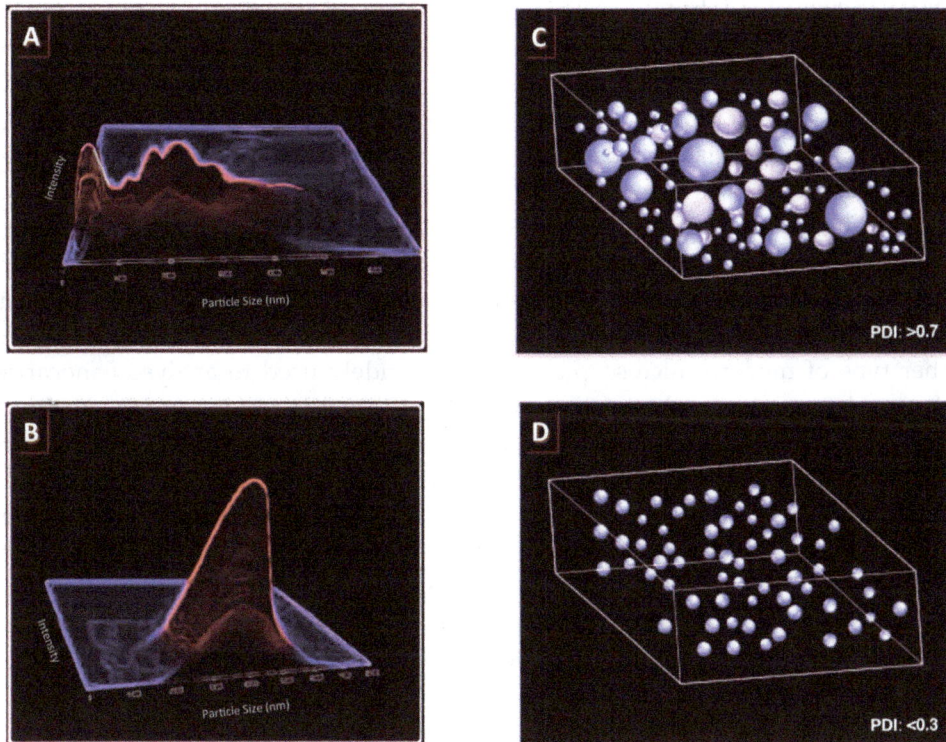

Figure 3. (**A**,**B**) schematic representation of typical particle size graphs indicating a polydisperse sample (composed of heterogeneous population of particles) (**A**); and a monodisperse sample (containing homogenous population of particles) (**B**); (**C**,**D**) representation of the particle size distribution of a sample containing a polydisperse population of particles (with a high PDI value) (**C**); and a sample containing a monodisperse population of particles (with a low PDI value) (**D**).

4. Methods of Analysis

The benefits of the delivery of therapeutics by nano-sized encapsulation systems is an area of much debate, and a better understanding of the possible mechanisms and opportunities to enhance tissue selective uptake could provide clues to obtaining more clinically significant delivery outcomes. Advances in approaches to the preparation of lipidic nanocarriers have provided new opportunities to fine-tune their particle size distributions and PDI. Various techniques of determining the size of the lipidic nanocarriers include microscopy (e.g., optical microscopy, negative stain electron microscopy, cryo-transmission electron microscopy, scanning electron microscopy, confocal microscopy and scanning probe microscopy), diffraction and scattering techniques (laser light scattering and photon correlation spectroscopy) and hydrodynamic techniques (field flow fractionation, gel permeation chromatography, ultracentrifugation and centrifugal sedimentation). The other available techniques for size analysis of nanoliposomal formulations are fluorescence microscopy, coulter counter, flow cytometry and the optical density method [15,77,87–92]. There are many reports on the usefulness of these techniques in providing complementary information regarding liposomes and nanoliposomes, as well as characterization of other lipid-based structures [90–93]. Ideally, methods of characterization of nanocarriers have to be meaningful, reproducible and rapid. Microscopic methods are widely used in order to establish the morphology, lamellarity, surface characteristics, size and stability of nanocarriers. With respect to a statistically meaningful analysis of the size distribution of nanocarrier formulations, methods such as light scattering, which measures the size distribution of a large number of particles in an aqueous sample instantaneously, are more applicable than microscopic techniques [3,91]. DLS is a noninvasive technique, which offers good statistics with respect to the in situ measurements of the size and PDI of nanocarriers, and also, it allows particle sizing down to 1 nm in diameter [15,77,91]. However, it does not provide information regarding the morphology and shape of the lipidic system (e.g., oval, spherical, cylindrical), and it assumes any aggregation of several vesicles as one single particle. Microscopic techniques, on the other hand, give a more detailed view of the morphology of nanostructures. They make direct observation of the sample possible and as such provide information about the shape of the nanocarriers, as well as the presence/absence of any aggregation and/or fusion. Freeze fracture electron microscopy, for instance, can also make it possible to visualize the number of vesicle bilayers (lamellarity) and internal compartments. Some of the main disadvantages of the microscopic techniques, in general, are that the number of particles that can be analysed in the sample is limited and the sample preparation can be tedious. The general approach for the characterization of nanocarrier formulations should hence be to employ as many of the above-mentioned techniques as possible.

Another type of modern microscopic technique, widely used to analyse nanocarriers with high resolution, is scanning probe microscopy (SPM). SPM is a technique for imaging surfaces at the nanometre scale by rastering a fine probe (also known as a tip) across the surface and measuring the repulsive/attractive interactions between the tip and the surface. SPM is a general term comprising a wide variety of techniques based on different interactions between the tip and the surface. These techniques, defined by the type of interaction being measured, include atomic force microscopy (AFM), scanning tunnelling microscopy (STM), magnetic force microscopy (MFM), electrostatic force microscopy (EFM) and Kelvin probe force microscopy (KPFM). Unlike most of the other microscopic techniques, scanning probe microscopes do not require extensive sample preparation procedures [90,94,95]. SPM techniques can be used to study nanostructures in air or solution at ambient conditions with simple sample preparation procedures. The majority of other microscopic techniques involve sample manipulation procedures such as staining, labelling, fixation or vacuum, which may cause some alterations in the structure and/or size of the lipidic nanocarriers [88,96].

Small-angle X-ray scattering (SAXS) is another technique by which nanoscale density differences in a sample can be quantified. This method can determine size distributions and resolve the size and shape of (monodisperse) nanocarrier samples. SAXS provides complementary information about folding and unfolding of macromolecules in addition to extended conformations, flexibly linked domains, aggregation/fusion of particles, shape and assembly state of samples in solution, at the resolution range of approximately 10 A–50 A, without the size limitations encountered in the electron microscopy methods and NMR [97].

There are some other analytical techniques, which make the assessment of size and PDI of single individual nanocarriers, possible. One of these methods is "scanning ion occlusion sensing" (SIOS), which is a nanopore-based technology that can be used for single-particle analysis [98]. SIOS analyses lipid-based nanocarriers in the size range of 60 nm to a few micrometres [99]. The operation mechanism of SIOS is based on the conventional Coulter counter, where individual particles are measured as they traverse a nanopore. When an individual particle or vesicle passes through the tuneable nanopore, a current reduction occurs due to an increase in the electrical resistance. The extent of current reduction and the frequency of the pulses are related to the particle size and concentration of the nanocarrier sample, respectively. Particles are driven either by electrophoresis and electroosmosis or by pressure generated from a pressure module [100,101]. SIOS is a useful method to analyse multiple parameters of nanocarriers on a particle-by-particle basis. This technique has proven to possess higher resolution in comparison with techniques such as dynamic light scattering. Furthermore, SIOS was successfully used to measure changes in the size and surface charge of phospholipid vesicles as a result of incubation in plasma [98,100]. There are still some limitations and issues that need to be improved with SIOS analysis. For instance, it is problematic to choose a suitable elastic pore for polydisperse samples to avoid detecting several particles at the same time. Moreover, it is still difficult to detect only one particle at the time, and the data acquired with different nanopore sizes cannot be compared in parallel [101].

An established method for the assessment of a single nanocarrier diameter and size distribution is flow cytometry (FCM). This technology is widely employed in analysing and sorting cells, bacteria, and other cell-sized particles. FCM has been applied in the analysis of multilamellar and large unilamellar vesicles (MLV and LUV) [102]. It employs light scattering to measure particles and vesicles in a continuous flow system. Samples have to be fluorescently labelled in order to be distinguished from the impurities and noise signal. Consequently, the scattered light at a 10° angle, or side scattered light at a 90° angle, or the fluorescence of the sample is measured. FCM is a very quick, reliable, robust and reproducible method. However, when employing light scattering detection, its operation can be disturbed by noisy signals from buffers, optics or electronics [98,101,102].

Nanoparticle tracking analysis (NTA) is another technology that is able to track and measure a single nanocarrier moving under Brownian motion [103]. NTA is a high-resolution method and effective at measuring the size, size distribution and concentration of liposome and nanoliposome samples. It can be employed to measure the size of the vesicles and particles within a size range of 30–1000 nm [104]. For NTA analysis, samples are injected into the special cell and then illuminated by laser light (635 nm) that passes through a liquid layer on the optical surface [104,105]. Refraction occurs, and the region in which the lipid-based nanocarriers are present is illuminated and visualized under the microscope. A charge-coupled camera records a video (30 frames per second) in which the motion of nanocarriers (Brownian motion) could be observed. Computer software identifies and tracks the centre of each object throughout the length of the video and relates it to the size of the vesicles. The hydrodynamic size and size distribution of the nanocarriers can be calculated by the Stokes–Einstein equation using a particle diffusion coefficient. This method enables measurement of the size of both monodisperse and polydisperse samples. Furthermore, it is able to measure the surface charge of the lipid-based carriers and detect their fluorescence signals. The drawbacks of NTA method, however, include its requirement for complex optimization by a skilled operator and the difficulty to identify an appropriate concentration of the sample. Furthermore, characterization employing the NTA technique can be hindered by the refractive index of the sample [106,107].

5. Conclusions

The use of lipid-based nanocarriers in medicinal and non-medicinal formulations has been reported mainly at laboratory scales, and many resulting nanomedicines are in the transition phase towards clinical applications. Trends of the global market have been indicating strong growth of the nanotherapy sector in the next few years. The translation of nanomedicines to the clinical phase and subsequent commercialization requires research, development and characterization of new formulations to ensure the quality, safety and efficacy of such products. Size variations of nanocarrier systems over time must be seriously considered when formulating encapsulated therapeutic agents. Nanocarrier formulations with a constant and narrow size distribution are necessary to achieve optimum clinical outcomes. Moreover, particle size and size distribution are important factors for evaluating the stability of a colloidal dosage form upon storage. The size stability issue is more crucial for nanosystems than for microscale drug delivery systems. This is due to the fact that nanosystems have a large specific surface area compared to microsystems. A number of available techniques for the evaluation of the size and PDI of nanocarriers were described in this entry along with their advantages and limitations. The regulatory agencies will benefit from information on the performance of novel or modified particle characterization techniques, which can be applied to the research and development of the current and next generation of nanotherapeutic agents.

Funding: This research did not receive any specific grant from funding agencies in the public, commercial or not-for-profit sectors.

References

1. Mozafari, M.R. Liposomes: An overview of manufacturing techniques. *Cell. Mol. Biol. Lett.* **2005**, *10*, 711–719. [PubMed]

2. Maherani, B.; Arab-Tehrany, E.; Mozafari, M.R.; Gaiani, C.; Linder, M. Liposomes: A review of manufacturing techniques and targeting strategies. *Curr. Nanosci.* **2011**, *7*, 436–452. [CrossRef]

3. Mozafari, M.R.; Mortazavi, S.M. *Nanoliposomes: From Fundamentals to Recent Developments*; Trafford Pub. Ltd.: Oxford, UK, 2005.

4. Sharma, D.; Ali, A.A.; Trivedi, L.R. An Updated Review on: Liposomes as drug delivery system. *PharmaTutor* **2018**, *6*, 50–62. [CrossRef]

5. Amoabediny, G.; Haghiralsadat, F.; Naderinezhad, S.; Helder, M.N.; Akhoundi Kharanaghi, E.; Mohammadnejad Arough, J.; Zandieh-Doulabi, B. Overview of preparation methods of polymeric and lipid-based (niosome, solid lipid, liposome) nanoparticles: A comprehensive review. *Int. J. Poly. Mater. Poly. Biomater.* **2018**, *67*, 383–400. [CrossRef]

6. Tian, W.; Schulze, S.; Brandl, M.; Winter, G. Vesicular phospholipid gel-based depot formulations for pharmaceutical proteins: Development and in vitro evaluation. *J. Control. Release* **2010**, *142*, 319–325. [CrossRef] [PubMed]

7. Breitsamer, M.; Winter, G. Needle-free injection of vesicular phospholipid gels—A novel approach to overcome an administration hurdle for semisolid depot systems. *J. Pharm. Sci.* **2017**, *106*, 968–972. [CrossRef] [PubMed]

8. Mozafari, M.R.; Danaei, M.; Javanmard, R.; Raji, M.; Maherani, B. Nanoscale Lipidic Carrier Systems: Importance of Preparation Method and Solvents. *Glob. J. Nano* **2017**, *2*, 555593.

9. Nomura, S.I.; Yoshikawa, Y.; Yoshikawa, K.; Dannenmuller, O.; Chasserot-Golaz, S.; Ourisson, G.; Nakatani, Y. Towards Proto-Cells: "Primitive" Lipid Vesicles Encapsulating Giant DNA and Its Histone Complex. *ChemBioChem* **2001**, *2*, 457–459. [CrossRef]

10. Monnard, P.A.; Luptak, A.; Deamer, D.W. Models of primitive cellular life: Polymerases and templates in liposomes. *Philos. Trans. R. Soc. B Biol. Sci.* **2007**, *362*, 1741–1750. [CrossRef] [PubMed]

11. Rasti, B.; Erfanian, A.; Selamat, J. Novel nanoliposomal encapsulated omega-3 fatty acids and their applications in food. *Food Chem.* **2017**, *230*, 690–696. [CrossRef] [PubMed]

12. Rasti, B.; Jinap, S.; Mozafari, M.R.; Abd-Manap, M.Y. Optimization on preparation condition of polyunsaturated fatty acids nanoliposome prepared by Mozafari method. *J. Liposome Res.* **2014**, *24*, 99–105. [CrossRef] [PubMed]

13. Rasti, B.; Jinap, S.; Mozafari, M.R.; Yazid, A.M. Comparative study of the oxidative and physical stability of liposomal and nanoliposomal polyunsaturated fatty acids prepared with conventional and Mozafari methods. *Food Chem.* **2012**, *135*, 2761–2770. [CrossRef] [PubMed]

14. Livney, Y.D. Nanostructured delivery systems in food: Latest developments and potential future directions. *Curr. Opin. Food. Sci.* **2015**, *3*, 125–135. [CrossRef]

15. Maherani, B.; Wattraint, O. Liposomal structure: A comparative study on light scattering and chromatography techniques. *J. Dispers. Sci. Technol.* **2017**, *38*, 1633–1639. [CrossRef]

16. Aveling, E.; Zhou, J.; Lim, Y.F.; Mozafari, M.R. Targeting lipidic nanocarriers: Current strategies and problems. *Pharmakeftiki* **2006**, *19*, 101–109.

17. Kirpotin, D.B.; Drummond, D.C.; Shao, Y.; Shalaby, M.R.; Hong, K.; Nielsen, U.B.; Marks, J.D.; Benz, C.C.; Park, J.W. Antibody targeting of long-circulating lipidic nanoparticles does not increase tumor localization but does increase internalization in animal models. *Cancer Res.* **2006**, *66*, 6732–6740. [CrossRef] [PubMed]

18. Bahari, L.A.; Hamishehkar, H. The impact of variables on particle size of solid lipid nanoparticles and nanostructured lipid carriers; a comparative literature review. *Adv. Pharm. Bull.* **2016**, *6*, 143. [CrossRef] [PubMed]

19. Sadat, S.M.; Jahan, S.T.; Haddadi, A. Effects of size and surface charge of polymeric nanoparticles on in vitro and in vivo applications. *J. Biomater. Nanobiotechnol.* **2016**, *7*, 91. [CrossRef]

20. Zhao, F.; Zhao, Y.; Liu, Y.; Chang, X.; Chen, C.; Zhao, Y. Cellular uptake, intracellular trafficking, and cytotoxicity of nanomaterials. *Small* **2011**, *7*, 1322–1337. [CrossRef] [PubMed]

21. Blasi, P.; Giovagnoli, S.; Schoubben, A.; Ricci, M.; Rossi, C. Solid lipid nanoparticles for targeted brain drug delivery. *Adv. Drug Deliv. Rev.* **2007**, *59*, 454–477. [CrossRef] [PubMed]

22. Bertrand, N.; Leroux, J.C. The journey of a drug-carrier in the body: An anatomo-physiological perspective. *J. Control. Release* **2012**, *161*, 152–163. [CrossRef] [PubMed]

23. Townsley, M.I.; Parker, J.C.; Longenecker, G.L.; Perry, M.L.; Pitt, R.M.; Taylor, A.E. Pulmonary embolism: Analysis of endothelial pore sizes in canine lung. *Am. J. Physiol. Heart Circ. Physiol.* **1988**, *255*, H1075–H1083. [CrossRef] [PubMed]

24. Choi, C.H.; Zuckerman, J.E.; Webster, P.; Davis, M.E. Targeting kidney mesangium by nanoparticles of defined size. *Proc. Natl. Acad. Sci. USA* **2011**, *108*, 6656–6661. [CrossRef] [PubMed]

25. Kraft, J.C.; Freeling, J.P.; Wang, Z.; Ho, R.J. Emerging research and clinical development trends of liposome and lipid nanoparticle drug delivery systems. *J. Pharm. Sci.* **2014**, *103*, 29–52. [CrossRef] [PubMed]

26. Sarin, H. Physiologic upper limits of pore size of different blood capillary types and another perspective on the dual pore theory of microvascular permeability. *J. Angiogenes. Res.* **2010**, *2*, 14. [CrossRef] [PubMed]

27. Ogawa, S.; Ota, Z.; Shikata, K.; Hironaka, K.; Hayashi, Y.; Ota, K.; Kushiro, M.; Miyatake, N.; Kishimoto, N.; Makino, H. High-resolution ultrastructural comparison of renal glomerular and tubular basement membranes. *Am. J. Nephrol.* **1999**, *19*, 686–693. [CrossRef] [PubMed]

28. Mozafari, M.R.; Reed, C.J.; Rostron, C. Development of non-toxic liposomal formulations for gene and drug delivery to the lung. *Technol. Health Care* **2002**, *10*, 342–344.

29. Labiris, N.R.; Dolovich, M.B. Pulmonary drug delivery. Part I: Physiological factors affecting therapeutic effectiveness of aerosolized medications. *Br. J. Clin. Pharmacol.* **2003**, *56*, 588–599. [CrossRef] [PubMed]

30. Gerrity, T.R. Pathophysiological and disease constraints on aerosol deposition. In *Respiratory Drug Delivery*; Byron, P.R., Ed.; CRC Press Inc.: Boca Raton, FL, USA, 1990; pp. 1–38.

31. Effros, R.M. Measurements of pulmonary epithelial permeability in vivo. *Am. Rev. Respir.* **1983**, *127*, S59–S65.

32. Folkesson, H.G.; Westrom, B.R.; Karlsson, B.W. Permeability of the respiratory tract to different-sized macromolecules after intratracheal instillation in young and adult rats. *Acta Physiol.* **1990**, *139*, 347–354. [CrossRef] [PubMed]

33. Rytting, E.; Nguyen, J.; Wang, X.; Kissel, T. Biodegradable polymeric nanocarriers for pulmonary drug delivery. *Exp. Opin. Drug Deliv.* **2008**, *5*, 629–639. [CrossRef] [PubMed]

34. Gaul, R.; Ramsey, J.M.; Heise, A.; Cryan, S.A.; Greene, C.M. Nanotechnology approaches to pulmonary drug delivery: Targeted delivery of small molecule and gene-based therapeutics to the lung. In *Design of Nanostructures for Versatile Therapeutic Applications*; Elsevier Inc.: Amsterdam, The Netherlands, 2018; pp. 221–253.

35. Chow, A.H.; Tong, H.H.; Chattopadhyay, P.; Shekunov, B.Y. Particle engineering for pulmonary drug delivery. *Pharm. Res.* **2007**, *24*, 411–437. [CrossRef] [PubMed]

36. Mozafari, M.R.; Pardakhty, A.; Azarmi, S.; Jazayeri, J.A.; Nokhodchi, A.; Omri, A. Role of nanocarrier systems in cancer nanotherapy. *J. Liposome Res.* **2009**, *19*, 310–321. [CrossRef] [PubMed]

37. Aw-Yong, P.Y.; Gan, P.H.; Sasmita, A.O.; Mak, S.T.; Ling, A.P. Nanoparticles as carriers of phytochemicals: Recent applications against lung cancer. *Int. J. Res. Biomed. Biotechnol.* **2018**, *7*, 1–11.

38. Greish, K.; Fang, J.; Inutsuka, T.; Nagamitsu, A.; Maeda, H. Macromolecular therapeutics. *Clin. Pharmacokinet.* **2003**, *42*, 1089–1105. [CrossRef] [PubMed]

39. Maeda, H. Toward a full understanding of the EPR effect in primary and metastatic tumors as well as issues related to its heterogeneity. *Adv. Drug Deliv. Rev.* **2015**, *91*, 3–6. [CrossRef] [PubMed]

40. Caracciolo, G. Clinically approved liposomal nanomedicines: Lessons learned from the biomolecular corona. *Nanoscale* **2018**, *10*, 4167–4172. [CrossRef] [PubMed]

41. Gabizon, A.A.; Barenholz, Y.; Bialer, M. Prolongation of the circulation time of doxorubicin encapsulated in liposomes containing a polyethylene glycol-derivatized phospholipid: Pharmacokinetic studies in rodents and dogs. *Pharm. Res.* **1993**, *10*, 703–708. [CrossRef] [PubMed]

42. Proffitt, R.T.; Williams, L.E.; Presant, C.A.; Tin, G.W.; Uliana, J.A.; Gamble, R.C.; Baldeschwieler, J.D. Tumor-imaging potential of liposomes loaded with In-111-NTA: Biodistribution in mice. *J. Nucl. Med.* **1983**, *24*, 45–51. [PubMed]

43. Rocha, M.; Chaves, N.; Bao, S. Nanobiotechnology for Breast Cancer Treatment. In *Breast Cancer-From Biology to Medicine*; InTech: Winchester, UK, 2017. [CrossRef]

44. Sun, Q.; Zhou, Z.; Qiu, N.; Shen, Y. Rational design of cancer nanomedicine: Nanoproperty integration and synchronization. *Adv. Mater.* **2017**, *29*. [CrossRef] [PubMed]

45. Tefas, L.R.; Sylvester, B.; Tomuta, I.; Sesarman, A.; Licarete, E.; Banciu, M.; Porfire, A. Development of antiproliferative long-circulating liposomes co-encapsulating doxorubicin and curcumin, through the use of a quality-by-design approach. *Drug Des. Dev. Ther.* **2017**, *11*, 1605–1621. [CrossRef] [PubMed]

46. Li, M.; Shi, F.; Fei, X.; Wu, S.; Wu, D.; Pan, M.; Luo, S.; Gu, N.; Dou, J. PEGylated long-circulating liposomes deliver homoharringtonine to suppress multiple myeloma cancer stem cells. *Exp. Biol. Med.* **2017**, *242*, 996–1004. [CrossRef] [PubMed]

47. Beck-Broichsitter, M.; Merkel, O.M.; Kissel, T. Controlled pulmonary drug and gene delivery using polymeric nano-carriers. *J. Control. Release* **2012**, *161*, 214–224. [CrossRef] [PubMed]

48. Abdelaziz, H.M.; Gaber, M.; Abd-Elwakil, M.M.; Mabrouk, M.T.; Elgohary, M.M.; Kamel, N.M.; Kabary, D.M.; Freag, M.S.; Samaha, M.W.; Mortada, S.M.; et al. Inhalable particulate drug delivery systems for lung cancer therapy: Nanoparticles, microparticles, nanocomposites and nanoaggregates. *J. Control. Release* **2018**, *269*, 374–392. [CrossRef] [PubMed]

49. Gagnadoux, F.; Hureaux, J.; Vecellio, L.; Urban, T.; Le Pape, A.; Valo, I.; Montharu, J.; Leblond, V.; Boisdron-Celle, M.; Lerondel, S.; et al. Aerosolized chemotherapy. *J. Aerosol Med. Pulm. Drug Deliv.* **2008**, *21*, 61–70. [CrossRef] [PubMed]

50. Gratton, S.E.; Ropp, P.A.; Pohlhaus, P.D.; Luft, J.C.; Madden, V.J.; Napier, M.E.; DeSimone, J.M. The effect of particle design on cellular internalization pathways. *Proc. Natl. Acad. Sci. USA* **2008**, *105*, 11613–11618. [CrossRef] [PubMed]

51. Prausnitz, M.R.; Langer, R. Transdermal drug delivery. *Nat. Biotechnol.* **2008**, *26*, 1261–1268. [CrossRef] [PubMed]

52. Mezei, M.; Gulasekharam, V. Liposomes—A selective drug delivery system for the topical route of administration, I. Lotion dosage form. *Life Sci.* **1980**, *26*, 1473–1477. [CrossRef]

53. Mezei, M.; Gulasekharam, V. Liposomes—A selective drug delivery system for the topical route of administration: II. gel dosage form. *J. Pharm. Pharmacol.* **1982**, *34*, 473–474. [CrossRef] [PubMed]

54. Ho, N.F.; Ganesan, M.G.; Weiner, N.D.; Flynn, G.L. Mechanisms of topical delivery of liposomally entrapped drugs. *J. Control. Release* **1985**, *2*, 61–65. [CrossRef]

55. Vanic, Z.; Holaeter, A.M.; Skalko-Basnet, N. (Phospho) lipid-based nanosystems for skin administration. *Curr. Pharm. Des.* **2015**, *21*, 4174–4192. [CrossRef] [PubMed]

56. Du Plessis, J.; Ramachandran, C.; Weiner, N.; Muller, D.G. The influence of particle size of liposomes on the deposition of drug into skin. *Int. J. Pharm.* **1994**, *103*, 277–282. [CrossRef]

57. Verma, D.D.; Verma, S.; Blume, G.; Fahr, A. Particle size of liposomes influences dermal delivery of substances into skin. *Int. J. Pharm.* **2003**, *258*, 141–151. [CrossRef]

58. Verma, D.D.; Verma, S.; Blume, G.; Fahr, A. Liposomes increase skin penetration of entrapped and non-entrapped hydrophilic substances into human skin: A skin penetration and confocal laser scanning microscopy study. *Eur. J. Pharm. Biopharm.* **2003**, *55*, 271–277. [CrossRef]

59. Hua, S. Lipid-based nano-delivery systems for skin delivery of drugs and bioactives. *Front. Pharmacol.* **2015**, *6*, 219. [CrossRef] [PubMed]

60. Geusens, B.; Strobbe, T.; Bracke, S.; Dynoodt, P.; Sanders, N.; Van Gele, M.; Lambert, J. Lipid-mediated gene delivery to the skin. *Eur. J. Pharm. Sci.* **2011**, *43*, 199–211. [CrossRef] [PubMed]

61. Zeb, A.; Qureshi, O.S.; Kim, H.S.; Cha, J.H.; Kim, H.S.; Kim, J.K. Improved skin permeation of methotrexate via nanosized ultradeformable liposomes. *Int. J. Nanomed.* **2016**, *11*, 3813.

62. Benson, H.A. Transdermal drug delivery: Penetration enhancement techniques. *Curr. Drug Deliv.* **2005**, *2*, 23–33. [CrossRef] [PubMed]

63. Jain, A.K.; Kumar, F. Transfersomes: Ultradeformable vesicles for transdermal drug delivery. *Asian J. Biomater. Res.* **2017**, *3*, 1–3.

64. Yang, L.; Wu, L.; Wu, D.; Shi, D.; Wang, T.; Zhu, X. Mechanism of transdermal permeation promotion of lipophilic drugs by ethosomes. *Int. J. Nanomed.* **2017**, *12*, 3357. [CrossRef] [PubMed]

65. Gul, R.; Ahmed, N.; Shah, K.U.; Khan, G.M.; Rehman, A.U. Functionalised nanostructures for transdermal delivery of drug cargos. *J. Drug Target.* **2018**, *26*, 110–122. [CrossRef] [PubMed]

66. Mozafari, M.R.; Javanmard, R.; Raji, M. Tocosome: Novel drug delivery system containing phospholipids and tocopheryl phosphates. *Int. J. Pharm.* **2017**, *528*, 381–382. [CrossRef] [PubMed]

67. Reddy, Y.D.; Sravani, A.B.; Ravisankar, V.; Prakash, P.R.; Reddy, Y.S.; Bhaskar, N.V. Transferosomes a novel vesicular carrier for transdermal drug delivery system. *J. Innov. Pharm. Biol. Sci.* **2015**, *2*, 193–208.

68. Lesniak, M.S.; Brem, H. Targeted therapy for brain tumours. *Nat. Rev. Drug Discov.* **2004**, *3*, 499–508. [CrossRef] [PubMed]

69. Trompetero, A.; Gordillo, A.; del Pilar, M.C.; Cristina, V.; Bustos Cruz, R.H. Alzheimer's Disease and Parkinson's Disease: A Review of Current Treatment Adopting a Nanotechnology Approach. *Curr. Pharm. Des.* **2018**, *24*, 22–45. [CrossRef] [PubMed]

70. Pardridge, W.M. Drug and gene targeting to the brain with molecular Trojan horses. *Nat. Rev. Drug Discov.* **2002**, *1*, 131–139. [CrossRef] [PubMed]

71. Miller, G. Drug targeting. Breaking down barriers. *Science* **2002**, *297*, 1116–1118. [CrossRef] [PubMed]

72. Zong, T.; Mei, L.; Gao, H.; Cai, W.; Zhu, P.; Shi, K.; Chen, J.; Wang, Y.; Gao, F.; He, Q. Synergistic dual-ligand doxorubicin liposomes improve targeting and therapeutic efficacy of brain glioma in animals. *Mol. Pharm.* **2014**, *11*, 2346–2357. [CrossRef] [PubMed]

73. Zhang, Y.; Zhai, M.; Chen, Z.; Han, X.; Yu, F.; Li, Z.; Xie, X.; Han, C.; Yu, L.; Yang, Y.; et al. Dual-modified liposome codelivery of doxorubicin and vincristine improve targeting and therapeutic efficacy of glioma. *Drug Deliv.* **2017**, *24*, 1045–1055. [CrossRef] [PubMed]

74. Liu, C.; Liu, X.N.; Wang, G.L.; Hei, Y.; Meng, S.; Yang, L.F.; Yuan, L.; Xie, Y. A dual-mediated liposomal drug delivery system targeting the brain: Rational construction, integrity evaluation across the blood–brain barrier, and the transporting mechanism to glioma cells. *Int. J. Nanomed.* **2017**, *12*, 2407–2425. [CrossRef] [PubMed]

75. Bulbake, U.; Doppalapudi, S.; Kommineni, N.; Khan, W. Liposomal formulations in clinical use: An updated review. *Pharmaceutics* **2017**, *9*, 12. [CrossRef] [PubMed]

76. Dong, Y.D.; Tchung, E.; Nowell, C.; Kaga, S.; Leong, N.; Mehta, D.; Kaminskas, L.M.; Boyd, B.J. Microfluidic preparation of drug-loaded PEGylated liposomes, and the impact of liposome size on tumour retention and penetration. *J. Liposome Res.* **2017**, 1–9. [CrossRef] [PubMed]

77. Nobbmann, U.L. Polydispersity–What Does It Mean for DLS and Chromatography. 2014. Available online: http://www.materials-talks.com/blog/2014/10/23/polydispersity-what-does-it-mean-for-dls-and-chromatography/ (accessed on 14 March 2018).

78. Bera, B. Nanoporous silicon prepared by vapour phase strain etch and sacrificial technique. In Proceedings of the International Conference on Microelectronic Circuit and System (Micro), Kolkata, India, 11–12 July 2015; pp. 42–45.

79. Worldwide, M.I. *Dynamic Light Scattering, Common Terms Defined*; Inform White Paper; Malvern Instruments Limited: Malvern, UK, 2011; pp. 1–6.

80. Rane, S.S.; Choi, P. Polydispersity index: How accurately does it measure the breadth of the molecular weight distribution? *Chem. Mater.* **2005**, *17*, 926. [CrossRef]

81. Gooch, J.W. Polydispersity. In *Encyclopedic Dictionary of Polymers*; Springer: New York, NY, USA, 2011; p. 556.

82. Clarke, S. Development of Hierarchical Magnetic Nanocomposite Materials for Biomedical Applications. Ph.D. Thesis, Dublin City University, Northside, Dublin, 2013.

83. Badran, M. Formulation and in vitro evaluation of flufenamic acid loaded deformable liposome for improved skin delivery. *Digest J. Nanomater. Biostruct.* **2014**, *9*, 83–91.

84. Chen, M.; Liu, X.; Fahr, A. Skin penetration and deposition of carboxyfluorescein and temoporfin from different lipid vesicular systems: In vitro study with finite and infinite dosage application. *Int. J. Pharm.* **2011**, *408*, 223–234. [CrossRef] [PubMed]

85. Putri, D.C.; Dwiastuti, R.; Marchaban, M.; Nugroho, A.K. Optimization of mixing temperature and sonication duration in liposome preparation. *J. Pharm. Sci. Commun.* **2017**, *14*, 79–85. [CrossRef]

86. FDA—Liposome Drug Products; Chemistry, Manufacturing, and Controls; Human Pharmacokinetics and Bioavailability; Labeling Documentation. *Guidance for Industry*; April 2018 Pharmaceutical Quality/CMC.; U.S. Department of Health and Human Services Food and Drug Administration Center for Drug Evaluation and Research (CDER): Silver Spring, MD, USA, 2018.

87. Shekunov, B.Y.; Chattopadhyay, P.; Tong, H.H.; Chow, A.H. Particle size analysis in pharmaceutics: Principles, methods and applications. *Pharm. Res.* **2007**, *24*, 203–227. [CrossRef] [PubMed]

88. Ozer, A.Y. Applications of light and electron microscopic techniques in liposome research. In *Nanomaterials and Nanosystems for Biomedical Applications*; Springer: Dordrecht, The Netherlands, 2007; pp. 145–153.

89. Jones, M.N. The surface properties of phospholipid liposome systems and their characterisation. *Adv. Colloid Interface Sci.* **1995**, *54*, 93–128. [CrossRef]

90. Mozafari, M.R.; Reed, C.J.; Rostron, C.; Hasirci, V. A review of scanning probe microscopy investigations of liposome-DNA complexes. *J. Liposome Res.* **2005**, *15*, 93–107. [CrossRef] [PubMed]

91. Mozafari, M.R.; Reed, C.J.; Rostron, C. Prospects of anionic nanolipoplexes in nanotherapy: Transmission electron microscopy and light scattering studies. *Micron* **2007**, *38*, 787–795. [CrossRef] [PubMed]

92. Negussie, A.H.; Yarmolenko, P.S.; Partanen, A.; Ranjan, A.; Jacobs, G.; Woods, D.; Bryant, H.; Thomasson, D.; Dewhirst, M.W.; Wood, B.J.; et al. Formulation and characterisation of magnetic resonance imageable thermally sensitive liposomes for use with magnetic resonance-guided high intensity focused ultrasound. *Int. J. Hyperth.* **2011**, *27*, 140–155. [CrossRef] [PubMed]

93. Mozafari, M.R. Nanoliposomes: Preparation and analysis. In *Liposomes*; Humana Press: New York, NY, USA, 2010; pp. 29–50.

94. Jiang, Y.; Genin, G.M.; Pryse, K.M.; Elson, E.L. Atomic force microscopy of phase separation on ruptured, giant unilamellar vesicles. *BioRxiv* **2018**, 250944. [CrossRef]

95. Hasegawa, Y. Scanning Tunneling Microscopy. In *Compendium of Surface and Interface Analysis*; Springer: Singapore, 2018; pp. 599–604.

96. Khosravi-Darani, K.; Pardakhty, A.; Honarpisheh, H.; Rao, V.M.; Mozafari, M.R. The role of high-resolution imaging in the evaluation of nanosystems for bioactive encapsulation and targeted nanotherapy. *Micron* **2007**, *38*, 804–818. [CrossRef] [PubMed]

97. Putnam, C.D.; Hammel, M.; Hura, G.L.; Tainer, J.A. X-ray solution scattering (SAXS) combined with crystallography and computation: Defining accurate macromolecular structures, conformations and assemblies in solution. *Q. Rev. Biophys.* **2007**, *40*, 191–285. [CrossRef] [PubMed]

98. Chen, C.; Zhu, S.; Huang, T.; Wang, S.; Yan, X. Analytical techniques for single-liposome characterization. *Anal. Methods* **2013**, *5*, 2150–2157. [CrossRef]

99. Henriquez, R.R.; Ito, T.; Sun, L.; Crooks, R.M. The resurgence of Coulter counting for analyzing nanoscale objects. *Analyst* **2004**, *129*, 478–482. [CrossRef] [PubMed]

100. Yang, L.; Broom, M.F.; Tucker, I.G. Characterization of a nanoparticulate drug delivery system using scanning ion occlusion sensing. *Pharm. Res.* **2012**, *29*, 2578–2586. [CrossRef] [PubMed]

101. Kanasova, M.; Nesmerak, K. Systematic review of liposomes' characterization methods. *Monatshefte Chem. Chem. Mon.* **2017**, *148*, 1581–1593. [CrossRef]

102. Chen, C.; Zhu, S.; Wang, S.; Zhang, W.; Cheng, Y.; Yan, X. Multiparameter Quantification of Liposomal Nanomedicines at the Single-Particle Level by High-Sensitivity Flow Cytometry. *ACS Appl. Mater. Interfaces* **2017**, *9*, 13913–13919. [CrossRef] [PubMed]

103. Saveyn, H.; De Baets, B.; Thas, O.; Hole, P.; Smith, J.; Van Der Meeren, P. Accurate particle size distribution determination by nanoparticle tracking analysis based on 2-D Brownian dynamics simulation. *J. Colloid Interface Sci.* **2010**, *352*, 593–600. [CrossRef] [PubMed]

104. Filipe, V.; Hawe, A.; Jiskoot, W. Critical evaluation of Nanoparticle Tracking Analysis (NTA) by NanoSight for the measurement of nanoparticles and protein aggregates. *Pharm. Res.* **2010**, *27*, 796–810. [CrossRef] [PubMed]

105. Reshetov, V.; Zorin, V.; Siupa, A.; D'Hallewin, M.A.; Guillemin, F.; Bezdetnaya, L. Interaction of liposomal formulations of meta–tetra (hydroxyphenyl) chlorin (Temoporfin) with serum proteins: Protein Binding and Liposome Destruction. *Photochem. Photobiol.* **2012**, *88*, 1256–1264. [CrossRef] [PubMed]

106. De Morais Ribeiro, L.N.; Couto, V.M.; Fraceto, L.F.; de Paula, E. Use of nanoparticle concentration as a tool to understand the structural properties of colloids. *Sci. Rep.* **2018**, *8*, 982. [CrossRef] [PubMed]

107. Gioria, S.; Caputo, F.; Urban, P.; Maguire, C.M.; Bremer-Hoffmann, S.; Prina-Mello, A.; Calzolai, L.; Mehn, D. Are existing standard methods suitable for the evaluation of nanomedicines: Some case studies. *Nanomedicine* **2018**, *13*, 539–554. [CrossRef] [PubMed]

9

Skull Bone Regeneration Using Chitosan–Siloxane Porous Hybrids—Long-Term Implantation

Yuki Shirosaki [1],* (iD), Motomasa Furuse [2], Takuji Asano [3], Yoshihiko Kinoshita [3] and Toshihiko Kuroiwa [2] (iD)

[1] Faculty of Engineering, Kyushu Institute of Technology, 1-1 Sensui-cho, Tobata-ku, Kitakyushu 804-8550, Japan

[2] Department of Neurosurgery, Osaka Medical College, 2-7 Daigaku-machi, Takatsuki, Osaka 569-8686, Japan; neu054@poh.osaka-med.ac.jp (M.F.); neu040@poh.osaka-med.ac.jp (T.K.)

[3] Nikkiso Co., Ltd., Ebisu, Shibuya-ku, Tokyo 150-6022, Japan; takuji.asano@nikkiso.co.jp (T.A.); y.kinoshita@nikkiso.co.jp (Y.K.)

* Correspondence: yukis@che.kyutech.ac.jp

Abstract: Burr holes in craniotomy are not self-repairing bone defects. To regenerate new bone at the sites of these defects, a good scaffold is required. Biodegradable hybrids including silica or siloxane networks have been investigated as bone tissue scaffolds. This study examined skull bone regeneration using chitosan-siloxane hybrids after long-term implantation (two and three years). After implantation of the hybrids, the surrounding cells migrated and formed fibrous tissues and blood vessels. Then, bone formation occurred from the surrounding blood vessels. Addition of calcium ions and coating with hydroxyapatite improved bone regeneration. Finally, the regenerated tissue area became smaller than the initial hole, and some areas changed to completed bone tissues.

Keywords: skull bone regeneration; chitosan-siloxane porous hybrid; long-term implantation

1. Introduction

"Burr holes" are required in craniotomy to insert surgical tools for neurological and brain surgeries [1–3]. They often leave undesirable indentations in the area, and patients are unsatisfied after surgery, even in areas where there is abundant coverage by hair. To cover the holes, various materials have been used, such as metallic plates [4,5], hydroxyapatite buttons [6–9], calcium phosphate cements [10–12], and acrylic cements [13,14]. Chronic pain is caused by metallic plates, and thinning of the skin also occurs, leading to extrusion of the plate [15,16]. Moreover, the metallic plates interfere with magnetic resonance imaging. In the case of acrylic cement, irritation is caused by the exothermic heat of polymerization [13,14]. Hydroxyapatite buttons are good candidates for burr holes because of their osteocompatibility. However, they are not flexible, and it is difficult to adjust their shapes to the defects during the operation. Calcium phosphate cements are also compatible with bone formation, but they also have the risks of leakage into the brain before hardening because of their delayed setting time [17]. Thus far, many biomaterials have been used for facial bone regeneration [18].

Biodegradable organic-inorganic hybrids have been investigated as bone tissue scaffolds because of their controllable degradation and flexibility. Many studies have reported that hybrids including silica or silicate improve osteocompatibility and bone formation [19]. Hybrids with siloxane networks have also been investigated for their ability to promote bone formation. However, in vivo examination has been insufficient to clarify the effect of their structure on bone regeneration.

In previous studies [20–24], we investigated a chitosan-γ-glycidoxypropyltrimethoxysilane (GPTMS) hybrid prepared by the sol-gel method. The human osteosarcoma cell line MG63 adhered and proliferated on the hybrid membranes and showed high alkaline phosphatase activity compared with the chitosan membrane [20,21]. Moreover, human osteoblast bone marrow cells differentiated and formed a fibrillar extracellular matrix with numerous calcium phosphate globules [21]. MG63 cells also migrated and proliferated into the pores of porous hybrids prepared from the same sols [22]. These results indicate that hybrids have the potential for use as bone tissue scaffolds. We also prepared chitosan-GPTMS porous hybrids with hydroxyapatite (HAp) by soaking in an alkaline phosphate solution and observed skull bone formation in vivo [24]. The blood from burr holes infiltrated the pores and prevented overflowing. No inflammation occurred, calcium ions were incorporated into the hybrids, and the hydroxyapatite modified on their surfaces accelerated new bone formation during one year, however, the bone formation was not yet completed.

In this study, we observed bone formation in long-term implantations, i.e., for two and three years, to clarify the potential of chitosan–siloxane hybrids for skull bone regeneration.

2. Materials and Methods

2.1. Preparation of Porous Hybrids

The porous hybrids were prepared by previously published methods [24]. Chitosan (0.5 g, high molecular weight, deacetylation: 79.0%, Aldrich®, St. Louis, MO, USA) was dissolved in aqueous acetic acid (0.25 M, 25 mL). GPTMS (Lancaster, Lancashire, UK) and calcium chloride (Nacalai Tesque, Kyoto, Japan) were added to the chitosan solution to provide a molar ratios of chitosan-GPTMS (ChG) of 1.0:0.5 and chitosan-GPTMS-CaCl$_2$ (ChGCa) of 1.0:0.5:1.0. One mole of chitosan equates to one mole of deacetylated amino groups. The mixtures were stirred for 1 h at room temperature, and fractions of each resultant sol were poured into a polystyrene container and frozen at $-20\,^{\circ}$C for 24 h. The frozen sols were then transferred to a freeze dryer (FDU-506, EYELA, Tokyo, Japan) for 12 h until dry. The obtained porous ChG and ChGCa hybrids were then washed with NaOH (0.25 M) and distilled water to neutralize the remaining acetic acid and lyophilized again. Some ChGCa hybrids were not washed with NaOH but were soaked in aqueous Na$_2$HPO$_4$ (0.01 M, pH 8.8) at 80 $^{\circ}$C for 3 days (ChGCa_HAp). The hybrids were then washed with distilled water and lyophilized again. The compressive strength was measured by a creep meter (RE2-3305C, YAMADEN Co., Ltd., Tokyo, Japan). The compressive test was carried out at 0.5 mm/s to calculate the compressive stress at a 50% strain rate.

2.2. In Vivo Animal Experiments

The hybrids were sterilized by the ethylene oxide gas method and maintained for one week at room temperature to clear any ethylene oxide gas remnants. All surgical procedures were performed with the approval of the animal care and use committee of Osaka Medical College (Approval No. 26044). In brief, eight adult female beagles weighing around 10 kg were anesthetized with a mask, using isoflurane (Abbott, Tokyo, Japan) in oxygen. Tracheal intubation was performed after anesthesia induction. Anesthesia was maintained by isoflurane in oxygen delivered via a calibrated vaporizer (TEC3, Ohmeda, UK). The beagles were cleaned and draped in a standard manner with a longitudinal incision made over the scalp, and the pericranium was lifted off with a sharp periosteal elevator. Then, four 10 mm burr holes were created in each beagle dog using a drill to evacuate the liquefied hematoma. After evacuation of the hematoma, a small wound was created on the dura mater, and the hybrids were inserted into each burr hole. Commercial bone cement was also implanted as a control. The periosteal and skin were sutured. All of the above surgical procedures were performed in a sterile manner. Specimens of the parietal bones, including the cranioplasty, were harvested and examined histologically. After fixation in 10% buffered formaldehyde, the specimens were dehydrated in a series of ethanol solutions and soaked in xylene for defatting. Subsequently, the specimens were decalcified, and thin sections were prepared by a microtome and stained with hematoxyline-eosine (HE) and Azan-Mallory (AM) method. The AM staining method is commonly used to distinguish cells from extracellular components and stains muscle fibers red, while cartilage and bone matrix are stained blue [25].

3. Results and Discussion

The defect size (10 mm) is critical in the beagle dog skull and remains even after seven years, indicating slow self-healing. Figure 1 shows the appearance of the skull implanted with samples after three years. All beagles survived and no infection or auto-mutilation were observed. No inflammation was also observed visually. The dura mater recovered after implantation in all samples. The commercial bone cement performed the same as the hybrids after one year from the implantation [24], and the interface between the bone cement and bone tissue was very clear. Chitosan hybrids (ChG, ChGCa, and ChGCa_HAp) did not remain the same, and new tissues regenerated. In the case of the hybrids, the holes became smaller compared to their initial size, and a hollow in the implanted site was observed. The implanted site of ChGCa_HAp was harder than that of ChG and ChGCa upon palpation.

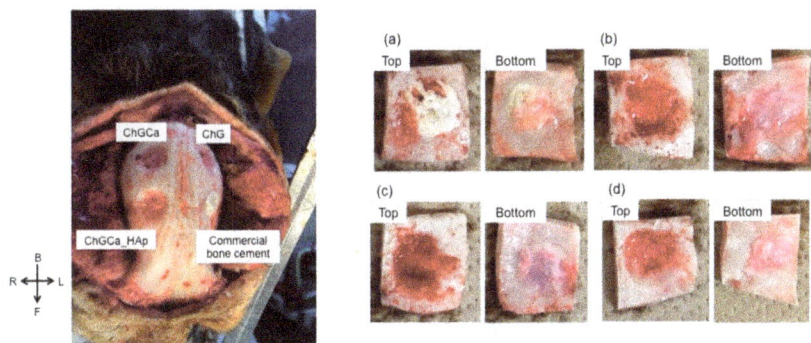

Figure 1. Photographs of Beagle skulls implanted with the samples after three years. On the left, the general appearance of a skull is shown, and, on the right, the appearance of each implanted position is shown. (**a**) commercial bone cement; (**b**) chitosan–γ-glycidoxypropyltrimethoxysilane (GPTMS) (ChG); (**c**) chitosan–GPTMS–CaCl$_2$ (ChGCa); and (**d**) chitosan–GPTMS with hydroxyapatite (HAp) (ChGCa_HAp).

Figures 2–8 show the histological results postoperatively. The commercial bone cement did not change the bone defect size even after three years, as shown in Figure 2. At the bottom of the cement, fibrous tissues had regenerated to reconstruct the dura mater. The bone cement inhibited the regeneration of new tissues, and the top of the implanted site was still open.

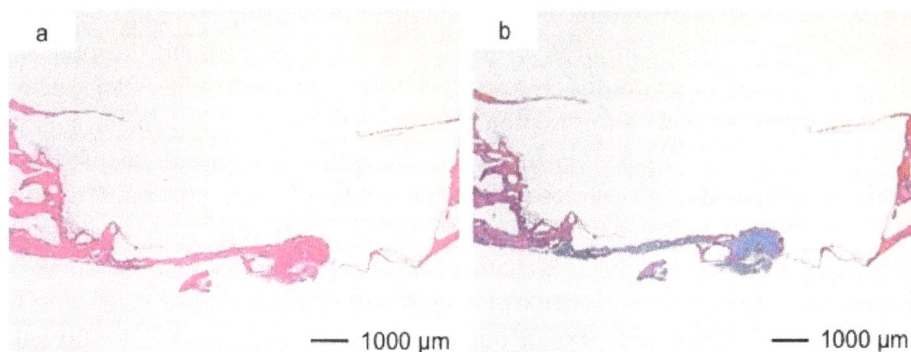

Figure 2. Light microscopic images of the commercial bone cement in cranioplasty at three years postoperatively stained by hematoxyline–eosine (HE) (**a**) and Light microscopic images of the commercial bone cement in cranioplasty at three years postoperatively stained by Azan-Mallory (AM) method (**b**).

Porous hybrid materials had degraded completely and were substituted by fibrous and bone tissues after one year [24]. No defect was observed at the implanted site in histological images (Figures 3–8), such as those observed in sites implanted with the commercial bone cement. The regenerated tissues in ChG and ChGCa implantations were about 1 mm in thickness, and the thickness did not increase after theee years (Figures 3–6). There were many blood vessels (*) with havers canals in the newly formed tissue, and osteoid tissue formation and new bone matrix ($\rightarrow$) were observed around the blood vessels. The defect size of ChG (Figures 3 and 4) and ChGCa (Figures 5 and 6) implantations did not change between two and three years after implantation. The formation of new bone matrix in the osteoid tissues of the ChGCa implantation was much more accelerated than that in the site of the ChG implantation. New bone formation occurred even in the middle and upper area of the implanted site (Figure 5c).

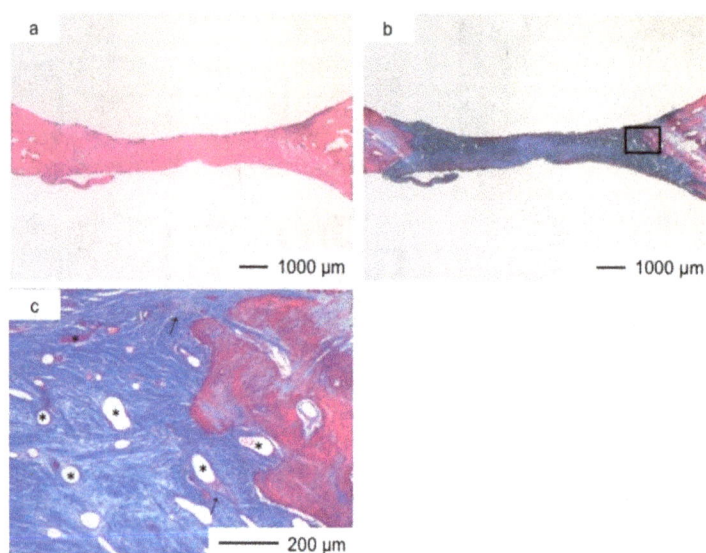

Figure 3. Light microscopic images of ChG in cranioplasty two years after implantation, stained by HE (**a**); and AM (**b**); (**c**) Magnification of the inset in (**b**).

In previous studies [20,21], we confirmed that human osteosarcoma cells and bone marrow cells proliferated on or into a chitosan–siloxane hybrid (ChG) and showed good alkaline phosphate activity. Other studies have reported that porous chitosan has healing properties [26,27] because it takes up wound exudates and forms blood vessels to promote tissue regeneration. In general, connective tissue regeneration follows fibroblast proliferation and extracellular matrix synthesis [28]. Connective tissues regenerated at the implanted sites of chitosan-siloxane hybrids. Tissue regeneration induced by the hybrids occurred as follows; (1) blood filtrated into the pores of the hybrids; (2) fibroblast proliferation was stimulated in the hybrids; (3) fibroblasts synthesized extracellular matrix; (4) blood vessels formed in the regenerated tissues; (5) osteoblasts in the tissues secreted osteoid; (6) osteoid became mineralized to form new bone tissues. Soluble silica and calcium ions stimulate bone growth [29]. The silicon species released from the hybrids also affect osteoblast differentiation [30] and lead to osteoid production in ChG. The higher new bone formation of ChGCa depends on calcium ions released from the hybrids. However, the connective tissues size was unchanged, indicating that calcium ions released from the hybrids promoted the formation of new bone matrix by the osteoblasts in the connective tissue.

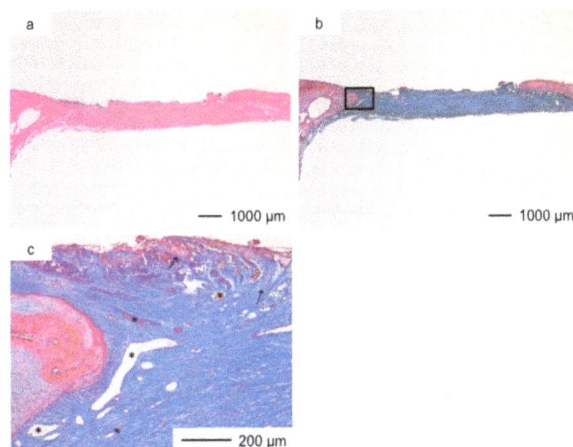

Figure 4. Light microscopic images of ChG in cranioplasty three years after implantation, stained by HE (**a**) and Light microscopic images of ChG in cranioplasty three years after implantation, stained by AM (**b**); (**c**) Magnification of the inset in (**b**).

The thickness of the tissues regenerated by ChGCa_HAp increased, and the defected size became smaller. The thicknesses after two and three years were about 1.5 and 2.0 mm, respectively (Figures 7 and 8). High new bone formation in osteoid tissues was found in ChGCa_HAp implantations. Not only the pre-existing bone tissues migrated to the implanted site, but also new bone formation (★) occurred in the newly formed tissues (Figure 8c,d). ChGCa_HAp has low crystalline needle-like apatite deposits on the surface of pores [31]. The low crystalline apatite dissolves in vivo, and the released calcium and phosphate ions accelerate bone formation. As a result, bone formation in the ChGCa_HAp implantation was observed in the connective tissue. The decrease in the defect size indicated that the surrounding bone also migrated into the hybrids.

Although the defects were filled by the newly generated tissue with blood vessels, osteoid, and new bone formation, and the size became smaller, even ChGCa_HAp could not achieve completed bone formation after three years. Engler et al. showed that the elasticity of materials affects mesenchymal stem cell differentiation [32]. Soft matrices are neurogenic, stiffer matrices are myogenic, and rigid matrices induce osteogenesis. In this study, ChGCa_HAp (compressive stress: 0.099 ± 0.007 MPa) was more rigid than the other hybrids (ChG: 0.024 ± 0.008 MPa; ChGCa: 0.034 ± 0.007 MPa). However, it was not stiffer than the natural skull bone. To form completed new bone earlier, the hybrid stiffness should be controlled by crosslinking between chitosan, GPTMS, and hydroxyapatite deposits.

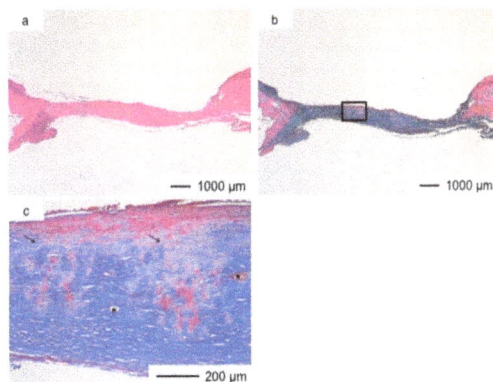

Figure 5. Light microscopic images of ChGCa in cranioplasty two years after implantation, stained by HE (**a**) and Light microscopic images of ChGCa in cranioplasty two years after implantation, stained by AM (**b**); (**c**) Magnification of the inset in (**b**).

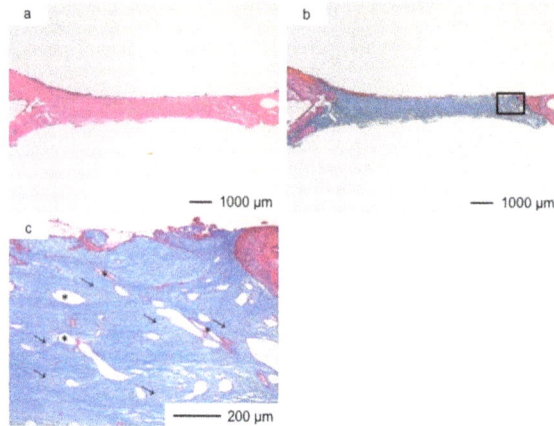

Figure 6. Light microscopic images of ChGCa in cranioplasty three years after implantation, stained by HE (**a**) and Light microscopic images of ChGCa in cranioplasty three years after implantation, stained by AM (**b**); (**c**) Magnification of the inset in (**b**).

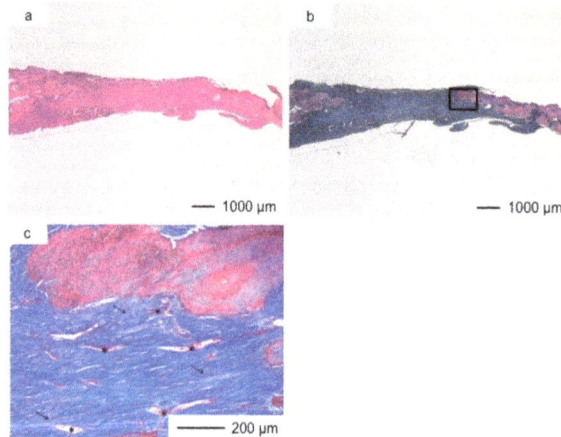

Figure 7. Light microscopic images of ChGCa_HAp in cranioplasty two years after implantation, stained by HE (**a**) and Light microscopic images of ChGCa_HAp in cranioplasty two years after implantation, stained by AM (**b**); (**c**) Magnification of the inset in (**b**).

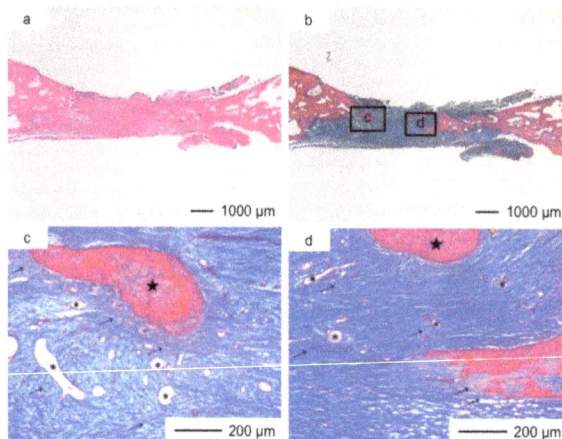

Figure 8. Light microscopic images of ChGCa_HAp in cranioplasty three years after implantation, stained by HE (**a**) and Light microscopic images of ChGCa_HAp in cranioplasty three years after implantation, stained by AM (**b**); (**c**,**d**) Magnifications of the insets in (**b**).

4. Conclusions

Long-term skull bone regeneration was observed using chitosan–siloxane porous hybrids. After two and three years from implantation, commercial bone cement was still present. The hybrids were substituted with new regenerated tissues that were completely closed the holes. Incorporated calcium ions and the inclusion of hydroxyapatite accelerated the new bone formation. However, the thickness of the regenerated skull bone was lower than the normal thickness, and depressions were observed. The results in this study may facilitate the design of new bone tissue scaffolds using hybrids including siloxane units.

Author Contributions: Y.S. conceived and designed the project, performed the experiments, analyzed data, interpreted the results, and prepared the manuscript. M.F., T.A. and Y.K. performed the experiments and interpreted the results. T.K. interpreted the results.

Acknowledgments: This work was supported by the programs in "Improvement of Research Environment for Young Researchers (Kojinsenbatsu)", Ministry of Education Culture, Sports, Science and Technology (MEXT), and the Foundation for the Promotion Ion Engineering.

References

1. Sanan, A.; Haines, S.J. Repairing holes in the head: A history of cranioplasty. *Neurosurgery* **1997**, *40*, 588–603. [PubMed]
2. Czirjak, S.; Szeifert, G.T. Surgical experience with frontolateral keyhole craniotomy through a superciliary skin incision. *Neurosurgery* **2001**, *48*, 145–150. [PubMed]
3. Lindert, E.V.; Perneczky, A.; Fries, G.; Pierangeli, E. The supraorbital keyhole approach to supratentorial aneurysms; concept and technique. *Surg. Neurol.* **1998**, *49*, 481–490. [CrossRef]
4. Karl-Dieter, L. Reliability of cranial flap fixation techniques: Comparative experimental evaluation of suturing, titanium miniplates, and a new rivet-like titanium clamp (CranioFix). *Neurosurgery* **1999**, *44*, 902–905.
5. Ohata, K.; Haque, M.; Tsuruno, T.; Morino, M.; Soares, S.B., Jr.; Hakuda, A. Craniotomy repair with titanium miniplates. *J. Clin. Neurosci.* **1998**, *5*, 81–86. [CrossRef]
6. Waite, P.D.; Morawetz, R.B.; Zeiger, E.; Pincock, J.L. Reconstruction of cranial defects with porous hydroxyapatite blocks. *Neurosurgery* **1989**, *25*, 214–217. [CrossRef] [PubMed]
7. Yamashita, T. Reconstruction of surgical skull defects with hydroxyapatite ceramic buttons and granules. *Acta Neurochir.* **1988**, *90*, 157–162. [CrossRef]
8. Kobayashi, S.; Hara, H.; Okudera, H.; Takemae, T.; Sugita, K. Usefulness of ceramic implants in neurosurgery. *Neurosurgery* **1987**, *21*, 751–755. [CrossRef] [PubMed]
9. Easwer, H.V.; Rajeev, A.; Varma, H.K.; Vijayan, S.; Bhattacharya, R.N. Cosmetic and radiological outcome following the use of synthetic hydroxyapatite porous-dense bilayer burr-hole buttons. *Acta Neurochir.* **2007**, *149*, 481–485. [CrossRef] [PubMed]
10. Dujovny, M.; Aviles, A.; Agner, C. An innovative approach for cranioplasty using hydroxyapatite cement. *Surg. Neurol.* **1997**, *48*, 294–297. [CrossRef]
11. Constantino, P.D.; Friedman, C.D.; Jones, K.; Chow, L.C.; Sisson, G.A. Experimental hydroxyapatite cement cranioplasty. *Plat. Reconstr. Surg.* **1992**, *90*, 174–185. [CrossRef]
12. Verheggen, R.; Merten, H.A. Correction of skull defects using hydroxyapatite cement (HAC)—Evidence derived from animal experiments and clinical experience. *Acta Neurochir.* **2001**, *143*, 919–926. [CrossRef] [PubMed]
13. Cabanela, M.E.; Coventry, M.D.; MacCarty, C.S.; Miller, W.E. The fate of patients with methyl methacrylate cranioplasty. *J. Bone Joint Surg.* **1972**, *54*, 278–281. [CrossRef] [PubMed]
14. Linder, L. Tissue reaction to methyl methacrylate monomer: A comparative study in the rabbit's ear on the toxicity of methyl metacrylate of varying composition. *Acta Orthop. Scand.* **1976**, *47*, 3–9. [CrossRef] [PubMed]

15. Yoon, S.H.; Burm, J.S.; Yang, W.Y.; Kang, S.Y. Vascularized bipedicled pericranial flaps for reconstruction of chronic scalp ulcer occurring after cranioplasty. *Arch. Plast. Surg.* **2013**, *40*, 341–347. [CrossRef] [PubMed]

16. Sanus, G.Z.; Tanriverdi, T.; Ulu, M.O.; Kafadar, A.M.; Tanriover, N.; Ozien, F. Use of Cortoss as an alternative material in calvarial defects: The first clinical results in cranioplasty. *J. Craniofac. Surg.* **2008**, *19*, 88–95. [CrossRef] [PubMed]

17. Nakano, M.; Hirano, N.; Ishihara, H.; Kawaguchi, Y.; Matsuura, K. Calcium phosphate cement leakage after percutaneous vertebroplasty for osteoporotic vertebral fractures: Risk factor analysis for cement leakage. *J. Neurosurg.* **2005**, *2*, 27–33. [CrossRef] [PubMed]

18. Cicciù, M.; Cervino, G.; Herford, A.S.; Famà, F.; Bramanti, E.; Fiorillo, L.; Lauritano, F.; Sambataro, S.; Troiano, G.; Laino, L. Facial bone reconstruction using both marine or non-marine bone substitutes: Evaluation of current outcomes in a systematic literature review. *Mar. Drugs* **2018**, *16*, 27. [CrossRef] [PubMed]

19. Jones, J.R. Reprint of: Review of bioactive glass: From Hench to hybrids. *Acta Biomater.* **2015**, *23*, S58–S82. [CrossRef] [PubMed]

20. Shirosaki, Y.; Tsuru, K.; Hayakawa, S.; Osaka, A.; Lopes, M.A.; Santos, J.D.; Fernandes, M.H. Cytocompatibility of MG63 cells on chitosan-organosiloxane hybrid membranes. *Biomaterials* **2005**, *26*, 485–493. [CrossRef] [PubMed]

21. Shirosaki, Y.; Tsuru, K.; Hayakawa, S.; Osaka, A.; Lopes, M.A.; Santos, J.D.; Costa, M.A.; Fernandes, M.H. Physical, chemical and in vitro biological profile of chitosan hybrid membrane as a function of organosiloxane concentration. *Acta Biomater.* **2009**, *5*, 346–355. [CrossRef] [PubMed]

22. Shirosaki, Y.; Okayama, T.; Tsuru, K.; Hayakawa, S.; Osaka, A. Synthesis and cytocompatibility of porous chitosan-silicate hybrids for tissue engineering scaffold application. *Chem. Eng. J.* **2008**, *137*, 122–128. [CrossRef]

23. Shirosaki, Y. Preparation of organic-inorganic hybrids with silicate network for the medical applications. *J. Ceram. Soc. Jpn.* **2012**, *120*, 555–559. [CrossRef]

24. Shirosaki, Y.; Furuse, M.; Asano, T.; Kinoshita, Y.; Miyazaki, T.; Kuroiwa, T. Use of chitosan-siloxane porous hybrid scaffold as novel burr hole covers. *Lett. Appl. NanoBioSci.* **2016**, *5*, 342–345.

25. Kiernan, J.A. *Histological and Histochemical Methods. Theory and Practice*; Cold Spring Harbor Laboratory Press: Bloxham, UK, 2008.

26. Ueno, H.; Mori, T.; Fujinaga, T. Topical formulations and wound healing applications of chitosan. *Adv. Drug Deliv. Rev.* **2001**, *52*, 102–115. [CrossRef]

27. Ueno, H.; Yamada, H.; Tanaka, I.; Kaba, N.; Matsuura, M.; Okumura, M.; Kadosawa, T.; Fujinaga, T. Accelerating effects of chitosan for healing at early phase of experimental open wound in dogs. *Biomaterials* **1999**, *20*, 1407–1414. [CrossRef]

28. Ueno, H.; Nakamura, F.; Murakami, M.; Okumura, M.; Kadosawa, T.; Fujinaga, T. Evaluation effects of chitosan for the extra-cellular matrix production by fibroblasts and the growth factors production by macrophages. *Biomaterials* **2001**, *22*, 2125–2130. [CrossRef]

29. Xynos, I.D.; Edgar, A.J.; Buttery, L.D.K.; Hench, L.L.; Polak, J.K. Ionic products on bioactive glass dissolution increase proliferation of human osteoblasts and induce insulin-like growth factor II mRNA expression and protein synthesis. *Biochem. Biophys. Res. Commun.* **2000**, *276*, 461–465. [CrossRef] [PubMed]

30. Shirosaki, Y.; Tsuru, K.; Moribayashi, H.; Hayakawa, S.; Nakamura, Y.; Gibson, I.R.; Osaka, A. Preparation of osteocompatible Si(IV)-enriched chitosan-silicate hybrids. *J. Ceram. Soc. Jpn.* **2010**, *118*, 989–992. [CrossRef]

31. Shirosaki, Y.; Okamoto, K.; Hayakawa, S.; Osaka, A.; Asano, T. Preparation of porous chitosan-siloxane hybrids coated with hydroxyapatite particles. *BioMed Res. Int.* **2014**. [CrossRef] [PubMed]

32. Engler, A.J.; Sen, S.; Sweeney, H.L.; Discher, D.E. Matrix elasticity directs stem cell lineage specification. *Cell* **2006**, *126*, 677–689. [CrossRef] [PubMed]

10

Formulation, Development, and In Vitro Evaluation of a CD22 Targeted Liposomal System Containing a Non-Cardiotoxic Anthracycline for B Cell Malignancies

Nivesh K. Mittal [1],*(ID), Bivash Mandal [1], Pavan Balabathula [1,2], Saini Setua [2], Dileep R. Janagam [1], Leonard Lothstein [3], Laura A. Thoma [2] and George C. Wood [2]

[1] Plough Center for Sterile Drug Delivery Solutions, University of Tennessee Health Science Center, Memphis, TN 38163, USA; bmandal@uthsc.edu (B.M.); bpavan18@gmail.com (P.B.); dileep.janagam@gmail.com (D.R.J.)

[2] Department of Pharmaceutical Sciences, College of Pharmacy, University of Tennessee Health Science Center, Memphis, TN 38163, USA; ssetua@uthsc.edu (S.S.); lthoma@uthsc.edu (L.A.T.); gwood@uthsc.edu (G.C.W.)

[3] Department of Pathology, College of Medicine, University of Tennessee Health Science Center, Memphis, TN 38163, USA; llothstein@uthsc.edu

* Correspondence: nmittal@uthsc.edu

Abstract: Doxorubicin cardiotoxicity has led to the development of superior chemotherapeutic agents such as AD 198. However, depletion of healthy neutrophils and thrombocytes from AD 198 therapy must be limited. This can be done by the development of a targeted drug delivery system that delivers AD 198 to the malignant cells. The current research highlights the development and in vitro analysis of targeted liposomes containing AD 198. The best lipids were identified and optimized for physicochemical effects on the liposomal system. Physiochemical characteristics such as size, ζ-potential, and dissolution were also studied. Active targeting to CD22 positive cells was achieved by conjugating anti-CD22 Fab' to the liposomal surface. Size and ζ-potential of the liposomes was between 115 and 145 nm, and -8 to -15 mV. 30% drug was released over 72 h. Higher cytotoxicity was observed in CD22+ve Daudi cells compared to CD22$-$ve Jurkat cells. The route of uptake was a clathrin- and caveolin-independent pathway. Intracellular localization of the liposomes was in the endolysosomes. Upon drug release, apoptotic pathways were activated partly by the regulation of apoptotic and oncoproteins such as caspase-3 and c-myc. It was observed that the CD22 targeted drug delivery system was more potent and specific compared to other untargeted formulations.

Keywords: AD 198; B-cell malignancy; liposome; nanoparticle; CD22 targeting

1. Introduction

Nanomedicines have seen significant advancements in the past few decades and have been actively pursued as a means of providing alternative drug delivery systems for disease targeted therapies. In 1995, Doxil® established the foundation for the potential of nanomedicines being approved by the United States Food and Drug Administration (FDA) [1]. Since then there has been a rapid increase in research on nanoparticulate drug delivery systems [2]. This has led to the FDA's approval of Abraxane® [3], DaunoXome® [4] and most recently, Marquibo® [5,6]. Nanoparticles have provided researchers with the tools to overcome some of the drawbacks of conventional drug delivery systems, most common of which are adverse effects due to non-specific actions of the drug or the drug delivery system [7,8]. Specific binding nature of ligands can be exploited to target these types of drug carriers to the target tissues or cells [9–14]. Antibodies are one such type of ligand that can be conjugated to nanoparticles to aid in targeted drug delivery. Liposomes are by far one of the most commonly used of the nanoparticulate drug delivery systems, commercially and in clinical trials [15–17]. Liposomes are biodegradable in nature and are versatile in the drug that can be carried as well as the ligands that can be conjugated to their surface for targeted drug delivery [18,19].

Cancer therapy is one field in which researchers have been consistently exploring for breakthroughs using nanotechnology as their primary tool for targeted drug delivery [20,21]. Current medications are still not sufficient to treat the numerous variations of cancers [21], primarily because each variation of cancer needs customized therapies for each patient [20]. Nanotechnology is an adaptable science that can be used to create tailor-made drug delivery systems for specific malignancies.

B cell malignancies are a type of hematological malignancy that have almost 80,000 new cases every year and claim the lives of almost a third of these [22,23]. The standard therapy for B cell malignancies is CHOP [24], of which doxorubicin is an integral part. The treatment of hematological malignancies presents considerable differences from solid cancers in that a large population of the cancer cells are circulating. In a previous review [25] we had discussed the potential of nanoparticles, such as targeted liposomes, being utilized for targeted therapies for B cell cancers. Drug delivery scientists have worked towards the development of a targeted nanoparticulate system for the treatment of B cell cancers [11,13,14,23,26–31]. Most of these groups have utilized doxorubicin [11,14,23,32,33] or vincristine [5,6,34] as the drug of choice. Although nanoparticulate systems for both these drugs are already approved by the FDA [1,6], significant enhancements are still needed in view of the adverse effects associated with the non-specific action of the drug delivery system [20] as well as the inherent toxicity of the drug [35]. This has supported the use of novel molecules that would exhibit more desirable properties than currently approved drugs.

Several strategies have been investigated to reduce adverse effects such as the cardiotoxic potential of doxorubicin. One strategy is designing less toxic anthracycline analogues such as epirubicin and idarubicin. However, these analogues only succeeded in delaying cardiotoxic events to higher doses, later stages of therapy or by producing lesser acute cardiotoxicity [36–38]. Valrubicin however, is one anthracycline analogue which lacks cardiotoxicity [39]. N-Benzyladriamycin-14-valerate (AD 198) is another anthracycline that displays no dose-dependent cardiotoxic properties along with an added cardioprotective action from the damage caused by doxorubicin [40–42]. It is a protein kinase C (PKC) activating agent that displays superiority over doxorubicin [41]. It functions by a completely different mechanism of action compared to doxorubicin which has been or is under study by four groups, Cekanova et al., Xie et al., He et al. and Lothstein et al. [40,43–45]. AD 198 does not display any significant organ toxicities and is less myelosuppressive compared to doxorubicin [39]. Myelosuppression, even in reduced forms, is debilitating for the patients undergoing prolonged treatment. To cope with the adverse effects such as neutropenia and thrombocytopenia, we have developed long circulating CD22 targeted liposomes loaded with AD 198 (LCCTLA) and have compared their efficacy with long circulating untargeted liposomal AD 198 (LCLA) and free drug [46]. Consequently, the development of a targeted drug delivery system was expected to impose specificity and considerably moderate adverse effects compared to the other two formulations. Figure 1 gives a schematic representation of the developed LCCTLA drug delivery system.

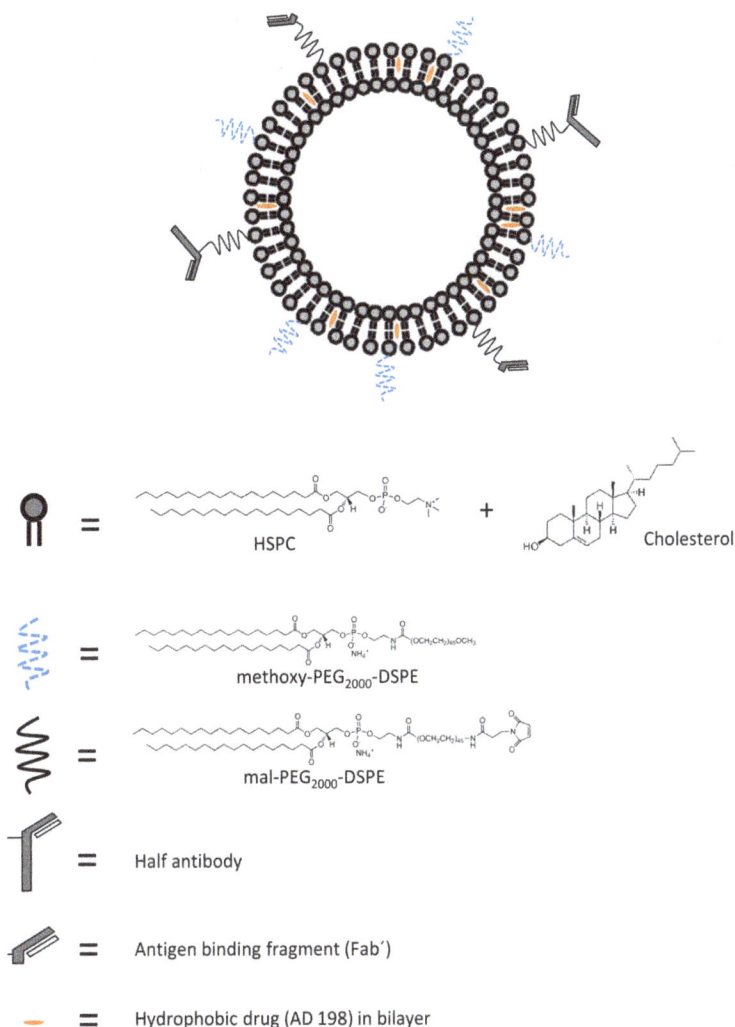

Figure 1. Components of developed long circulating CD22 targeted liposomal AD 198 drug delivery system (HSPC: hydrogenated soy phosphatidylcholine, methoxy-PEG$_{2000}$-DSPE: 1,2-distearoyl-*sn*-glycero-3-phosphoethanolamine-*N*-[methoxy(polyethylene glycol)-2000], mal-PEG$_{2000}$-DSPE: 1,2-distearoyl-*sn*-glycero-3-phosphoethanolamine-*N*-[maleimide(polyethylene glycol)-2000].

2. Materials and Methods

2.1. Materials

HSPC (hydrogenated soy phosphatidylcholine), EPC (egg phosphatidylcholine), mal-PEG2000-DSPE (1,2-distearoyl-*sn*-glycero-3-phosphoethanolamine-*N*-[maleimide(polyethylene glycol)-2000]), mPEG2000-DSPE (1,2-distearoyl-sn-glycero-3-phosphoethanolamine-*N*-[methoxy(polyethylene glycol)-2000]) and NBD-PC (12-[*N*-(nitrobenz-2-oxa-1,3-diazol-4-yl) amino] dodecanoyl phosphatidylethanolamine) were purchased from Avanti Polar Lipids, Alabaster, AL, USA, cholesterol, MTT (3-(4, 5-dimethylthiazol-2-yl)-2, 5-diphenyltetrazolium bromide), amiloride, genistein, M-β-CD (methyl-β-cyclodextrin) and chlorpromazine were purchased from Sigma-Aldrich Co. LLC, St. Louis, MI, USA, chloroform, methanol, Whatman® Nucleopore track etched polycarbonate membranes, 200 proof ethanol, 10× PBS (phosphate buffered saline) and HPLC (high pressure liquid chromatography) grade water, Slide-A-Lyzer® MINI Dialysis Devices, 3.5 kD MWCO (molecular weight cut off), 0.5 mL capacity, ammonium hydroxide and 80% formic acid, immobilized pepsin, Thermo Scientific™ CL-XPosure™ Film (X-ray Film), Sepharose CL4B gel filtration gel, anhydrous citric acid, empty PD-10 columns, SDS (sodium dodecyl sulfate), DMF (dimethylformamide), DMSO (dimethyl sulfoxide), 80% acetic acid 1 N HCl (hydrochloric acid) and LysoTracker® Deep Red were purchased from Thermo Fisher Scientific, Waltham, MA, USA, ultrapure nitrogen was purchased from Nexair, Memphis, TN, USA, Sephadex G50 pre-filled macro SpinColumns® and empty macro SpinColumns® were purchased from Harvard Apparatus, Holliston, MA, USA, Total Recovery® HPLC vials were purchased from Waters, Milford, MA, USA, anti-CD22 monoclonal antibody (RFB4) was a generous gift from the lab of Ellen Vitetta, University of Texas, Southwestern Medical Center, Dallas, TX, USA, Amicon® Ultra—0.5 mL centrifugal filters, Ultracel®—100 K and Ultracel®—30 K were purchased from Millipore, Bellericka, MA, Laemmli buffer and polyacrylamide gels were purchased from Bio-Rad, Hercules, CA, USA, Daudi and Jurkat cells were purchased from ATCC, Manassas, VA, and Vectashield® cell mounting medium with DAPI (4',6-diamidino-2-phenylindole) was purchased from Vector Labs, Burlingame, CA, USA, Iron oxide nanoparticles were purchased from Ocean NanoTech, San Diego CA, USA, antibodies for c-myc #5605, pAKT #4058, caspase-3 #9662 and anti-mouse secondary #7076 were purchased from Cell Signaling Technologies, Danvers, MA, USA and antibodies for pJNK (sc-571), β-actin (sc-130065) and anti-rabbit secondary (sc-2357) were purchased from Santa Cruz Biotechnology, Dallas, TX, USA. TEM (transmission electron microscopy) sample preparation materials were generously provided by the Imaging Center at the Neuroscience Institute at UTHSC, Memphis, TN, USA.

2.2. Preparation and Formulation Optimization of LCLA (Untargeted Long Circulating Liposomal AD 198)

The liposomes were prepared by the Bangham method [47] followed by extrusion via polycarbonate membranes [12,14,48]. Briefly, the lipids and drug (AD 198 free base) were weighed accurately and dissolved in 3 mL 9:1 solvent mixture of chloroform:methanol in a round bottom flask. A thin lipid film was formed at the bottom of the flask by evaporating the solvent using a BUCHI Rotavapor®. Rotations were maintained at rotation speed no 3 and temperature was maintained at 40 °C using a BUCHI heating bath. This step was carried out for 1 h following which the vacuum was released, and the water bath heated to 65 °C. Simultaneously, $1 \times$ PBS was prepared from the $10 \times$ PBS and added to the thin lipid film for hydration. Rotations were maintained at the number 3 setting. Hydration was carried out for 1 h which gave MLVs (multi-lamellar vesicles). The MLVs were extruded through polycarbonate filters in two steps to give SUVs (small unilamellar vesicles). Extrusion was carried out using LIPEX® Extruders purchased from Northern Lipids, Burnaby, BC, Canada, connected to a high pressure ultrapure nitrogen tank. In the first step of extrusion, polycarbonate membranes of two sizes, 100 nm (nanometers) and 200 nm, were stacked and the drug loaded liposomes extruded only once using 450 psi pressure. In the second step, the resulting liposomes were extruded three times via 80 nm and 100 nm stacked membranes again using 450 psi pressure. Since there was some loss of volume during the rehydration and extrusion process, the final volume was made up to 3 mL with $1 \times$ PBS. The size and ζ-potential (zeta potential) of the final liposomes was measured using a Malvern Zetasizer Nano ZS.

2.3. Removal of Un-Encapsulated AD 198

The unencapsulated drug was removed using Sephadex—G50 prefilled macro-column [49,50]. Briefly, the powdered G50 gel was rehydrated using $1 \times$ PBS for 15 min and centrifuged using a Thermo Scientific IEC CL31R centrifuge at 4 °C for 4 min at 1500 rpm. The resulting gel was washed three times using 150 µL of blank liposomes containing no AD 198, under the same centrifugation conditions as mentioned above. This was to block any non-specific retention of drug loaded liposomes in the column. Then 150 µL of the AD 198 loaded liposomes were passed through the treated column. The final eluate was reconstituted to 150 µL.

2.4. Analysis of Liposomal Encapsulated Drug Content

Encapsulated AD 198 content in the liposomes was calculated using a Waters Alliance e2695 HPLC coupled to a Waters 2998 UV Photodiode Array Detector. Samples were prepared at a dilution factor of 20. Briefly, 50 μL of the purified liposomes were dissolved in 950 μL of 1:1 methanol:ethanol. Samples were briefly vortexed to give a clear solution and 300 μL transferred to Waters total recovery HPLC vials. These vials were loaded into the autosampler of the HPLC separations module. Conditions for HPLC analysis were adapted from previously optimized methods [51]. The column used for separation was Waters Nova-Pak® C18 4 μm, 3.9 × 150 mm and was maintained at 30 °C throughout the separation process. The mobile phase was a 70:30 acetonitrile:pH 4.0 ammonium formate buffer. The ammonium formate buffer was prepared by adding 3.85 mL of ammonium hydroxide to 950 mL of HPLC grade water. The pH was adjusted to 4.0 using 80% formic acid and the volume was made up to 1 L. The flow rate for the mobile phase was maintained at 1.2 mL/ min, the injection volume was 20 μL and the run time for each injection was 7 min. AD 198 eluted between 3 and 4 min and was detected at a wavelength (λ) of 254 nm.

2.5. Determination of Phospholipid Concentration

To calculate the amount of HSPC retained in the final formulation of LCLA, total phospholipids were estimated using a procedure adapted from Stewart et al. [52]. 2.703 g (grams) ferric chloride hexahydrate and 3.04 g ammonium thiocyanate was dissolved in 100 mL distilled water and mixed to give ferrithiocyanate reagent. To determine the concentration of HSPC in the LCLA dispersion, an HSPC standard curve was made ranging from 10 to 60 μg/mL. Analysis of these standards was done as follows. A mixture of 2 mL chloroform, 2 mL ferrithiocyanate reagent and 100 μL of the standard solution was made for each standard and vortexed vigorously for exactly one min each. The mixture was allowed to settle and the lower layer containing chloroform was aspirated carefully and transferred to a 1 mL quartz cuvette. The absorbance for each standard was measured at λ 488 against a chloroform blank. Samples of LCLA were prepared in the same method and the absorbance measured. Absorbance of the standard vs. HSPC concentration was plotted for each standard concentration and the unknown amount of HSPC in the LCLA sample was determined.

2.6. LCLA AD 198 Release Study

Drug release in 1× PBS at pH 7.4 and 37 °C was tested for the LCLA's as described by Zhang et al. [53]. Briefly, 100 μL of the LCLA's were placed in Slide-A-Lyzer® MINI Dialysis Devices, 3.5 K MWCO, 0.5 mL capacity [54,55]. 5 time points were tested; 6, 12, 24, 48 and 72 h. Each sample was tested in triplicates. The sample loaded dialysis devices were loaded into floats introduced into a 3000 mL beaker containing 3000 mL of 1× PBS preheated to 37 °C and dissolution started. Samples were taken out at the pre-determined time points and the drug content measured by HPLC as stated earlier.

2.7. Fab' (Antigen Binding Fragment) Generation from Whole Anti-CD22 Antibody

The anti-CD22 whole antibody was first purified by passing through a G50 prefilled macro column. The Fc (constant fragment) region was first digested using immobilized pepsin. Briefly, the immobilized pepsin was first separated from the vehicle by loading the immobilized pepsin suspension into an empty macro column and centrifuging it for 2 min at 5000 g and 4 °C. The purified anti-CD22 monoclonal antibody was then incubated with the immobilized pepsin at pH 3.0, 37 °C for 6 h. pH 3.0 was adjusted using 1M citric acid solution. After the given time, the antibody was collected by centrifuging the immobilized pepsin and antibody digest in an empty macro spin column at 5000 g for 2 min at 4 °C. The collected antibody digest was then incubated with 10μl of 5 mM TCEP (tris(2-carboxyethyl)phosphine) at room temperature (RT) for 1 h. This gave 2Fab' fragments from each molecule of antibody. The resulting digest mix was purified by filtration using two filters 100 kD and 30 kD MWCO and the appropriate fraction containing the 50 kD Fab' was collected and used for conjugation. A schematic or this reaction is given in Figure 2A.

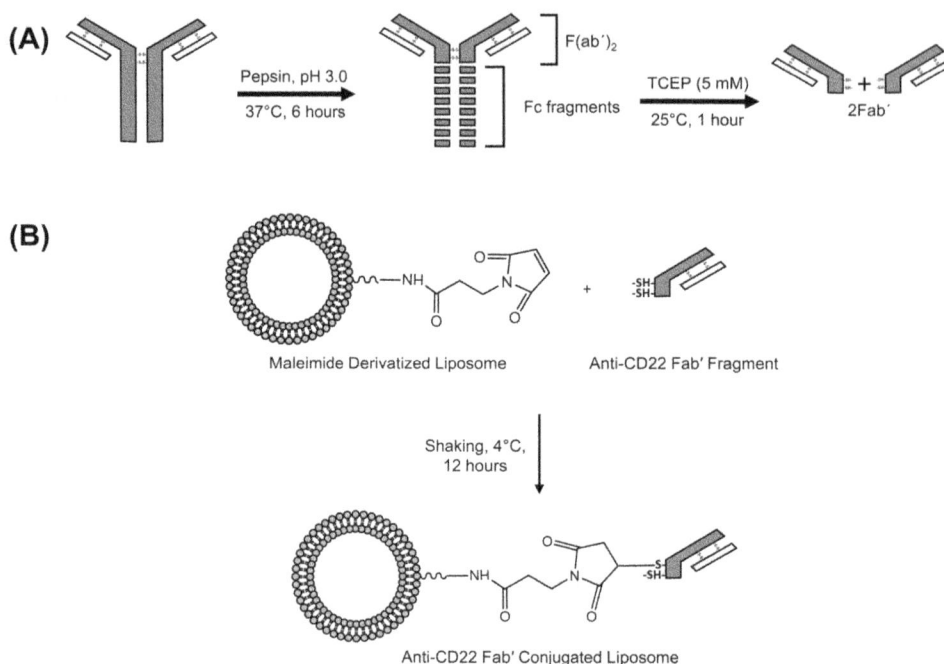

Figure 2. (**A**) Schematic for generation of anti-CD22 Fab′ fragments; and (**B**) Conjugation of anti-CD22 Fab′ to maleimide derivatized LCLA (untargeted long circulating liposomal AD 198).

2.8. Conjugation of Fab′ to Liposomes to Give Long Circulating CD22 Targeted Liposomal AD 198 (LCCTLA)

For conjugation with antibody, liposomes were prepared by the same method as mentioned above, only 50% of m-DSPE-PEG2000 was replaced with mal-PEG2000-DSPE to serve as an anchor for the antibody. 100 μL of the Fab′ was incubated with an equal volume of the maleimide derivatized liposomes at 4 °C for 12–15 h. Following incubation, unconjugated antibody fragments were removed by gel filtration chromatography using Sepharose CL4B gel. Briefly, the 70% gel slurry in ethanol was filled in an empty PD-10 column and centrifuged at 1000 g for 150 s at 4 °C to remove the ethanol. Three 1× PBS washes followed the removal of ethanol. The column was the saturated with placebo liposomes in three separate runs and then the 200 μL of targeted liposomes were passed through the column. The final reaction for the conjugation between the maleimide derivatized liposomes is depicted in Figure 2B. The resulting solution was analyzed for proof of conjugation by western blotting.

2.9. Verification of Conjugation

Conjugation of the 50 kD Fab′ fragment to the liposomes was verified by western blotting as done by Oliveira et al. [56]. Briefly, 4 samples were studied: the targeted liposomes, the fraction higher than 100 kD, the fraction below 50 kD and the whole antibody were quantified for total protein by the BCA assay and 20 μL (10 μL sample and 10 μL Laemmli buffer) of an equal concentration sample of protein (250 ng) were loaded into a 4–15% polyacrylamide gel. Samples were run at 100 V for approximately one hour (until the Laemmli dye reached the end of the gel). The protein bands were then transferred from the gel onto a PVDF (polyvinylidene fluoride) membrane. The membrane was probed with a mouse secondary antibody and the blot was developed on an X-ray film.

2.10. Calculation of Number of Antibody Molecules per Liposome

The number of anchors (maleimide groups) and the number of antibody molecules per liposome were calculated by first calculating the number of liposomes as previously discussed. Then number of antibody molecules and maleimide were calculated in one mL of the LCCTLA by using Avogadro's number and substituting the values in Equations (1) to (7).

2.11. Cellular Uptake of LCLA and LCCTLA by Flow Cytometry

To determine and compare cellular uptake in CD22$^+$ Daudi and CD22$^-$ Jurkat cells CD22 targeted liposomes were prepared by the same method as specified previously only 0.125 mole % of the HSPC was substituted with an equal mole percent of NBD-PC for fluorescence imaging. Six time points were tested ranging from 5 min to 4 h [57]. 10 ml each of Daudi and Jurkat cells at a cell density of 7×10^5 cells/mL were grown in T25 flasks for each time point. At each time point, both cell types were treated with two types of 1 μM AD 198 formulations, LCLA and LCCTLA separately. At the end of each time point the cells were centrifuged at 4 °C and 100 g for 4 min. The pellet obtained was washed with 1× PBS thrice and the final cell pellet was re-suspended in 1 mL of 1× PBS and tested for fluorescence intensity for NBD-PC per 10,000 cells using the BD Accuri™ C6 flow cytometer (BD Biosciences, San Jose, CA, USA).

2.12. Evaluation of LCCTLA Cytotoxicity

To determine cellular cytotoxicity, the MTT assay was used [58]. Briefly, Daudi and Jurkat cells were grown to the required cell density. The assay was set up in 96 well plates. Three different formulations of AD 198 were tested; LCCTLA, LCLA and free AD 198. Free AD 198 was prepared in DMSO such that the final concentration of DMSO was less than 3% in any treatment well. Two time points were prepared for each treatment, 24 h and 48 h. For the 24-h treatment 17,500 cells per well were plated and for the 48-h treatment 8750 cells per well were plated. Treatment was done for 10 concentrations of each of the three AD 198 formulations ranging from 0.01 μM to 3 μM and the control was cells with no drug treatment. These plates were incubated at 37 °C and 5% CO$_2$ for the study time period. At the end of the study time (24 or 48 h) 15 μL of 5 mg/mL concentration of MTT dye was added to each well of study and incubated under the same conditions mentioned above for 4 more h at 37 °C. Following the 4-h incubation the insoluble formazan dye formed as a result of the reaction was dissolved in 100 μL of solubilization buffer (20% SDS in 50% DMF, 0.5% of 80% acetic acid and 0.4% 1N HCl) and incubated for 3 h at 37 °C. After incubation absorbance was read at λ 570 nm using the SpectraMax M2e® microplate reader (Molecular Devices, San Jose, CA, USA).

2.13. Energy Dependent or Independent Pathway for LCCTLA Internalization

To confirm that the mechanism of uptake of LCCTLA particles into Daudi cells was by receptor-mediated endocytosis cellular association studies were performed [56]. Briefly, 10 mL of Daudi cells at a cell density of 7×10^5 cells/mL were grown in two separate T25 flasks. One was pre-cooled to 4 °C and then treated with 1 μM fluorescent LCCTLA for one hour and the other was treated with 1 μM fluorescent LCCTLA at 37 °C for one hour. At the end of the time point, the cells were centrifuged at 4 °C and 100 g for 4 min. The pellet obtained was washed with 1× PBS thrice and the final cell pellet was re-suspended in 1 mL of 1× PBS and tested for fluorescence intensity for NBD-PC per 10,000 cells using the BD Accuri™ C6 Flow cytometer.

2.14. Route of Uptake of LCCTLA into Daudi Cells

To determine the mechanism of entry of LCCTLA into the Daudi cells, various inhibitors were used to block specific pathways and then the uptake analyzed as done in the determination of CD22 targeted liposomal drug uptake in cells by flow cytometry. As per Douglas et al. [59] four specific inhibitors were used; amiloride for micropinocytosis, genistein or M-β-CD for caveolae and related structures mediated endocytosis and chlorpromazine for clathrin-mediated endocytosis. 10 mL Daudi cells at a concentration of 7×10^5 cells/mL were incubated with the inhibitors for one hour at the following specific concentrations; amiloride 10 μM, genistein 0.2 μM and chlorpromazine 10 μg/mL. Following this the inhibitor treated cells were treated with 1 μM fluorescent CD22 targeted liposomal AD 198 and incubated for 1 h at 37 °C. At the end of the treatment the cells were processed in the same method as for the determination of LCCTLA uptake in Daudi cells by flow cytometry.

2.15. Intracellular Trafficking of LCCTLA by TEM

2.15.1. MLV Preparation and Treatment of Daudi Cells

To view the intracellular localization of LCCTLA in the Daudi cells [60,61], 15 nm sized magnetic iron oxide nanoparticles in water (with carboxylic acid functional group) were processed into the liposomes [62]. Briefly, 1% w/w iron oxide nanoparticles were added to the 1× PBS that was used to rehydrate the dried lipid film. The MLV's thus obtained were sonicated for 5 s with 5 min intervals (extrusion was initially tried as the size reduction technique, however the liposomes failed to extrude). During the sonication and the interval, the liposomal suspension was kept in ice. The sonication was repeated three times to give magnetic LCLA (MLCLA). The anti-CD22 Fab' was conjugated as specified previously to give MLCCTLA (magnetic LCCTLA). 10 mL Daudi cells at a density of 7×10^5 cells/mL were treated with 1 µM of the MLCCTLA for 4 h. After treatment, the cells were centrifuged at 100 g for 5 min at 4 °C. The pellet was washed with ice cold 1× PBS thrice and suspended in 1 mL 2.5% glutaraldehyde in 1× PBS.

2.15.2. TEM Sample Preparation

Once the cells were fixed in 2.5% glutaraldehyde overnight they were spun down at 100 g for 5 min and washed with 10× PBS thrice for 20 min each. Then the cells were stained with a 4% osmium tetroxide in PBS solution for 1 h at RT and excess stain washed off using 10× PBS thrice for 20 min each. The cell sample was then dehydrated in an ethanol series gradually increasing from 50% ethanol to 100% ethanol in four steps. Each dehydration cycle was done once for 10 min and the 100% ethanol thrice. The cells were then infiltrated with 50% Spurr's resin in ethanol under rotation overnight. Infiltration was continued with 100% Spurr's resin the next day thrice for 2 h periods. With the 100% Spurr's resin, the centrifugation was done at 800 g for 20 min. The cells were then embedded in fresh Spurr's resin in a mold and cured at 65 °C for 48 h. Once the resin hardened the sample block was placed in an ultramicrotome and approximately 80 nm sections cut using a diamond knife. Chloroform was used to smoothen the sections. The sections were loaded onto copper grids and stained with uranyl acetate and lead citrate to increase contrast and electron density. The grids were then inserted into the TEM for viewing. The TEM used was the JEOL 2000EX with a high resolution digital camera and monitor (JEOL, Peabody, MA, USA).

2.16. Intracellular Trafficking of LCCTLA by CLSM

To confirm that the intracellular vesicles the magnetic liposomes were observed in were endolysosomes, cells were stained with endolysosome specific dye [63–65]. Briefly, 10 mL Daudi cells were cultured to a cell density of 7×10^5 cells/mL and treated with 10 µL of placebo fluorescent CD22 targeted liposomes (prepared by substituting 0.125 mole % of HSPC with an equal mole % of NBD-PC, and not loading any drug) for 1 h. During the final 5 min of treatment, 50 nM LysoTracker® Deep Red was added to the treated cell culture. The media was then removed by centrifugation and the cell pellet thus obtained was washed 3 times using 1× PBS. The final cell pellet was suspended in a single drop of Vectashield® cell mounting medium with DAPI. This final cell suspension was mounted onto a microscope slide and covered by a Fisherbrand number 1 coverslip. The slide was allowed to dry in a fume hood for approximately 30 min and the edges were sealed using a transparent nail polish. The nail polish was also allowed to dry in a fume hood for another 30 min after which the slide was viewed under a Nikon Eclipse E800 confocal scanning laser microscope (Nikon Instruments, Melville, NY, USA). The lasers were set at the wavelength for NBD-PC, LysoTracker® Deep Red and DAPI and images were obtained.

2.17. Effect of LCCTLA on Cell Cycle Regulatory Molecules by Western Blot

To study the efficacy of the drug delivery system on induction of apoptosis in the cancer cells, the cells were treated with the LCCTLA and the expression of 4 proteins was monitored, Caspase 3, c-myc, p-JNK, pAKT. β-actin was used as a control to signify equal loading. The process [66] has been briefly outlined below.

2.17.1. Sample preparation

10 mL of Daudi cells at a density of 7×10^5 cells/mL were treated with 1 µM of LCCTLA at three separate time points, 2, 4 and 6 h. The control was the same density and volume of cells but without any drug treatment. At the end of the treatment, cells were centrifuged in a Thermo Scientific Sorvall Legend X1 centrifuge (Thermo Fisher Scientific, Waltham, MA, USA) at 100 g for 4 min at 4 °C. The pellet obtained was washed with $1\times$ PBS thrice and then suspended in 70 µL whole cell lysis buffer [Tris HCl 50 mM, NaCl (sodium chloride) 150 mM, Triton X-100 1%, SDS 0.1%, EDTA (ethylene diamine tetra acetic acid) 5 mM, Na_2HPO_4 (disodium phosphate) 30 mM, NaF (sodium fluoride) 50 mM, $NaVO_4$ (sodium orthovandate) 0.5 mM, PMSF (phenylmethylsulfonylfluoride) 2 mM and protease inhibitor] at 1 µL/10^6 cells. This cell suspension was sonicated using a Virtis Virsonic® Ultrasonic Cell Disrupter. The samples were sonicated thrice for 5 s each with 5 min intervals. During the intervals, the cell debris suspension was placed on ice. The cell debris suspension was then centrifuged at 1000 rpm at 4 °C for 10 min and the supernatant collected. The pellet obtained was discarded.

2.17.2. Polyacrylamide Gel Electrophoresis (PAGE)

The protein content in the supernatant collected was quantified using the microplate BCA (bicinchoninic acid) protein assay. A volume of protein was calculated such that all samples had an equal concentration of protein. These whole cell protein samples were then mixed with an equal volume of $2\times$ Laemmli sample buffer and boiled for 5 min. Samples were then cooled to RT for 3 min and loaded onto a 4–15% polyacrylamide gel of 50 µL well capacity. The buffer reservoir was filled up with electrode running buffer to the given mark. The electrodes were connected to a Bio-Rad power pack and samples were electrophoresed at 100 V for approximately one hour (until the Laemmli sample dye reached near the bottom of the gel).

2.17.3. Blotting

The gel was then loaded onto a transfer cassette to transfer the protein bands onto a PVDF membrane. The sized membrane was first soaked in 100% methanol followed by transfer buffer. It was then placed over the gel in the cassette and the transfer apparatus set up. A stir bar was placed at the bottom of the buffer reservoir along with a freezer pack. Transfer buffer was then poured into the reservoir to a level such that the freezer pack was fully submerged and covered the cassette completely. The electrodes were connected to a Bio-Rad power pack and the transfer was done at 100 V for one hour.

2.17.4. Primary and Secondary Antibody Probing

Once the bands were transferred to the membrane, the membrane was blocked using either 5% powdered milk or 5% BSA (bovine serum albumin) in TBST (Tris-buffered saline and Tween® 20). The blocking was done at RT for 1 h on a shaker. After the blocking was complete, excess milk or BSA was washed off the membrane with TBST (a quick wash) and the primary antibody for a specific protein was added at a dilution of 1:1000 (only β-actin 1:40,000) in TBST. The blot was incubated with the primary antibody for 12–15 h at 4 °C on a rocker. At the end of the incubation period, the excess primary antibody was washed off the membrane using TBST. The wash was done thrice for 5 min each. Then, the membrane was incubated with secondary antibody specific for the particular antibody used (anti-rabbit for c-myc, pJNK, pAKT and caspase-3 and anti-mouse for β-actin) at a dilution of 1:25,000 for 1 h at RT. The excess secondary antibody was then washed off the membrane using TBST thrice for 15 min each.

2.17.5. Analysis

Once the secondary antibody was probed onto the membrane, the substrate (hydrogen peroxide + luminol) was added and briefly incubated for 1–2 min. The membrane was then loaded onto an X-ray film cassette and covered with a fresh X-ray film. This film was then developed, and the results recorded.

2.17.6. Membrane Stripping

The membrane was reused for probing another protein with another antibody. For this, the previous antibody was removed by a process called stripping and was done by a stripping buffer. The membrane already bound with the primary and secondary antibody was incubated with the stripping buffer for 5 min at 45 °C following which it was washed with TBST and was reused for probing the next protein.

2.18. Statistical Methodology

All work was performed in triplicates ($n = 3$). Data are expressed as mean $\pm$ standard deviation (SD). Student's t-test was used for data analysis; p-values ≤ 0.05 were considered statistically significant.

3. Results

3.1. This Section Effect of Lipid Composition in the Bilayer

EPC and HSPC were studied for their effects on the physico-chemical properties of the liposomes such as liposomal encapsulation of AD 198, size and ζ-potential. Both lipids are derived from natural sources and are biodegradable. However, HSPC and EPC differ in their composition such that EPC is a crude mixture of saturated and unsaturated lipids of varying chain lengths, whereas HSPC is primarily composed of saturated lipids of a fixed chain length. The effect that this has on the lipid bilayer is that the longer chain length lipids in EPC increase the thickness of the bilayer (not the size of the liposome) [67]. The more saturated a lipid is, the higher is its transition temperature, thus imparting lesser fluidity and possibly increased stability [67]. A variable length between the two tail group chains also reduces the order of packing in the liposomal bilayer. Liposomes with saturated lipids such as HSPC also have higher circulation half-lives compared to liposomes with unsaturated lipids such as EPC [68,69].

Studies were performed using HSPC and EPC at various ratios to optimize the physico-chemical properties of LCLA. Figure 3A shows EPC and HSPC formulations studied in various ratios for their effect on AD 198 encapsulation, liposomal size, and ζ-potential. It was observed that the size of the liposomes was not related to the lipid composition in any definitive manner. One hundred percent HSPC gave the smallest liposomal size. Liposomal AD 198 concentration was also not associated with the lipid composition in a significant manner with 100% HSPC giving highest AD 198 encapsulation. Dependence of ζ-potential on the lipid composition however displayed a trend compared to size and drug encapsulation. As the percentage of HSPC was increased, ζ-potential became more electronegative with an average value of -19.3 mV at 100% HSPC concentration. Although the other formulations containing some percentage of EPC produced liposomes of size, ζ-potential and AD 198 encapsulation comparable to the formulation with 100% HSPC, the latter was selected as the formulation of choice this point forward due to the difficulty of working with EPC which can be attributable to its lesser stable nature which makes for a very hygroscopic powder and lesser stable formulations due to the unsaturation in its structure.

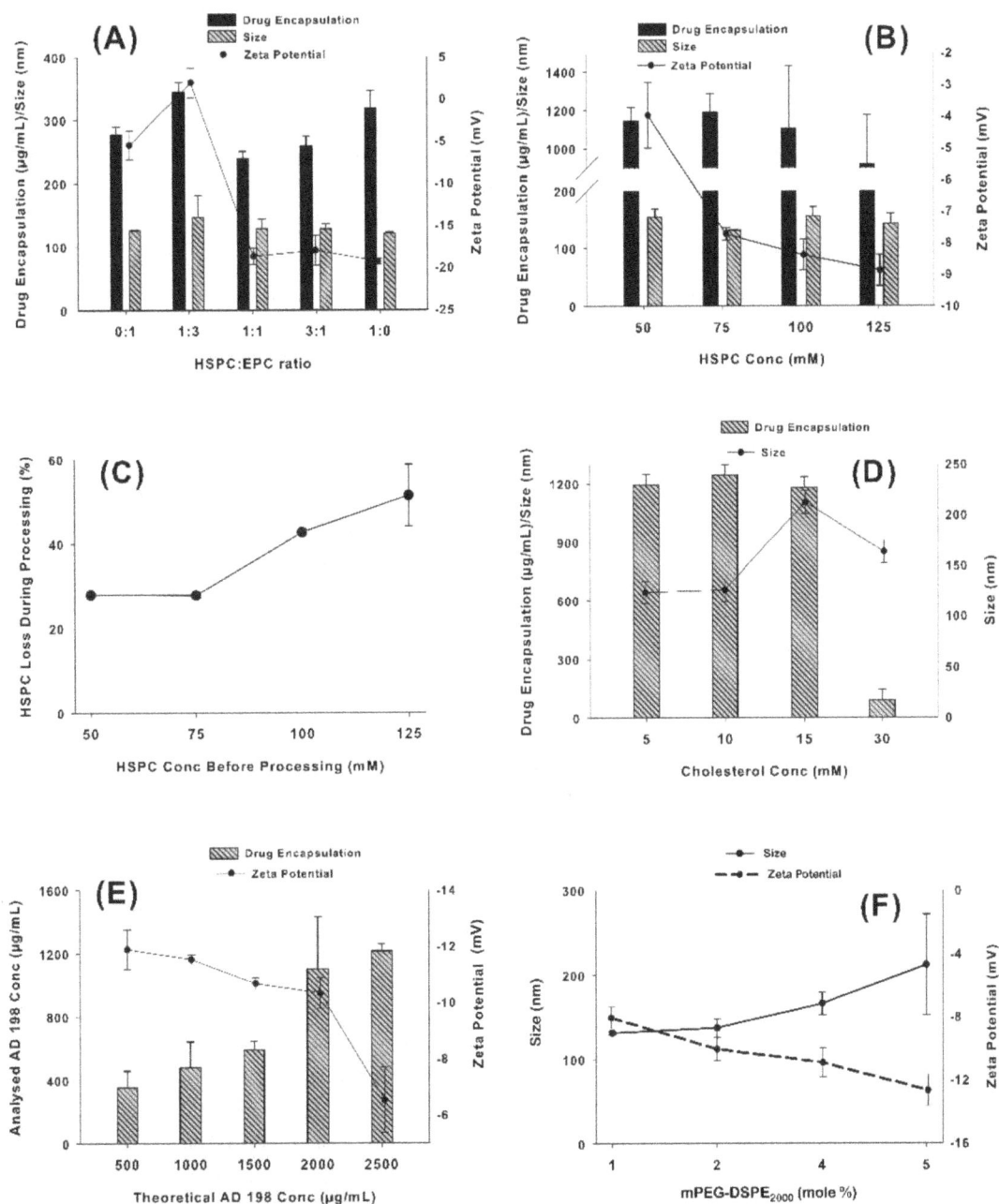

Figure 3. (**A**) Effect of lipid composition on AD 198 encapsulation and liposomal size; (**B**) Effect of total phospholipid concentration on liposome size, ζ-potential and AD 198 encapsulation; (**C**) Optimization of HSPC concentration; (**D**) Effect of cholesterol concentration on AD 198 encapsulation and liposome size; (**E**) Effect of AD 198 concentration on AD 198 encapsulation and ζ-potential; and (**F**) Effect of mPEG2000-DSPE concentration on ζ-potential and liposome size.

3.2. *Effect of Total Phospholipids on AD 198 Encapsulation, Liposomal Size and ζ-Potential*

Optimum concentration of HSPC was tested by comparing liposomes with 5 different concentrations of HSPC: 25, 50, 75, 100 and 125 mM. The drug concentration was kept constant at 2000 μg/mL. The batch with 25 mM HSPC failed to extrude. This may be attributed to the excess amount of drug in the system that the little amount of carrier (HSPC) would need to encapsulate. As seen from experiments, it is speculated that the un-encapsulated drug forms a thin layer on the membrane thus preventing the liposomes from extruding. The results for 50–125 mM HSPC are shown in Figure 3B. It would be logical to believe that with increase in the amount of HSPC in the system, which is the major encapsulating material, the amount of encapsulated drug would tend to increase. However, the results suggest that the amount of drug encapsulated may not necessarily be related to the amount of lipid in the system. This result can be explained with Figure 3C which indicates that during processing, a considerable amount of phospholipid was being lost as the total lipid content was increased beyond 75 mM. As portrayed in Figure 3C it was observed that the amount of HSPC loss during processing at 75 mM HSPC is approximately 25% (almost the same as 50 mM). However, at 100 mM and 125 mM the amount of phospholipid loss was more than 40%, whereas the benefits in terms of AD 198 encapsulation and liposomal size were negligible (Figure 3B). Although there was a pronounced increase in the net negative charge on the liposomal surface, as depicted in Figure 3B, the size of the liposome increased considerably which allowed the conclusion of total phospholipid concentration at 75 mM to be optimum for development purposes. An additional justification was that the extrusion time with total phospholipid concentration higher than 75 mM increased considerably (more than 10 times).

There was an increase in the negative charge of the liposomes when the phospholipid concentration was increased from 50 mM to 75 mM. This was followed by a reduced degree of increase from 75 mM to 100 mM and 125 mM can possibly be explained by the excess amount of AD 198 that remains un-encapsulated. Since AD 198 has a cationic nature and HSPC an anionic nature, the excess AD 198 in the dispersion could be adsorbed onto the liposomal surface thus shielding the anionic nature of HSPC.

3.3. Effect of Cholesterol Concentration on AD 198 Encapsulation and Liposomal Size

Cholesterol is incorporated into the membrane to obtain an optimum bilayer fluidity [67,70]. However, with encapsulation of hydrophobic drugs in the bilayer it is important to consider effects of cholesterol concentrations on the encapsulation of the drug even before bilayer fluidity is considered. This is shown in Figure 3D which depicts the results from a study on the effects of increasing cholesterol concentrations. Four concentrations of cholesterol ranging from 5 mM to 30 mM were studied. Liposomal size was relatively similar for 5 and 10 mM cholesterol concentrations. However, the size increased considerably at 15 and 30 mM cholesterol. This may be attributed to the liposomal bilayer trying to accommodate both the AD 198 and the increasing cholesterol molecules which could possibly increase the liposomal size. AD 198 concentration reduced more than 10-fold from approximately 1000 μg/mL to 90 μg/mL, when cholesterol concentration was increased from 15 mM to 30 mM. Since part of the cholesterol molecular structure is similar to that of AD 198, the excess cholesterol molecules trying to occupy volume within the bilayer may be pushing out AD 198. This was also in agreement with the liposomal size results. Once excess AD 198 was pushed out, the liposomal size reduced by approximately 50 nm. These results suggested that in view of AD 198 encapsulation and liposomal size, 10 mM cholesterol concentration was optimum for LCLA. It should also be noted that with increasing cholesterol concentrations bilayer permeability decreases as demonstrated by Hu et al. [71], which is an advantage for long circulating liposomes.

3.4. Effect of AD 198 Concentration on AD 198 Encapsulation and ζ-Potential

Five concentrations of AD 198 ranging from 500 μg/mL to 2500 μg/mL were tested to determine their effect on AD 198 encapsulation and ζ-potential. Figure 3E shows that as the AD 198 concentration was increased from 500 to 1500 μg/mL the AD 198 encapsulation increased steadily. However, when the AD 198 concentration was increased from 1500 to 2000 μg/mL, the AD 198 encapsulation almost doubled. However, if the AD 198 concentration was increased any further, there was not a considerable increase in AD 198 encapsulation. The ζ-potential was relatively constant up to 2000 μg/mL. However, once the AD 198 concentration reached 2500 μg/mL, the electronegativity of the particles reduced. Again, this can be attributed to the excess un-encapsulated cationic AD 198 adsorbing onto the predominantly anionic HSPC liposomes, which will shield the negative charge due to HSPC. Hence,

2000 µg/mL was selected as the optimum AD 198 concentration and hereon this was the concentration used for further studies.

3.5. Optimization of mPEG2000-DSPE Concentration

To determine the optimum amount of mPEG2000-DSPE, four concentrations of mPEG2000-DSPE ranging from 1 to 5 mole % were studied. Figure 3F represents the effect of mPEG2000-DSPE concentration on liposomal size and ζ-potential. The liposomal size was observed to increase with increasing concentrations of mPEG2000-DSPE. Conversely, ζ-potential was observed to turn more electronegative with an increase in mPEG2000-DSPE concentration which may be attributable to the anionic nature of mPEG2000-DSPE. mPEG2000-DSPE is a large molecule (MW = 2805.497). The increase in the number of mPEG2000-DSPE molecules may cause the net size of the liposome to increase as justified by Woodle and co-workers [72]. However, the 2 mole % mPEG2000-DSPE imparted optimum size and ζ-potential to the formulation and this was selected for further studies.

3.6. LCLA Drug Release

LCLA was tested for its release characteristics in $1\times$ PBS at 37°C. Figure 4 shows that approximately 30% AD 198 release was observed over the first 12 h following which only about 10% more AD 198 was released over the next 48 h. This may be due a biphasic release mechanism in which the drug is released in two separate phases. Initially the drug was released in a burst mode from drug simply adhered to the liposomal surface, followed by the release of drug from the liposomal bilayer. Possibly there may be micelles formed from the monomer lipid molecules which were not incorporated into liposomes. If these monomer lipids are above their critical micelle concentration (CMC), they will form micelles. Micelles are less stable compared to liposomes and may release drug faster than liposomes. Once micelle drug release is over the liposomal AD 198 release predominantly determines the kinetics. The release pattern is necessary with the theory of active targeting in which the liposome requires a certain period of time before it encounters a CD22$^+$ malignant B cell, binds to it and is internalized. The drug must largely be released once the liposome is inside the malignant cell. Therefore, the delayed release of AD 198 over >72 h is beneficial for the LCLA drug delivery system.

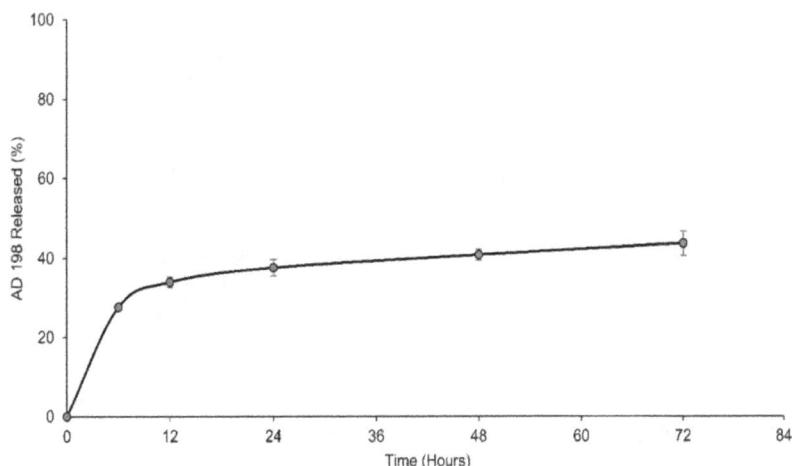

Figure 4. AD 198 release profile from LCLA at 37 °C.

3.7. Number of AD 198 Molecules/Liposome

The number of average HSPC molecules per mL of the LCLA was calculated by using the Avogadro's number, 6.023×10^{23} molecules/mole. This gave an average of 3.25×10^{22} HSPC molecules/mL of LCLA as per the analyzed concentration of HSPC, 54 mM from the HSPC assay results. The number of average AD 198 molecules/mL of LCLA were calculated similarly from the analyzed concentration of AD 198 to be 1250 µg/mL. This gave an average of 1.05×10^{21} AD 198 molecules/mL of LCLA. The outer surface area of the liposomal bilayer was calculated from Equation (1).

$$\text{Outer Surface Area} = 4\pi r^2 \tag{1}$$

Here 'r' was the average outer radius of the liposome. The thickness of the bilayer was denoted 'h' and is 5 nm [73]. Then the inner surface area was calculated from Equation (2).

$$\text{Inner Surface Area} = 4\pi(r - h)^2 \tag{2}$$

The cross-sectional area of a phosphatidylcholine headgroup was denoted as 'a' with a value of 0.71 nm^2 [74] and the number of HSPC molecules per liposome calculated from Equation (3).

$$\text{Number of HSPC molecules/liposome} = \frac{4\pi\left[r^2 + (r - h)^2\right]}{a} \tag{3}$$

$$\text{Number of HSPC molecules/liposome} = \frac{17.69\left[60^2 + (60 - 5)^2\right]}{0.71} = 117196$$

This gave us the number of liposomes/mL from Equation (4).

$$\text{Number liposomes/mL} = \frac{\text{Number of HSPC molecules/mL}}{\text{Number of HSPC molecules/liposome}} \tag{4}$$

$$\text{Number liposomes/mL} = \frac{3.25 \times 10^{22}}{117196} = 2.77 \times 10^{17}$$

Number of average AD 198 molecules per liposome were calculated from Equation (5).

$$\text{Number of AD 198 molecules/liposome} = \frac{\text{Number of AD 198 molecules/mL}}{\text{Number of liposomes/mL}} \tag{5}$$

$$\text{Number of AD 198 molecules/liposome} = \frac{1.05 \times 10^{21}}{2.77 \times 10^{17}} = 3790$$

3.8. Verification of Anti-CD22 Fab' Conjugation

A western blot of the LCCTLA was run with pure antibody digest fractions and the whole antibody. The results are shown in Figure 5. The whole antibody gave a very intense band at the 150 kD region whereas the concentration of protein for the fraction below 50 kD was very low and bands relatively faint. Figure 5A shows the possible combinations of the antibody digests that may be produced and may show up on the blot. Fab' would be 50 kD each, F(ab')$_2$ would be 100 kD, the Fc region has been digested by pepsin thus would be broken into very small peptides possible smaller than 10 kD, and undigested antibody would be 150 kD.

In Figure 5B in the first three lanes are for pure antibody and digests. Lane 1 is undigested whole antibody, lane 2 is the digested Fab' fragment and lane 3 is the fraction above 100 kD. The last lane is LCCTLA and here we observed a clear band at approximately 50 kD. Since we had removed other fragments such as the Fc pepsin digests and whole antibody from the 50 to 100 kD fraction, this was possibly the band for the anti-CD22 Fab'. The whole antibody is shown beside the LCCTLA lane for reference purposes. The appearance of a strong band at 50 kD in the LCCTLA sample proved that conjugation between the liposomes and the Fab' was successful.

(A)   **(B)**

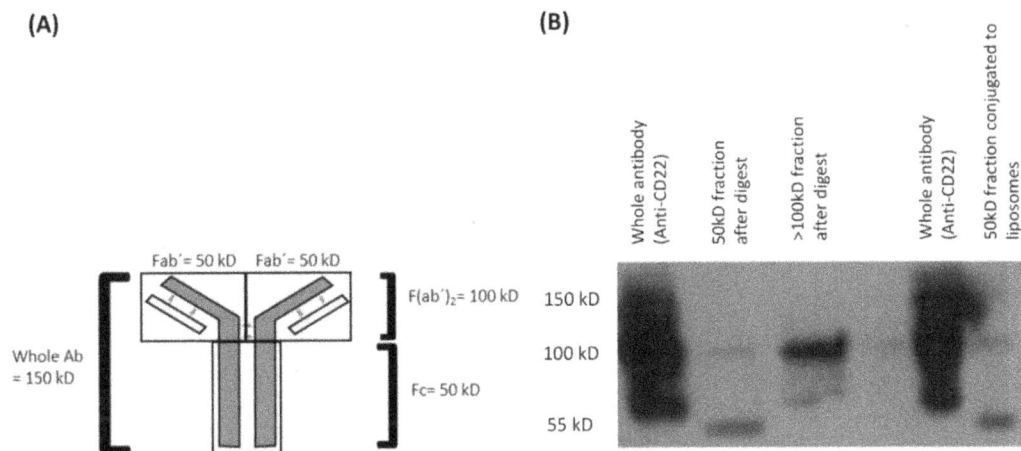

Figure 5. (**A**) Verification of anti-CD22 Fab′ conjugation; (**B**) Verification of conjugation of anti-CD22 Fab′ by western blotting.

3.9. Number of Anti-CD22 Fab′ and Maleimide per LCCTLA

2.2 mg/mL of mal-PEG2000-DSPE was added to make LCCTLA particles. This equals 748 μM of mal-PEG2000-DSPE. Using Avogadro's number, we got an average of 4.5×10^{20} mal-PEG2000-DSPE molecules/mL. As specified in the method, the number of maleimide's per liposome can be calculated by Equation (6).

$$\text{No. of maleimide molecules/liposome} = \frac{\text{No. of maleimide molecules/mL}}{\text{No. of liposomes/mL}} \tag{6}$$

$$\text{Number of maleimide molecules/liposome} = \frac{4.5 \times 10^{20}}{2.77 \times 10^{17}} \approx 1626$$

The average number of anti-CD22 Fab′ molecules were calculated in a similar method. The analyzed concentration of Fab′ fragments in LCCTLA was 313 μg/mL which equals 6.26 μM. Using Avogadro's number, the number of anti-CD22 Fab′ molecules/mL were calculated to be 3.77×10^{18} molecules/mL. Substituting these numbers into Equation (7):

$$\text{Number of Fab}'/\text{liposome} = \frac{\text{Number of Fab}'/\text{mL}}{\text{Number of liposomes/mL}} \tag{7}$$

$$\text{Number of Fab}'/\text{liposome} = \frac{3.77 \times 10^{18}}{2.77 \times 10^{17}} \approx 13 \text{ antiCD22 Fab}'/\text{liposome}$$

The physicochemical properties of the liposomes after anti-CD22 Fab′ conjugation was as follows: mean size was 148.6 ± 4 nm, mean ζ-potential was −10.7 ± 2 mV and average drug encapsulation was about 400 μg/mL.

3.10. Cellular Uptake of LCLA and LCCTLA

Flow cytometry and confocal laser scanning microscopy (CLSM) were utilized to determine the uptake of LCLA and LCCTLA in CD22 expressing Daudi and CD22 non-expressing Jurkat cells. Figure 6A summarizes the results for cellular uptake of both formulations in both Daudi and Jurkat cells. It was observed that the maximum uptake at each time point was for LCCTLA in Daudi cells. The least uptake was seen with LCLA treated Jurkat cells at every time point. Daudi cells treated with LCLA and Jurkat cells treated with LCCTLA had intermediate uptake. Maximum uptake in Daudi cells treated with LCCTLA was understandable due to the CD22 receptor being overexpressed on the Daudi cells and the LCCTLA having the antibody for this overexpressed receptor. However, the Jurkat cells having higher uptake with LCCTLA than LCLA is more complicated to explain. One theory we suggest is that the Jurkat cells may have some receptor on their surface with which the anti-CD22 Fab' non-specifically interacts, thus causing higher uptake. Also, it was seen for Daudi cells treated with LCCTLA, the uptake plateaued at approximately one hour. Therefore, maximum uptake had already taken place by one hour.

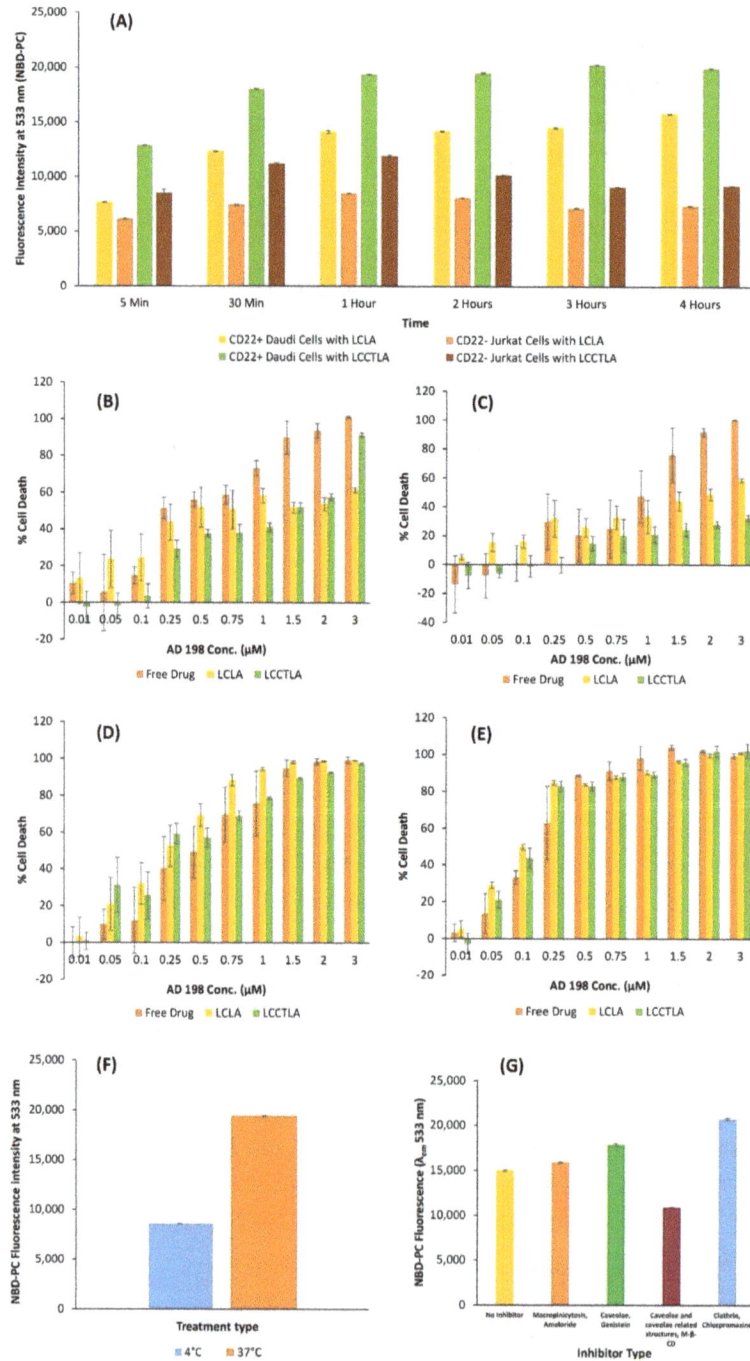

Figure 6. (**A**) Time-dependent cell uptake of LCLA and LCCTLA (long circulating CD22 targeted liposomal AD 198) in Daudi and Jurkat cells; (**B**) 24 h Daudi AD 198 cytotoxicity; (**C**) 24 h Jurkat AD 198 cytotoxicity; (**D**) 48 h Jurkat cytotoxicity; (**E**) 48 h Daudi cytotoxicity; (**F**) Cell association of LCCTLA in Daudi cells; and (**G**) LCCTLA uptake in Daudi cells under different inhibitors.

3.11. Analysis of Cytotoxicity of LCCTLA

Three formulations of AD 198 (free AD 198, LCLA and LCCTLA) were tested in Daudi and Jurkat cells. The study was performed to test the cytotoxic effect of the formulations at two lengths of exposure, 24 and 48 h. Figure 6B to 6E depict the results of this study. Figure 6B exhibits the cytotoxic effects of the three formulations, free drug, LCLA and LCCTLA over 24 h in Daudi cells. The difference in cytotoxicity between different formulations is clearly pronounced. From 0.01 μM to 3 μM AD 198 concentration, free AD 198 is most cytotoxic, with an IC_{50} of approximately 0.25 μM, as shown in Table 1 below. LCLA has an IC_{50} at about 0.5 μM, but LCCTLA have an IC_{50} of about 1.5 μM. Up to 1 μM LCLA was more cytotoxic than LCCTLA and almost equally cytotoxic at 1.5 μM. At 2 μM and 3 μM, LCCTLA displayed higher cytotoxicity. This may be attributable to the process of receptor-mediated endocytosis which may possibly require additional time to endocytose the targeted liposomes. The Jurkat cells are devoid of the CD22 receptors and thus we observed the results as displayed in Figure 6C, which are the results of the 24-h study in Jurkat cells. Since the CD22 receptor is absent in Jurkat cells, LCCTLA was not as cytotoxic as LCLA or free AD 198.

Table 1. IC50 values for the formulation in Daudi and Jurkat cells.

Study Duration	24 h			48 h		
Formulation Type	Free Drug	LCLA	LCCTLA	Free Drug	LCLA	LCCTLA
Cancer Cell Type						
Daudi	0.243	0.481	1.443	0.199	0.101	0.114
Jurkat	1.054	2.046	4.608*	0.509	0.238	0.438

LCLA: Untargeted long circulating liposomal AD 198; LCCTLA: Long circulating CD22 targeted liposomal AD 198.

In the 48-h study, a steadily increasing cell death pattern was noticed in both Jurkat (Figure 6D) and Daudi cells (Figure 6E) from 0.01 μM to 0.5 μM for all formulations. Then from 0.75 μM up to 3 μM, there is not much of a pronounced difference between concentrations and between the formulations. This result may be attributed to the overburdening of the cells with the drug in all types of formulations. Since the drug is not being cleared as in in vivo systems, all the drug from the formulation eventually enters the cells and kills them. This may be controlled by developing a system that would mimic blood circulation as in whole animals. One such model was developed by Budha et al. at the University of Tennessee Health Science Center [75]. Nevertheless, in vivo models would give more accurate representations of how the drug would behave in clinical settings.

3.12. Cellular Association

Figure 6F shows the results of the cellular association studies. It was observed that the LCCTLA uptake in Daudi cells was significantly reduced when the uptake study was being performed at 4 °C compared to when it was done at 37 °C. Receptor-mediated endocytosis is a specific process that requires ATP for appropriate functioning and is also temperature dependent (with optimum temperature being 37 °C) [76]. It may be possible that the reduced uptake in the 4 °C study group was due to the uptake mechanism for the LCCTLA being receptor-mediated endocytosis. Since the mechanism is greatly reduced and even possible halted, the uptake seen may be a result of the receptor associated LCCTLA being internalized before the washes were done. This result suggests that the mechanism of uptake of LCCTLA into CD22 expressing Daudi cells is receptor-mediated endocytosis.

3.13. LCCTLA Particles Are Endocytosed into Cells by a Clathrin- and Caveolae-Independent Pathway

Figure 6G shows the results for LCCTLA uptake under the effect of inhibitors for certain specific pathways. The control data is for uptake results under no inhibitor use. Compared to the control, the only pathway that was significantly inhibited was caveolae and caveolae related structures. All other pathways, macropinocytosis, caveolae-mediated internalization and clathrin-mediated internalization, LCCTLA uptake seems to have somewhat increased significantly. The results are not clear as to why the uptake is increasing in most pathways under inhibitor use and decreasing in one (similar to caveolae mediated uptake, in which the uptake increased). It is possible that none of these pathways is the mechanism for uptake of LCCTLA in CD22 expressing Daudi cells, which suggests that LCCTLA uptake could be via the fourth pathway which is independent of clathrin and caveolin proteins and that the uptake of LCCTLA was not affected in the presence of these inhibitors because its uptake was not dependent on those pathways [77]. This complete mechanism of this pathway is not yet fully understood especially during the late stage of vesicle formation.

3.14. LCCTLA Nanoparticles Were Localized Intracellularly in Endosomes

Figure 7A shows a whole Daudi cell image acquired by TEM post-MLCCTLA treatment. Two parts of the image have been enlarged in Figure 7B,C. As in Figure 7B an MLV inside an endocytotic vesicle can be observed. The size of each of the three dark structures inside the vesicle are approximately 70 nm in diameter, indicating that these are the SUV's inside the outer, larger MLV. In Figure 7C another endocytotic vesicle carrying SUV's was observed. These SUV's are approximately 50 nm in diameter. The size of these vesicles corresponds with the size of the MLCCTLA (data not shown here). This data confirms that the intracellular localization of the MLCCTLA is in endosomes. Later, these endosomes must fuse with lysosomes to form endolysosomes to release AD 198 [78].

3.15. The Endosomes Fuse with Lysosomes to Give Endolysosomes

Figure 7D shows the images for the study to determine if the endosome in which the LCCTLA were localized were endolysosomes. The cells shown here are Daudi cells treated with 10 μL of placebo LCCTLA and LysoTracker® Deep Red (a dye that binds to late endolysosomes). After washing off the excess placebo LCCTLA, the images showed red circular structures inside the Daudi cells (white arrows). Since the dye for tagging the endolysosomes was red, it was deduced that these circular red structures were the endolysosomes. The liposomes were processed with NBD-PC, a fluorescent green lipid, which also show up in the images as bright green (green arrows). When these two images were overlaid, it was observed that the endolysosomes and the LCCTLA were co-localized inside the cells (yellow arrows). This establishes that the LCCTLA were intracellularly localized in endosomes (as from Figure 7B,C) and these endosomes were later fusing with the lysosomes to give endolysosomes (Figure 7D).

3.16. LCCTLA Activates Classical Apoptotic Pathways

With LCCTLA treatment in Daudi cells, it was observed that expression of oncogenic markers decreased, and apoptotic markers increased. Figure 8B shows the proteins that were affected along with their functions and Figure 8A gives a comparison of their expressions with the control. C-myc is a marker for Burkitt's lymphoma and is a regulator gene that codes for a transcription factor [79]. The protein is multi-functional playing roles in apoptotic inhibition and cell cycle progression. Treatment with LCCTLA reduced the expression of c-myc in a time-dependent manner as shown in Figure 8A. Similar results were also demonstrated by Edwards et al. [45].

LCCTLA, once internalized is believed to release drug due to pH reduction in the endolysosomes. The intracellularly released AD 198 binds to PKC holoenzyme. Later the catalytic segment (CS) dissociates. The CS activates PLS3 which depolarizes the mitochondria releasing Cyt C. The Cyt C activates caspase 3. Caspase 3 being an apoptotic protein eventually results in apoptosis [40]. Thus, we observed a time-dependent increase in the concentration of caspase 3 as depicted in Figure 8A, which is a hallmark of cell death via apoptosis. There is a possibility for AD 198 to activate caspase-3 by other pathways but these are not well understood yet.

Protein kinase B also known as Akt is a serine-threonine specific protein kinase which plays a key role in multiple process in the cell such as cell proliferation, transcription, and apoptosis. It is capable of initiating cell survival via growth factor dependent and independent pathways [80]. Phosphorylated Akt is the activated form of Akt which is necessary for it to activate or deactivate its substrates [81,82]. In Figure 8A, we observed the expression of pAKT decreasing in a time-dependent manner compared to the control, which means that LCCTLA also inhibited cell proliferation via suppression of pAKT. JNK's or c-Jun N-terminal kinases are master protein kinases that regulate many processes in the cell such as inflammation, cell proliferation and differentiation and apoptosis. They belong to the mitogen-activated protein kinase family. Their active role in cancer development is now well-established [83]. JNK is activated by phosphorylation (pJNK). pJNK in turn phosphorylates multiple protein depending on its isoform. Figure 8A shows a time-dependent suppression of pJNK by treatment of Daudi cells with LCCTLA, thus proving that cell proliferation is also inhibited by suppression of pJNK.

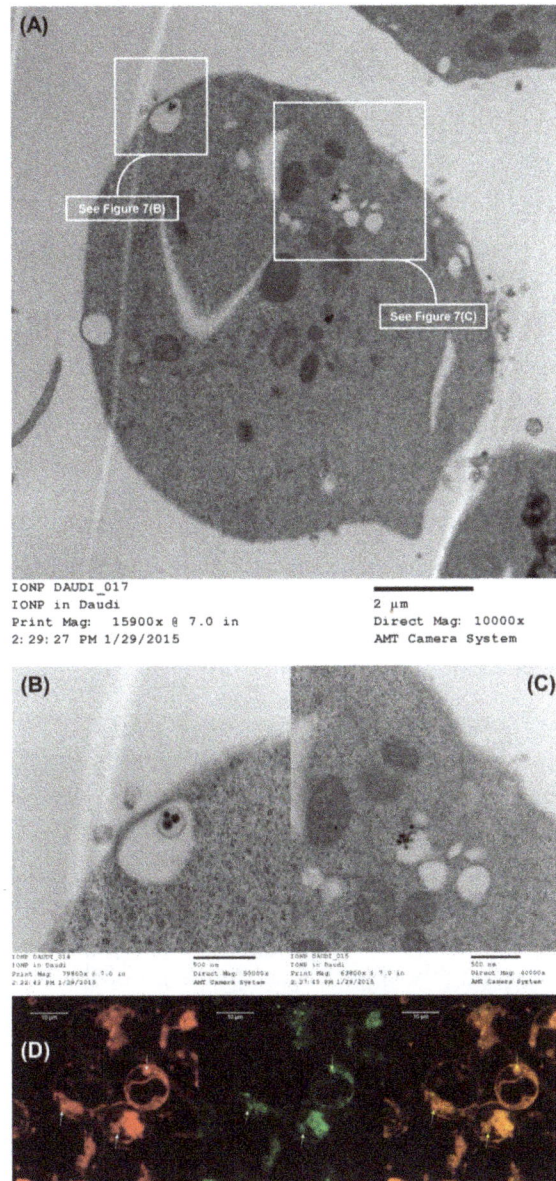

Figure 7. (**A**) TEM image of LCCTLA intracellular localization in Daudi cells; (**B**) Enlarged from Figure 7A showing an MLV of MLCCTLA inside an endosomal structure; (**C**) Enlarged from Figure 7A showing SUV's of MLCCTLA inside an endosomal structure; and (**D**) CLSM image of intracellular localization of LCCTLA in endolysosomes.

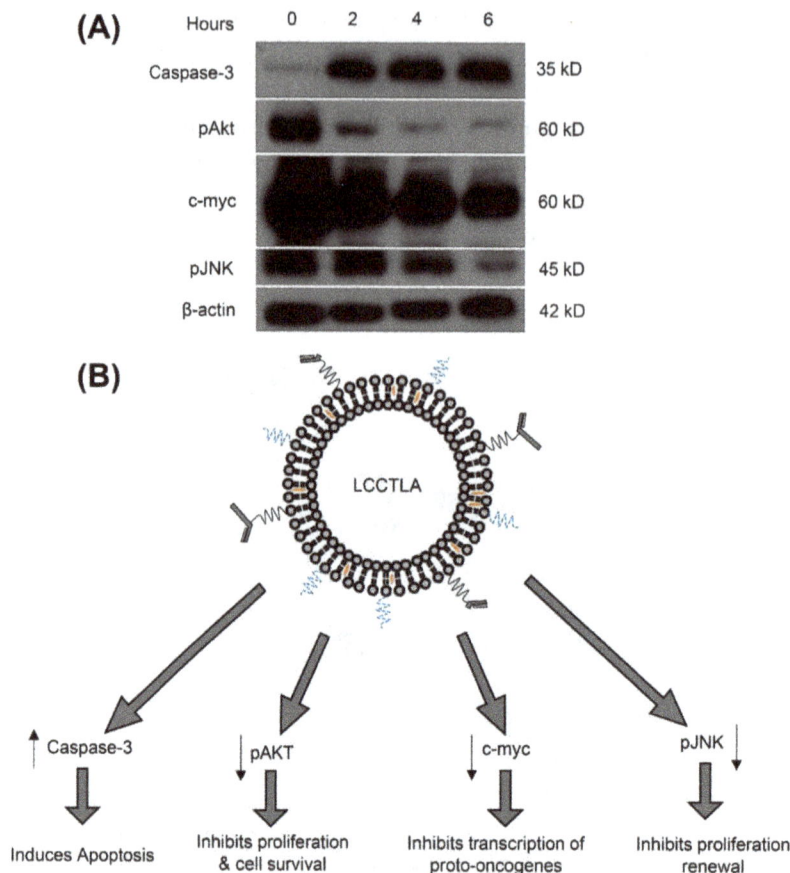

Figure 8. (**A**) Western blot results for the expression patterns post LCCTLA treatment for 3 time points, 2, 4 and 6 h; and (**B**) Effect of LCCTLA on the expression of caspase-3, pAKT, c-myc and pJNK.

4. Summary and Conclusions

A prototype formulation of AD 198 loaded liposomes (LCLA) was developed that would be able to encapsulate maximum AD 198 and have optimum parameters for effective delivery of the encapsulated drug. The optimized composition of LCLA was as follows. HSPC was the lipid of choice and was used at 75 mole %, mPEG2000-DSPE 2 mole %, cholesterol 10 mole % and AD 198 2 mg/mL. The physicochemical parameters of the optimized formulation were as follows; size 115–145 nm, ζ-potential -8 to -15 mV, AD 198 encapsulation 1000–1500 µg/mL and dissolution of not more than 30% AD 198 occurred for 72 h. The size of the LCLA as per TEM was found be in the range of 80–90 nm. TEM micrographs indicated a roughly spherical morphology of the liposomes. It was calculated that the number of HSPC molecules per liposome were approximately 117,196 and the number of AD 198 molecules were approximately 3790 per liposome.

To achieve active targeting, it was necessary to conjugate a ligand for a specific receptor on the surface of the malignant B cells. For this purpose, CD22 was selected as the receptor to be targeted on the malignant B cells. CD22 was selected due to its property of receptor mediated endocytosis upon interaction with the ligand and because it was overexpressed in malignant B cells. The anti-CD22 monoclonal antibody, RFB4, was selected as the targeting ligand. Since earlier studies by other research groups had proven that the circulating half-life of targeted liposomal systems was higher if targeted using just the Fab′ conjugated to the liposomes rather than the whole antibody, only the anti-CD22 Fab′ conjugation was optimized. Numerous methods for conjugating a ligand to the liposome exist. The one selected for conjugating the anti-CD22 Fab′ to the LCLA was with the thioether bond. The reason for selecting this strategy was its minimum use of harsh reagents and provision of a strong covalent chemical bond ensuring the stability of the targeted liposomal system. Proof of conjugation by the thioether bonding was provided by a western blot of the targeted liposomes which evidently portrayed a band at the 50 kD region which was the molecular weight of the anti-CD22 Fab'. It was calculated that every liposome displayed an average of approximately 13 anti-CD22 Fab' molecules.

Whether or not the 13 anti-CD22 Fab' molecules were sufficient to effectively target and deliver the liposomal AD 198 to the malignant B cells was determined by testing the long-circulating CD22 targeted liposomal AD 198 (LCCTLA), in vitro in CD22 overexpressing Daudi cells and comparing this result with non-CD22 expressing Jurkat cells. It was seen that Daudi cells had a significantly higher uptake of the LCCTLA compared to Jurkat cells, which confirmed specificity of the delivery system. The MTT assay results for cell cytotoxicity suggested a delay in cell kill for Daudi cells treated with LCCTLA, but this could be explained by the method of endocytosis that they underwent which would take more time compared to the diffusion mechanism for LCLA and solution AD 198. Nevertheless, cytotoxicity by the LCCTLA in Daudi cells was highest for a 24-h study. However, the results from the 48-h study suggest that studies in animals need to be performed in which unbound drug would be cleared faster, and this would mimic clinical settings better.

The functioning of LCCTLA was explained by the several studies performed in vitro. Cellular association studies determined that the endocytotic mechanism was an energy dependent mechanism and it was further ascertained that the mechanisms of endocytosis possibly were a clathrin- and caveolin-independent pathway. This pathway has not been fully understood yet particularly the later stages of internalization. However, it was successfully determined that after endocytosis, the liposomes were localized in endolysosomes. This result suggested that the drug release would take place due to liposomal breakdown by the low lysosomal pH. Once the drug was released into the cytosol, it functioned via the activation of apoptotic proteins such as caspase-3 and the suppression of oncoproteins such as c-myc. These verifications were deduced by protein expression studies performed in Daudi cells post-LCCTLA treatment.

In conclusion, targeted drug delivery with AD 198 was more potent and specific compared to other untargeted formulations. Further studies in small animal models are necessary to ascertain the efficacy of the system in more clinically relevant models.

Acknowledgments: The authors would like to acknowledge The University of Tennessee Health Science Center, College of Pharmacy, Department of Pharmaceutical Sciences, Plough Center for Sterile Drug Delivery Systems, and all supporting labs for their constant support of this work. The authors would also like to acknowledge the lab of Ellen Vitetta, University of Texas, Southwestern Medical Center, for providing valuable molecules from their lab without which this study would not have been possible.

Author Contributions: This original research has been conceived and designed by Nivesh K. Mittal, with valuable inputs from the rest of the authors. Experiments were conducted by Nivesh K. Mittal, Pavan Balabathula, Bivash Mandal, Saini Setua and Dileep R. Janagam, under the guidance of George C. Wood, Leonard Lothstein and Laura Thoma. Data Analysis was performed by all authors. Laura Thoma, George C. Wood and Leonard Lothstein provided materials and equipment for the experiments and Nivesh K. Mittal wrote the paper.

References

1.   Barenholz, Y.C. Doxil®—The first FDA-approved nano-drug: Lessons learned. *J. Control. Release* **2012**, *160*, 117–134. [CrossRef] [PubMed]

2.   Venditto, V.J.; Szoka, F.C., Jr. Cancer nanomedicines: So many papers and so few drugs! *Adv. Drug Deliv. Rev.* **2013**, *65*, 80–88. [CrossRef] [PubMed]

3.   Green, M.R.; Manikhas, G.M.; Orlov, S.; Afanasyev, B.; Makhson, A.M.; Bhar, P.; Hawkins, M.J. Abraxane, a novel cremophor-free, albumin-bound particle form of paclitaxel for the treatment of advanced non-small-cell lung cancer. *Ann. Oncol.* **2006**, *17*, 1263–1268. [CrossRef] [PubMed]

4.   Petre, C.E.; Dittmer, D.P. Liposomal daunorubicin as treatment for kaposi's sarcoma. *Int. J. Nanomed.* **2007**, *2*, 277–288.

5. Deitcher, O.R.; O'Brien, S.; Deitcher, S.R.; Thomas, D.A.; Kantarjian, H.M. Single-agent vincristine sulfate liposomes injection (marqibo®) compared to historical single-agent therapy for adults with advanced, relapsed and/or refractory philadelphia chromosome negative acute lymphoblastic leukemia. *Blood* **2011**, *118*, 2592.

6. Rodriguez, M.; Pytlik, R.; Kozak, T.; Chhanabhai, M.; Gascoyne, R.; Lu, B.; Deitcher, S.R.; Winter, J.N. Vincristine sulfate liposomes injection (marqibo) in heavily pretreated patients with refractory aggressive non-hodgkin lymphoma. *Cancer* **2009**, *115*, 3475–3482. [CrossRef] [PubMed]

7. Bharali, D.J.; Mousa, S.A. Emerging nanomedicines for early cancer detection and improved treatment: Current perspective and future promise. *Pharmacol. Ther.* **2010**, *128*, 324–335. [CrossRef] [PubMed]

8. Davis, M.E.; Chen, Z.G.; Shin, D.M. Nanoparticle therapeutics: An emerging treatment modality for cancer. *Nat. Rev. Drug Discov.* **2008**, *7*, 771–782. [CrossRef] [PubMed]

9. Torchilin, V.P. Immunoliposomes and pegylated immunoliposomes: Possible use for targeted delivery of imaging agents. *ImmunoMethods* **1994**, *4*, 244–258. [CrossRef] [PubMed]

10. Allen, T.M. Ligand-targeted therapeutics in anticancer therapy. *Nat. Rev. Cancer* **2002**, *2*, 750–763. [CrossRef] [PubMed]

11. Allen, T.M.; Mumbengegwi, D.R.; Charrois, G.J.R. Anti-CD19-targeted liposomal doxorubicin improves the therapeutic efficacy in murine b-cell lymphoma and ameliorates the toxicity of liposomes with varying drug release rates. *Clin. Cancer Res.* **2005**, *11*, 3567–3573. [CrossRef] [PubMed]

12. Allen, T.M.; Sapra, P.; Moase, E. Use of the post-insertion method for the formation of ligand-coupled liposomes. *Cell. Mol. Biol. Lett.* **2002**, *7*, 217–219. [PubMed]

13. Cheng, W.W.; Allen, T.M. Targeted delivery of anti-CD19 liposomal doxorubicin in b-cell lymphoma: A comparison of whole monoclonal antibody, fab' fragments and single chain fv. *J. Control. Release* **2008**, *126*, 50–58. [CrossRef] [PubMed]

14. De Menezes, D.E.L.; Kirchmeier, M.J.; Gagne, J.F.; Pilarski, L.M.; Allen, T.M. Cellular trafficking and cytotoxicity of anti-CD19-targeted liposomal doxorubicin in b lymphoma cells. *J. Liposome Res.* **1999**, *9*, 199–228. [CrossRef]

15. Pillai, G. Nanomedicines for cancer therapy: An update of fda approved and those under various stages of development. *SOJ Pharm. Pharm. Sci.* **2014**, *1*, 1–13.

16. Allen, T.M.; Cullis, P.R. Liposomal drug delivery systems: From concept to clinical applications. *Adv. Drug Deliv. Rev.* **2013**, *65*, 36–48. [CrossRef] [PubMed]

17. Bulbake, U.; Doppalapudi, S.; Kommineni, N.; Khan, W. Liposomal formulations in clinical use: An updated review. *Pharmaceutics* **2017**, *9*, 12. [CrossRef] [PubMed]

18. Torchilin, V.P. Recent advances with liposomes as pharmaceutical carriers. *Nat. Rev. Drug Discov.* **2005**, *4*, 145–160. [CrossRef] [PubMed]

19. Heger, Z.; Polanska, H.; Rodrigo, M.A.M.; Guran, R.; Kulich, P.; Kopel, P.; Masarik, M.; Eckschlager, T.; Stiborova, M.; Kizek, R. Prostate tumor attenuation in the nu/nu murine model due to anti-sarcosine antibodies in folate-targeted liposomes. *Sci. Rep.* **2016**, *6*, 33379. [CrossRef] [PubMed]

20. Dothager, R.S.; Piwnica-Worms, D. Nano in cancer: Linking chemistry, biology, and clinical applications in vivo. *Cancer Res.* **2011**, *71*, 5611–5615. [CrossRef] [PubMed]

21. Ali, I.; Salim, K.; Rather, M.A.; Wani, W.A.; Haque, A. Advances in nano drugs for cancer chemotherapy. *Curr. Cancer Drug Targ.* **2011**, *11*, 135–146. [CrossRef]

22. Siegel, R.L.; Miller, K.D.; Jemal, A. Cancer statistics, 2015. *CA A Cancer J. Clin.* **2015**, *65*, 5–29. [CrossRef] [PubMed]

23. Chen, W.C.; Completo, G.C.; Sigal, D.S.; Crocker, P.R.; Saven, A.; Paulson, J.C. In vivo targeting of b-cell lymphoma with glycan ligands of cd22. *Blood* **2010**, *115*, 4778–4786. [CrossRef] [PubMed]

24. Tirelli, U.; Errante, D.; Van Glabbeke, M.; Teodorovic, I.; Kluin-Nelemans, J.; Thomas, J.; Bron, D.; Rosti, G.; Somers, R.; Zagonel, V. Chop is the standard regimen in patients > or= 70 years of age with intermediate-grade and high-grade non-hodgkin's lymphoma: Results of a randomized study of the european organization for research and treatment of cancer lymphoma cooperative study group. *J. Clin. Oncol.* **1998**, *16*, 27–34. [CrossRef] [PubMed]

25. Mittal, N.K.; Bhattacharjee, H.; Mandal, B.; Balabathula, P.; Thoma, L.A.; Wood, G.C. Targeted liposomal drug delivery systems for the treatment of b cell malignancies. *J. Drug Targ.* **2014**, *22*, 372–386. [CrossRef] [PubMed]

26. Binsky, I.; Haran, M.; Starlets, D.; Gore, Y.; Lantner, F.; Harpaz, N.; Leng, L.; Goldenberg, D.M.; Shvidel, L.; Berrebi, A.; et al. Il-8 secreted in a macrophage migration-inhibitory factor- and cd74-dependent manner regulates b cell chronic lymphocytic leukemia survival. *Proc. Natl. Acad. Sci. USA* **2007**, *104*, 13408–13413. [CrossRef] [PubMed]

27. DiJoseph, J.F.; Dougher, M.M.; Kalyandrug, L.B.; Armellino, D.C.; Boghaert, E.R.; Hamann, P.R.; Moran, J.K.; Damle, N.K. Antitumor efficacy of a combination of cmc-544 (inotuzumab ozogamicin), a cd22-targeted cytotoxic immunoconjugate of calicheamicin, and rituximab against non-hodgkin's b-cell lymphoma. *Clin. Cancer Res.* **2006**, *12*, 242–249. [CrossRef] [PubMed]

28. Du, X.; Beers, R.; Fitzgerald, D.J.; Pastan, I. Differential cellular internalization of anti-cd19 and -cd22 immunotoxins results in different cytotoxic activity. *Cancer Res* **2008**, *68*, 6300–6305. [CrossRef] [PubMed]

29. Loomis, K.; Smith, B.; Feng, Y.; Garg, H.; Yavlovich, A.; Campbell-Massa, R.; Dimitrov, D.S.; Blumenthal, R.; Xiao, X.; Puri, A. Specific targeting to b cells by lipid-based nanoparticles conjugated with a novel cd22-scfv. *Exp. Mol. Pathol.* **2010**, *88*, 238–249. [CrossRef] [PubMed]

30. Sapra, P.; Allen, T.M. Improved outcome when b-cell lymphoma is treated with combinations of immunoliposomal anticancer drugs targeted to both the cd19 and cd20 epitopes. *Clin. Cancer Res.* **2004**, *10*, 2530–2537. [CrossRef] [PubMed]

31. Tuscano, J.M.; Martin, S.M.; Ma, Y.; Zamboni, W.; O'Donnell, R.T. Efficacy, biodistribution, and pharmacokinetics of cd22-targeted pegylated liposomal doxorubicin in a b-cell non–hodgkin's lymphoma xenograft mouse model. *Clin. Cancer Res.* **2010**, *16*, 2760–2768. [CrossRef] [PubMed]

32. O'Donnell, R.T.; Martin, S.M.; Ma, Y.; Zamboni, W.C.; Tuscano, J.M. Development and characterization of cd22-targeted pegylated-liposomal doxorubicin (il-pld). *Investig. New Drugs* **2010**, *28*, 260–267. [CrossRef] [PubMed]

33. Sapra, P.; Allen, T.M. Internalizing antibodies are necessary for improved therapeutic efficacy of antibody-targeted liposomal drugs. *Cancer Res.* **2002**, *62*, 7190–7194. [PubMed]

34. Sapra, P.; Moase, E.H.; Ma, J.; Allen, T.M. Improved therapeutic responses in a xenograft model of human b lymphoma (namalwa) for liposomal vincristine versus liposomal doxorubicin targeted via anti-cd19 igg2a or fab' fragments. *Clin. Cancer Res.* **2004**, *10*, 1100–1111. [CrossRef] [PubMed]

35. Frishman, W.H.; Sung, H.M.; Yee, H.C.M.; Liu, L.L.; Einzig, A.I.; Dutcher, J.; Keefe, D. Cardiovascular toxicity with cancer chemotherapy. *Curr. Probl. Cardiol.* **1996**, *21*, 233–286. [CrossRef]

36. Jensen, B.; Skovsgaard, T.; Nielsen, S. Functional monitoring of anthracycline cardiotoxicity: A prospective, blinded, long-term observational study of outcome in 120 patients. *Ann. Oncol.* **2002**, *13*, 699–709. [CrossRef] [PubMed]

37. Speyer, J.; Wasserheit, C. Strategies for reduction of anthracycline cardiac toxicity. *Semin. Oncol.* **1998**, *25*, 525–537. [PubMed]

38. Binaschi, M.; Bigioni, M.; Cipollone, A.; Rossi, C.; Goso, C.; Maggi, C.A.; Capranico, G.; Animati, F. Anthracyclines: Selected new developments. *Curr. Med. Chem. Anti-Cancer Agents* **2001**, *1*, 113–130. [CrossRef] [PubMed]

39. Teicher, B.A. *Cancer Therapeutics: Experimental and Clinical Agents*; Springer Science & Business Media: Berlin, Germany, 1996.

40. He, Y.; Liu, J.; Durrant, D.; Yang, H.S.; Sweatman, T.; Lothstein, L.; Lee, R.M. N-benzyladriamycin-14-valerate (AD198) induces apoptosis through protein kinase C-delta-induced phosphorylation of phospholipid scramblase 3. *Cancer Res.* **2005**, *65*, 10016–10023. [CrossRef] [PubMed]

41. Hofmann, P.A.; Israel, M.; Koseki, Y.; Laskin, J.; Gray, J.; Janik, A.; Sweatman, T.W.; Lothstein, L. N-benzyladriamycin-14-valerate (AD 198): A non-cardiotoxic anthracycline that is cardioprotective through pkc-epsilon activation. *J. Pharmacol. Exp. Ther.* **2007**, *323*, 658–664. [CrossRef] [PubMed]

42. Cai, C.; Lothstein, L.; Morrison, R.R.; Hofmann, P.A. Protection from doxorubicin-induced cardiomyopathy using the modified anthracycline N-benzyladriamycin-14-valerate (AD 198). *J. Pharmacol. Exp. Ther.* **2010**, *335*, 223–230. [CrossRef] [PubMed]

43. Lothstein, L.; Savranskaya, L.; Barrett, C.M.; Israel, M.; Sweatman, T.W. N-benzyladriamycin-14-valerate (AD 198) activates protein kinase c-δ holoenzyme to trigger mitochondrial depolarization and cytochrome c release independently of permeability transition pore opening and Ca^{2+} influx. *Anti-Cancer Drugs* **2006**, *17*, 495–502. [CrossRef] [PubMed]

44. Rathore, K.; Cekanova, M. A novel derivative of doxorubicin, AD198, inhibits canine transitional cell carcinoma and osteosarcoma cells in vitro. *Drug Des. Dev. Ther.* **2015**, *9*, 5323–5335.

45. Edwards, S.K.; Han, Y.; Liu, Y.; Kreider, B.Z.; Liu, Y.; Grewal, S.; Desai, A.; Baron, J.; Moore, C.R.; Luo, C. Signaling mechanisms of bortezomib in traf3-deficient mouse b lymphoma and human multiple myeloma cells. *Leuk. Res.* **2016**, *41*, 85–95. [CrossRef] [PubMed]

46. Mittal, N.K. Design, Development, Characterization and Testing of CD22 Targeted Long Circulating Liposomal Drug Delivery Systems for β Cell Malignancies. Ph.D. Thesis, University of Tennessee, Knoxville, TN, USA, 2015.

47. Bangham, A.; Horne, R. Negative staining of phospholipids and their structural modification by surface-active agents as observed in the electron microscope. *J. Mol. Biol.* **1964**, *8*, 660–668. [CrossRef]

48. Lopes de Menezes, D.E.; Pilarski, L.M.; Allen, T.M. In vitro and in vivo targeting of immunoliposomal doxorubicin to human b-cell lymphoma. *Cancer Res.* **1998**, *58*, 3320–3330. [PubMed]

49. Juliano, R.L.; Stamp, D. The effect of particle size and charge on the clearance rates of liposomes and liposome encapsulated drugs. *Biochem. Biophys. Res. Commun.* **1975**, *63*, 651–658. [CrossRef]

50. Haran, G.; Cohen, R.; Bar, L.K.; Barenholz, Y. Transmembrane ammonium sulfate gradients in liposomes produce efficient and stable entrapment of amphipathic weak bases. *Biochim. Biophys. Acta-Biomembr.* **1993**, *1151*, 201–215. [CrossRef]

51. Lothstein, L.; Rodrigues, P.J.; Sweatman, T.W.; Israel, M. Cytotoxicity and intracellular biotransformation of *N*-benzyladriamycin-14-yalerate (AD 198) are modulated by changes in 14-O-acyl chain length. *Anti-Cancer Drugs* **1998**, *9*, 58–66. [CrossRef] [PubMed]

52. Stewart, J.C.M. Colorimetric determination of phospholipids with ammonium ferrothiocyanate. *Anal. Biochem.* **1980**, *104*, 10–14. [CrossRef]

53. Zhang, L.; Chan, J.M.; Gu, F.X.; Rhee, J.-W.; Wang, A.Z.; Radovic-Moreno, A.F.; Alexis, F.; Langer, R.; Farokhzad, O.C. Self-assembled lipid-polymer hybrid nanoparticles: A robust drug delivery platform. *ACS Nano* **2008**, *2*, 1696–1702. [CrossRef] [PubMed]

54. Chan, J.M.; Zhang, L.; Yuet, K.P.; Liao, G.; Rhee, J.-W.; Langer, R.; Farokhzad, O.C. PLGA-lecithin-PEG core-shell nanoparticles for controlled drug delivery. *Biomaterials* **2009**, *30*, 1627–1634. [CrossRef] [PubMed]

55. Zhang, L.; Radovic-Moreno, A.F.; Alexis, F.; Gu, F.X.; Basto, P.A.; Bagalkot, V.; Jon, S.; Langer, R.S.; Farokhzad, O.C. Co-delivery of hydrophobic and hydrophilic drugs from nanoparticle–aptamer bioconjugates. *ChemMedChem* **2007**, *2*, 1268–1271. [CrossRef] [PubMed]

56. Oliveira, S.; Schiffelers, R.M.; van der Veeken, J.; van der Meel, R.; Vongpromek, R.; en Henegouwen, P.M.V.B.; Storm, G.; Roovers, R.C. Downregulation of EGFR by a novel multivalent nanobody-liposome platform. *J. Control. Release* **2010**, *145*, 165–175. [CrossRef] [PubMed]

57. Huth, U.S.; Schubert, R.; Peschka-Süss, R. Investigating the uptake and intracellular fate of pH-sensitive liposomes by flow cytometry and spectral bio-imaging. *J. Control. Release* **2006**, *110*, 490–504. [CrossRef] [PubMed]

58. Mosmann, T. Rapid colorimetric assay for cellular growth and survival: Application to proliferation and cytotoxicity assays. *J. Immunol. Methods* **1983**, *65*, 55–63. [CrossRef]

59. Douglas, K.L.; Piccirillo, C.A.; Tabrizian, M. Cell line-dependent internalization pathways and intracellular trafficking determine transfection efficiency of nanoparticle vectors. *Eur. J. Pharm. Biopharm.* **2008**, *68*, 676–687. [CrossRef] [PubMed]

60. Gao, H.; Yang, Z.; Zhang, S.; Cao, S.; Shen, S.; Pang, Z.; Jiang, X. Ligand modified nanoparticles increases cell uptake, alters endocytosis and elevates glioma distribution and internalization. *Sci. Rep.* **2013**, *3*. [CrossRef] [PubMed]

61. Suresh, D.; Zambre, A.; Chanda, N.; Hoffman, T.J.; Smith, C.J.; Robertson, J.D.; Kannan, R. Bombesin peptide conjugated gold nanocages internalize via clathrin mediated endocytosis. *Bioconjug. Chem.* **2014**, *25*, 1565–1579. [CrossRef] [PubMed]

62. Päuser, S.; Reszka, R.; Wagner, S.; Wolf, K.J.; Buhr, H.J.; Berger, G. Liposome-encapsulated superparamagnetic iron oxide particles as markers in an MRI-guided search for tumor-specific drug carriers. *Anticancer Drug Des.* **1997**, *12*, 125–135. [PubMed]

63. Wu, L.; Yu, X.; Feizpour, A.; Reinhard, B.M. Nanoconjugation: A materials approach to enhance epidermal growth factor induced apoptosis. *Biomater. Sci.* **2014**, *2*, 156–166. [CrossRef] [PubMed]

64. Jiang, M.; Gan, L.; Zhu, C.; Dong, Y.; Liu, J.; Gan, Y. Cationic core-shell liponanoparticles for ocular gene delivery. *Biomaterials* **2012**, *33*, 7621–7630. [CrossRef] [PubMed]

65. Zhao, Z.; Lou, S.; Hu, Y.; Zhu, J.; Zhang, C. A nano-in-nano polymer–dendrimer nanoparticle-based nanosystem for controlled multidrug delivery. *Mol. Pharm.* **2017**, *14*, 2697–2710. [CrossRef] [PubMed]

66. Jaggi, M.; Rao, P.S.; Smith, D.J.; Wheelock, M.J.; Johnson, K.R.; Hemstreet, G.P.; Balaji, K. E-cadherin phosphorylation by protein kinase D1/protein kinase Cµ is associated with altered cellular aggregation and motility in prostate cancer. *Cancer Res.* **2005**, *65*, 483–492. [PubMed]

67. Lian, T.; Ho, R.J. Trends and developments in liposome drug delivery systems. *J. Pharm. Sci.* **2001**, *90*, 667–680. [CrossRef] [PubMed]

68. Gregoriadis, G.; Senior, J. The phospholipid component of small unilamellar liposomes controls the rate of clearance of entrapped solutes from the circulation. *FEBS Lett.* **1980**, *119*, 43–46. [CrossRef]

69. Senior, J.H. Fate and behavior of liposomes in vivo: A review of controlling factors. *Crit. Rev. Ther. Drug Carr. Syst.* **1987**, *3*, 123–193.

70. Drummond, D.C.; Meyer, O.; Hong, K.; Kirpotin, D.B.; Papahadjopoulos, D. Optimizing liposomes for delivery of chemotherapeutic agents to solid tumors. *Pharmacol. Rev.* **1999**, *51*, 691–743. [PubMed]

71. Hu, Y.; Hoerle, R.; Ehrich, M.; Zhang, C. Engineering the lipid layer of lipid–PLGA hybrid nanoparticles for enhanced in vitro cellular uptake and improved stability. *Acta Biomater.* **2015**, *28*, 149–159. [CrossRef] [PubMed]

72. Woodle, M.C.; Matthay, K.K.; Newman, M.S.; Hidayat, J.E.; Collins, L.R.; Redemann, C.; Martin, F.J.; Papahadjopoulos, D. Versatility in lipid compositions showing prolonged circulation with sterically stabilized liposomes. *Biochim. Biophys. Acta* **1992**, *1105*, 193–200. [CrossRef]

73. Gramse, G.; Dols-Perez, A.; Edwards, M.A.; Fumagalli, L.; Gomila, G. Nanoscale measurement of the dielectric constant of supported lipid bilayers in aqueous solutions with electrostatic force microscopy. *Biophys. J.* **2013**, *104*, 1257–1262. [CrossRef] [PubMed]

74. Torre, L.G.; Carneiro, A.L.; Rosada, R.S.; Silva, C.L.; Santana, M.H.A. A mathematical model describing the kinetic of cationic liposome production from dried lipid films adsorbed in a multitubular system. *Br. J. Chem. Eng.* **2007**, *24*, 477–486. [CrossRef]

75. Budha, N.R.; Lee, R.B.; Hurdle, J.G.; Lee, R.E.; Meibohm, B. A simple in vitro PK/PD model system to determine time–kill curves of drugs against mycobacteria. *Tuberculosis* **2009**, *89*, 378–385. [CrossRef] [PubMed]

76. Schmid, S.L.; Carter, L.L. ATP is required for receptor-mediated endocytosis in intact cells. *J. Cell Biol.* **1990**, *111*, 2307–2318. [CrossRef] [PubMed]

77. Kou, L.; Sun, J.; Zhai, Y.; He, Z. The endocytosis and intracellular fate of nanomedicines: Implication for rational design. *Asian J. Pharm. Sci.* **2013**, *8*, 1–10. [CrossRef]

78. Luzio, J.P.; Pryor, P.R.; Bright, N.A. Lysosomes: Fusion and function. *Nat. Rev. Mol. Cell Biol.* **2007**, *8*, 622–632. [CrossRef] [PubMed]

79. Finver, S.N.; Nishikura, K.; Finger, L.R.; Haluska, F.G.; Finan, J.; Nowell, P.C.; Croce, C.M. Sequence analysis of the MYC oncogene involved in the t(8;14)(q24;q11) chromosome translocation in a human leukemia T-cell line indicates that putative regulatory regions are not altered. *Proc. Natl. Acad. Sci. USA* **1988**, *85*, 3052–3056. [CrossRef] [PubMed]

80. Nicholson, K.M.; Anderson, N.G. The protein kinase B/Akt signalling pathway in human malignancy. *Cell. Signal.* **2002**, *14*, 381–395. [CrossRef]

81. Sarbassov, D.D.; Guertin, D.A.; Ali, S.M.; Sabatini, D.M. Phosphorylation and regulation of Akt/PKB by the rictor-mtor complex. *Science* **2005**, *307*, 1098–1101. [CrossRef] [PubMed]

82. Edwards, S.K.; Moore, C.R.; Liu, Y.; Grewal, S.; Covey, L.R.; Xie, P. N-benzyladriamycin-14-valerate (AD 198) exhibits potent anti-tumor activity on TRAF3-deficient mouse b lymphoma and human multiple myeloma. *BMC Cancer* **2013**, *13*, 481. [CrossRef] [PubMed]

83. Bubici, C.; Papa, S. Jnk signalling in cancer: In need of new, smarter therapeutic targets. *Br. J. Pharmacol.* **2014**, *171*, 24–37. [CrossRef] [PubMed]

11

Ophthalmic Drug Delivery Systems for Antibiotherapy

Marion Dubald [1,2], **Sandrine Bourgeois** [1,3], **Véronique Andrieu** [4] **and Hatem Fessi** [1,3,*]

1   Univ Lyon, Université Claude Bernard Lyon 1, Centre National de la Recherche Scientifique (CNRS), Laboratoire d'Automatique et de GEnie des Procédés (LAGEP) Unité Mixte de Recherche UMR 5007, 43 boulevard du 11 novembre 1918, F-69100, Villeurbanne, France; Marion.Dubald@horus-pharma.fr (M.D.); sandrine.bourgeois@univ-lyon1.fr (S.B.)

2   Horus Pharma, Cap Var, 148 avenue Georges Guynemer, F-06700 Saint Laurent du Var, France

3   Univ Lyon, Université Claude Bernard Lyon 1, Institut des Sciences Pharmaceutiques et Biologiques (ISPB)—Faculté de Pharmacie de Lyon, 8 avenue Rockefeller, F-69008, Lyon, France

4   Unité de Recherche sur les Maladies Infectieuses et Tropicales Émergentes (URMITE), Unité Mixte de Recherche 6236 Centre National de la Recherche Scientifique (CNRS), Aix Marseille Université, Faculté de Médecine et de Pharmacie, F-13005 Marseille, France; veronique.andrieu@univ-amu.fr

*   Correspondence: hatem.fessi@univ-lyon1.fr

Abstract: The last fifty years, ophthalmic drug delivery research has made much progress, challenging scientists about the advantages and limitations of this drug delivery approach. Topical eye drops are the most commonly used formulation in ocular drug delivery. Despite the good tolerance for patients, this topical administration is only focus on the anterior ocular diseases and had a high precorneal loss of drugs due to the tears production and ocular barriers. Antibiotics are popularly used in solution or in ointment for the ophthalmic route. However, their local bioavailability needs to be improved in order to decrease the frequency of administrations and the side effects and to increase their therapeutic efficiency. For this purpose, sustained release forms for ophthalmic delivery of antibiotics were developed. This review briefly describes the ocular administration with the ocular barriers and the currently topical forms. It focuses on experimental results to bypass the limitations of ocular antibiotic delivery with new ocular technology as colloidal and in situ gelling systems or with the improvement of existing forms as implants and contact lenses. Nanotechnology is presently a promising drug delivery way to provide protection of antibiotics and improve pathway through ocular barriers and deliver drugs to specific target sites.

Keywords: antibiotics; ocular drug administration; nanoparticles; drug delivery

1. Introduction

Ophthalmic drug delivery presents major challenges for pharmaceutical and medicinal sciences. For several decades, progress has been achieved to improve the currently dosage forms. Ocular diseases are complicated to treat, and ocular forms need to be safe, non-allergic for the patient and sterile. Topical forms represent 90% of the marked formulation [1]. The tear fluid turnover, the nasolacrimal drainage, the corneal epithelium and the blood-ocular barriers are decreasing the local bioavailability of drugs and residence time on the ocular surface in topical application. Only 5%–10% of the drug crosses the corneal barriers. Anterior segment diseases as blepharitis, conjunctivitis, scleritis, keratitis and dry eye syndrome are resolved with topical or periocular administration. The delivery of drug to the posterior segment of the eye for glaucoma, endophthalmitis or uveitis and to the anterior segment has the same issue of poor bioavailability of the drug and barriers. However, intraocular administration might be preferred despite its risk of complication [2]. In addition, compared to the oral route, ocular drug delivery provided equivalent or better bioavailability in the eye [3]. Approaches have been made for the improvement of the bioavailability of the drug, the controlled release and the improvement of the therapeutic effect [4].

Antibiotics are group of medicines popularly used in ophthalmic delivery due to the multiples ocular diseases (microbial keratitis, conjunctivitis, Meibomian gland dysfunction and dry eye). Infectious disease is one of the most public health challenge [5]. Antibacterial therapies can be administrated in the eye by topical, subtenon, intraocular or subconjunctival administration. Tetracyclines, fluoroquinolones, aminoglycosides and penicillins are examples of antibiotics commonly used in the treatment of eye infections [6]. The antimicrobial resistance is the ability of bacteria to resist to the effect of an antibiotic administration. This limitation of efficacy is caused by the misuse of antibiotic, the overuse of this group of medicine and the adaptation of the bacteria to the effect. In fact, ophthalmic antibiotic delivery aims to decrease the frequency of administration and dosing by improving the current forms and developing new ones.

New ocular drug delivery forms are various; they included in situ gelling systems, liposomes, nanoparticles, niosomes, nanoemulsions and microemulsions. They are suitable for hydrophilic or lipophilic drugs, have the capacity of targeting a specific site and can be administrated in different routes. With the appropriate excipients, in situ gelling systems are able to increase the precorneal residence time and decrease the loss of drug due to the tear. Different polymers, methods of preparation and compositions allow the nanoparticles to respond to a need for mucoadhesion, topical, periocular or intraocular administration, and to obtain a stable, effective and non-irritating formulation for the patient.

The objective of this paper is to review the antibiotic formulations for an ophthalmic administration. First the ocular anatomy and physiology and the ocular barriers were described. Topical forms such as eye drops, ointments, hydrogels, contact lenses and ophthalmic inserts are developed in a second part to introduce the ocular administration and explain the currently marketed dosage form. Finally, recent advances on ocular antibiotic administration are reviewed. In vitro and in vivo studies explored the efficacy of antimicrobial formulations. Different compositions and forms are developed to improve the bioavailability of antibiotics, increase the residence time in the eye and the therapeutic response.

2. Anatomy and Physiology of the Eye for Ocular Drug Delivery

2.1. Anatomy and Physiology of the Eye

The eye has a spherical shape included in the orbital cavity and protected by lids. With a diameter of 24 mm and a volume of 6.5 cm^3, it weighs about 7.5 g.

Several layers with specifics structures compose the eyeball and divide it in two segments [3,7]: the anterior segment (cornea, conjunctiva, aqueous humor, iris, ciliary body and lens) and the posterior segment (retina, choroid, sclera and vitreous humor) as illustrated in Figure 1.

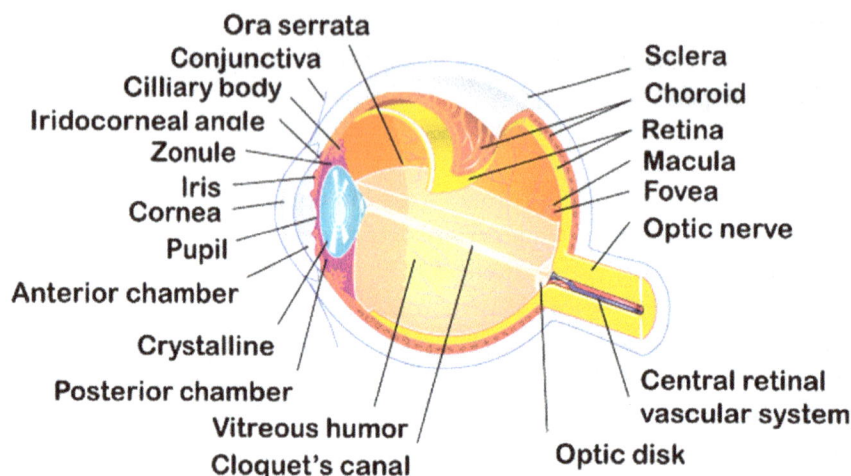

Figure 1. Schematic illustration of ocular structures and barriers.

2.1.1. Three Different Layers

The eye is surrounded by three different layers: the outer layer, the medium layer and the inner layer. The outer layer is composed by the cornea and the sclera. They are fibrous tissue and have a protective function for the eyeball. The sclera, continuous with the cornea, is an avascular, white, strong, and elastic tissue. It covers 80% of the eye's tunic. The cornea, joining the sclera at the limbus, is a thin (0.5 mm) [8], avascular and transparent layer which allows the light penetration to the globe. The anterior and posterior segments of the eye are anatomically separated by the sclera and the cornea (Figure 1).

The middle layer is a vascular envelope also called uvea, formed by the iris, the choroid and the ciliary body. The iris is a contractile, circular membrane opened at its center by the pupil. It is the color part of the eye located to the posterior region of the cornea. At the posterior of the uvea, the choroid is a highly vascularized membrane. It supplies nutriments and oxygen to the iris and retinal photoreceptors. Between the sclera and the retina, the ciliary body secrets the aqueous humor with the ciliary processes and contains smooth muscles that control the shape of the lens.

The innermost tissue is the retina. It is the neuronal tissue responsible of the vision composed of two types of tissues. The retina as the choroid, cover the inside of the posterior segment from the optic nerve to the *ora serrata*. The neural tissue is composed by the photoreceptor (rods for the night and the peripheral vision and cones for the color and the details), the bipolar cells and the ganglion cells.

2.1.2. Inside the Globe

The inside of the eye is composed of three major compounds: the crystalline, the aqueous humor and the vitreous humor.

The crystalline is a biconvex, transparent lens located behind the iris and the pupil. It is an avascular, elastic organ connected to the optical layer by the ciliary body. The crystalline separates the aqueous humor from the vitreous humor. Its function is to allow the accommodation by concentrating the light on the retina with its contraction.

The aqueous humor is a clear optical fluid with low viscosity. Located in the anterior and the posterior chambers of the eye, the aqueous humor is continuously formed by the ciliary body (2.4 ± 0.6 μL/min in humans) [9]. The anterior chamber and the posterior chamber contain 0.250 mL and 0.060 mL of aqueous humor respectively. Composed by 99% of water the aqueous humor supplies nutriments to the iris, the crystalline and the cornea [10]. It also maintains the intraocular pressure of the eye and the convex form of the lens.

The vitreous body, also called vitreous humor, is located between the crystalline and the retina. It is a transparent and gelatinous liquid, which represents 90% of the volume of the eye (4.0 mL).

Composed of 99% of water, it helps to maintain the structure of the eyeball and plays the role of a lens in the delivery of the light ray.

2.1.3. Ocular Annexes

Ocular annexes represent the external anatomic parts of the eye necessary for the proper functioning of the ocular apparatus as the muscles, the eyelids and the lacrimal apparatus.

The six extraocular muscles induce the movement of the eye in the orbit and the control of the superior eyelid movement. The eyelids are the first protection for the eye. They are movable folds of skin that covers the ocular surface, hydrate the cornea and clean the surface of the eye from debris. The superior eyelid regulates the light reaching the eye using extraocular muscles.

Located on the inside of the eyelid, the Meibomian glands are small, oily and sebaceous annexes secreting lipids and proteins to cover and protect the surface of the eye and reduce the evaporation of water contained in the tears.

The lacrimal apparatus is responsible of the tear secretion, which allows the evacuation of the debris from the ocular surface and the hydration of the eye. The lacrimal fluid is continuously formed (0.1 mL/hour) by the lacrimal glands and evacuated from the eye by the lacrimal canaliculus. At the end, all of the fluid and the debris are cleared out by the nasolacrimal duct. Human tears have a mean osmolarity of 310 mOsm/kg and a tonicity equivalent to that of 0.9% sodium chloride solution [8].

2.2. Blood-Ocular Barriers

The blood ocular barriers are composed of the blood-aqueous and the blood-retinal barriers. They are physical barriers between the blood and the eye that has a main function in the penetration, the elimination of ophthalmic route's drugs and the maintenance of the homeostatic control [11].

The blood retinal barrier is a posterior segment barrier forming an inner barrier in the endothelial membrane of the retinal vessel and an outer barrier in the retinal pigment epithelium [11,12]. It prevents diffusion of the drugs in the posterior part of the eye and is responsible for the homeostasis of the neuroretina, composed of nonleaky tight junctions. These junctions have a high degree of control of solute and fluid permeability. The retinal pigment epithelium controls exchange of nutriments with colloidal vessels. Retinal capillary endothelial cells and retinal pigment epithelial cells are connected to one other with tight junctions.

The blood aqueous barrier is an anterior segment barrier. It is a nano-porous (104 Å) and isotonic membrane (Dernouchamps and Heremans 1975; Dernouchamps and Michiels 1977) composed by the ciliary epithelium and the capillaries of the iris. The blood aqueous barrier produces aqueous humor and prevents access of large plasma albumin molecules and many other molecules such antibiotics for example, into the aqueous humor. The aqueous humor is secreted by the non-pigmented epithelium from the ciliary body [13]. The permeability of the blood-aqueous barrier is controlled by the osmotic pressure due to the sodium, chlorine and bicarbonate transport and by the physical-chemical characteristics of the drugs. Passages from the aqueous humor to the blood of lipophilic molecules are passive and active for hydrophilic molecules. The blood-aqueous barrier is composed of an epithelial barrier and an endothelial barrier. The epithelial barrier is composed of tight junctions between the non-pigmented ciliary epithelial cells and forms a pathway for the free diffusion of molecules. Iris vessels contain proteins similar to the epithelial tight junctions and form the endothelial barrier.

These barriers restricted the entry of drugs from systemic circulation to the posterior eye segment and conversely. Acute inflammation caused by intraocular surgery, induced ocular hypotony, and the use of inflammatory mediators can occur the breakdown of blood-ocular barrier. The reversal of this situation is made by the self-limited action of the inductive drug, the administration of anti-inflammatory or anti-hypotensive drug.

The ocular surface is directly exposed to the environment and to pathogens or allergens. It is an epithelial barrier composed of corneal epithelium connected with intercellular. These junctions are tight junctions, desmosomes, adherent junctions and gap junctions. The tears film is the first line of the entire ocular barrier. It washes the surface of the eye from the debris and protects the eye from the desiccation. Ocular inflammation, intraocular surgery, trauma and vascular disease can alter the ocular barrier.

3. Ophthalmic Forms

Firstly, the choice of the drug administration route depends of the target tissue. Different routes are described for the ophthalmic administration: topical ocular and subconjunctival administration are used to target the anterior segment; intravitreal and systemic administration are used to reach the posterior segment.

Two types of drug permeation after topical administration can be described: the transcorneal permeation from the lachrymal fluid to the anterior chamber and the transconjonctival and transscleral permeation from the external ocular surface to the anterior uvea-ciliary body and iris. Lipophilic drugs permeability is higher via the transcorneal route than for hydrophilic drugs because of the lipidic composition of the corneal epithelium [14]. In contrast, the transconjonctival pathway is suited to hydrophilic drugs and large molecules. Topical administration is used for the treatment of anterior chamber pathologies as inflammation, allergy, keratoconjunctivitis, infection or corneal ulceration. The topical forms must satisfy the criteria of efficacy, sterility, stability and ocular tolerance.

3.1. Eye Drops

Eye drops are sterile and mainly isotonic solution containing drugs or only lubricating or tears replacing solution. This conventional dosage form for ocular administration represents 90% of the marketed formulations due to its simplicity of development and production. Eye drops are cheaper than the other forms and have a good acceptance by patient [2]. Unfortunately, 95% of the drugs are eliminated with the lachrymal apparatus and the different barriers in 15 to 30 s after the instillation [14]. Moreover, a secondary eye infection may be caused by a microbiological contamination with multidoses packaging. The pH must be ideally around 7.4 which the pH of the tears [15] and the osmolarity around 310 mOsm/kg. Despite a little burning sensation after administration, responsible for lacrimation and cell desquamation, eye drops, single or multidose, are the most common dosage forms for the eyes.

However, the ocular bioavailability can be improved by increasing drug permeation through the cornea and the eye drop residence time at the eye surface. For this purpose, excipients as permeation enhancers, viscosifiant agents and cyclodextrins are used to improve the efficiency formulations [15]. Permeation enhancer modifies the corneal integrity and decreases barrier resistance [3]. Examples of permeation enhancers include polyoxyethylene glycol ester and ethylenediaminetetra acetic acid sodium salt [15]. Benzalkonium chloride is popularly used as preservative but could also plays the role of penetration enhancer due to its surfactant properties [16,17]. Viscosity enhancers by increasing the viscosity of solution allow the improvement of the residence time on the eye and the local bioavailability of the drug. To increase residence time of eye drops viscosifiant are used such as polyvinylalcohol (PVA) [18], hydroxylmethylcellulose, hydroxylethylcellulose [15]. Cyclodextrins (CD) are polysaccharides with a hydrophobic internal cavity and a hydrophilic external surface [19]. Sigurdsson et al. used CD to form inclusion complex with lipophilic molecules such as steroids or cyclosporine [20]. CD also allow the stabilization of drugs in aqueous solutions, the decrease of a local irritation after administration and the increase of the permeation of the drug through the ophthalmic barrier [21].

3.2. Ointments

Ophthalmic ointments are sterile, semi-solid, homogeneous preparations intended for application to the eye (conjunctiva or eyelid). Non-aqueous excipients are mainly used for this preparation and it must be non-irritating for the eye. Four types of ointment are described: oleaginous base, absorption base, water-removable base and water soluble base [22]. The oleaginous base is a lipophilic ointment, immiscible with water avoiding moisture evaporation. Composed of petrolatum and white ointment in a large amount, it can remain on skin or mucus for long period without drying out (Sterdex® , Thea, Clermont-Ferrand, France). The adsorption base may be used as emollient and contains lanolin, fatty alcohol and petrolatum (Maxidrol®, Norvatis, Bazel, Swizerland). It can adsorb a quantity of water and is difficult to wash. A water-soluble base is composed only of water soluble excipients as macrogol with high molecular weight. This hydrophilic ointment is easy to wash but its use is limited due to the possible discomfort from the osmotic effect. Water removable base is an oil in water emulsion, easy to wash and easily miscible with water. It facilitates the contact between the skin and the drug but of the presence of hydrophilic surfactant (such as lauryl sulfate) in formulation can be irritating for the eye.

Unlike eye drops, this form slows down the elimination of the drug by the tears flow and increases the corneal residence time by prolonging surface time residence. Ointment application is responsible for blurred vision and its administration is advised in the evening. The packaging can be single dose or multidose and the content is limited to 5 g of preparation.

3.3. Hydrogels

In ocular administration, hydrogels are used to increase residence time of drugs on the eye. Hydrogels are three-dimensional water-swollen structure, composed of a viscosity agent dispersed in water or hydrophilic liquid. Hydrogels are retained in the eye and well better tolerated than ointment by patient by decreasing the side effects induced by the systemic absorption. There are two types of hydrogel, the preformed gels and the in situ gels. Gels are usually composed of hydrophilic polymers. Research focus on the development of new materials and hydrogel has many potential applications in ocular drug delivery. Applications of hydrogels were recently described in a review [23]. The main disadvantage of this form can be the quantity and the homogeneity of the drug loading in the hydrogel which can be limited, specifically in the case of hydrophobic drug. Moreover, the viscosity of gels must be stable over time to maintain the physical properties and the efficacy of the product.

The preformed gels are simple viscous solution administered on the eye. This type of polymeric gels is commonly used as bioadhesive hydrogel to improve residence time on the eye and reduce dosing frequency [2]. Mucoadhesion is the adhesion of a drug delivery system to the mucosal surface for releasing drugs in a controlled way method. Various mucoadhesive polymers were described in the literature [24,25], such as methylcellulose, hydroxylethylcellulose, sodium hyaluronate, sodium alginate, povidone, polyvinylalcohol. Sodium hyaluronate is frequently used as a bioadhesive polymer in gel formulation [26–28] due to it viscoelastic properties and its water retention capacity. This polysaccharide is used in the treatment of dry eye disease such as Vismed® (Horus Pharma, Saint-Laurent-du-Var, France), Aqualarm® (Bausch + Lomb, Bridgewater, NJ, USA) Hylo™ (Candorvision, Montreal, QC, Canada).

In situ hydrogels are instilled as drops into the eye and undergo a sol-to-gel transition in the cul-de-sac with external changes (pH, temperature or ions). This formulation improved ocular bioavailability by increasing the duration of contact with corneal layer and reducing the frequency of administration [29]. In situ gelling delivery systems for the ocular administration of drugs improve the treatment of diseases of the anterior segment of the eye by simple, safe, and reproducible drug administration. Examples of in situ gelling polymers are shown in Table 1.

Table 1. Examples of thermosensitive, pH-sensitive and ion-sensitive polymers used for ophthalmic hydrogel formulations.

Type	Polymers	References
Thermosensitive gels	Negative: Pluronics, poly(N-isopropyl acrylamide) Positive: poly(acrylic acid), polyacrylamide, Reversible: poloxamer, chitosan, hydroxyl propyl méthyl cellulose	[30–33]
pH-sensitive gels	Cellulose acetate and derivatives Carbomer Magrogol Pseudolatex Polymethacrylic acid	[29] [34] [35]
Ion-sensitive gels	Alginate sodium gellan gum (Gelrite®)	[3] [29]

Thermosensitive gels are polymeric solutions that change from solution to gel with temperature modification. Three types of thermosensitive hydrogels can be described: negative gels, positive gels and reversible gels. The first is characterized by a decrease of the volume of the gel when the temperature increases. For the positive gels, the volume of the gel increases when the temperature increases [36]. Finally, the reversible gel [37] is characterized by a transition from solution to gel with an increase of the temperature due to a physical reticulation instead of a chemical reticulation. One of the most used polymers is poloxamer [38]; [34,39–42], a nonionic triblock copolymer composed of a central hydrophobic chain of polypropylene oxide and two chains of polyethylene oxide (Ikervis®, Santen, Evry, France). Several polymers can be used to accurately define the appropriate gelation temperature. For example, some researchers [43] demonstrated that the combination of poloxamer/chitosan in concentration of 16/1.0% w/w showed an optimal temperature gelation (32°C) and improved retention time. Disadvantage of thermosensitive hydrogel is the high concentration of polymer.

The pH-dependent system is induced by pH changes. pH-sensitive polymers are composed of acidic (anionic) or basic (cationic) groups. They accept or release proton and change the external pH. This change induces the swelling of the formulation and the release of the drugs. When polymers are composed of acidic groups, the solution turned to a gel by raising the pH. In contrast, polymers with basic group are converted to a gel with a pH decrease. Carbomer (Carbopol®, Lubrizol, Wickliffe, OH, USA) is frequently used in the formulation of in situ pH-dependent gels (Geltim® LP, Thea, Clermont-Ferrand, France). For example, studies performed with a combination of carbomer (Carbopol® 940) and hydroxylpropylmethylcellulose (HPMC-Methocel® E50 LV, Dow Chemical, Midland, MI, USA) resulted in an improvement of the stability, non-irritability and sustained ofloxacin release (more than 8 h) [44]. Another study using carbomer 940 and different HPMC obtained a satisfactory pH between 6.0 and 7.4 for an ocular administration after gelation [45]. The hydrogel obtained enhances contact time and controlled release of norfloxacin, increased the therapeutic efficacy of the drug and reduced frequency of administration. The disadvantage of this form is the risk of damaging the surface of the eye if the pH of the hydrogel is too low.

The ion triggered system is based on a change in ionic strength of external environment. The ionic hydrogel is formed and releases its drug content after a swelling induced by the change of concentration of ions inside the solution. The cations (Na^+, Mg^{2+}, Ca^{2+}) present in the tear fluid of the eye come in contact with the electrolytes of the solution and the solution turned into a viscous clear gel. For example, sodium alginate is a polymer which converts into a gel due to formation of Ca-alginate by interaction with divalent cation (Ca^{2+}). Ionic polymers are often used in combination with viscosity enhancers to increase the effect. The combination of sodium alginate as ionic polymer and HPMC as a viscosity enhancer improves patient compliance due to its easy instillation in the eye [46]. In another study, this combination was used to form a pH 6.5 gel which improved the release time of the drug over a period of 10 h and is non irritating [47]. Gelrite® is a linear anionic polysaccharide, a deacetylate gellan gum approved as pharmaceutical excipient. The elasticity of the gel depends of the concentration of Gelrite® in the formulation. A study shows that eye contact can be prolonged up to 20 h [48]. Others prove that Gelrite® in situ gels have a shelf life of more than two years and a better efficacy compared with standard eye drops [49]. This combination of different polymers is used to decrease the total polymer content in the formulation and to improve gelling properties [50]. The mixture of Gelrite® and alginate solution formed a hydrogel with the optimum concentration of 0.3% w/w for the Gelrite® and 1.4% w/w for the alginate. These concentrations made a non-irritant in situ gelling vehicle to enhance ocular retention for the delivery of drug [51]. Limitations of this type of gel are the possibility of interference with other ion and a low precision of the gelification process.

3.4. Emulsions

Emulsions are a clear, transparent and thermodynamically stable system of two immiscible fluids. This system is a dispersion of oil in water stabilized by a surfactant and sometimes a co-surfactant. There are interests for this emulsion because of the improvement of drug solubilization (hydrophilic and lipophilic) and dissolution efficiency of poorly water-soluble drugs. However, they are some limitations to this form such as a blurred vision after the instillation of the product which can decrease the patient compliance. Moreover, the homogeneity of the form is related to the uniformity of drug content and the emulsion must be stable to deliver the right dosage.

Its long shelf life, easy preparation (spontaneous formation) and improvement of bioavailability make it a potential ocular drug delivery system [52,53]. In ocular administration, micro- and nanoemulsions are privileged due to the small size of the droplets. They are structured as follow: an aqueous phase, a lipophilic phase and a surfactant phase. A co-surfactant may be required in some cases. This dispersed system has the advantages of not requiring much energy because of its spontaneously formation [54]. This carrier has natural biodegradability and can be sterilized. In 2002, FDA approved a lipid anionic (zeta potential < −40mV) emulsion containing 0.05% of cyclosporine; Restasis™ (Allergan, Irvine, CA, USA) [55].

Mucosal surface of the eye is negatively charged. Cationic nanoemulsions are positively charged formulations with a nanosize structure. They are useful in prolonging the residence time of the formulation in the eye because of the electrostatic attraction of the formulation and the surface of the eye. Novasorb® (Novagali Pharma, Evry, France) is a cationic (+10 mV) lipid nanoemulsion containing benzalkonium chloride or cetalkonium chloride as cationic agent [56]. Cationic agent is known to be the most toxic surfactants [57]. These surfactants are considering irritating for the skin and the eye due to their ability to solubilize lipid membrane. Formulation of cationic nanoemulsion required to find an appropriate cationic agent with high positive charge, low toxicity and good ocular acceptance. Cationic nanoemulsions containing palmatine were prepared with the emulsifying/high pressure homogenization method. The researchers obtained a particle size of 190 nm, a zeta potential of +45 mV. They demonstrated an improvement of the ocular residence time and concluded on a predominant cellular uptake and an internalization in the corneal epithelial cells [58].

3.5. Ophthalmic Insert

Ocular inserts are flexible polymeric materials placed in the cul-de-sac of the conjunctiva between the sclera of the eyeball and the lid. Discovered in 1971 [59], they are biologically inert, insoluble in tears fluid, sterile and non-allergic. This form was developed in order to attempt better ocular bioavailability and sustained drug action by increasing the contact time between drug and tissue of the eye. They also reduce systemic absorption and improve compliance of patients. Ocular inserts are exempt of preservative [60] and must be removed if necessary when they are no longer needed. However, they also present some drawbacks as the patient discomfort due to the solidity of this form, difficulty in placement, unintentional loss. It is also an expensive form and it can have some reluctance of the patient to use unfamiliar type of ophthalmic medication.

Different types of ocular inserts are defined: soluble inserts, bioerodible inserts and insoluble inserts. Soluble inserts are made of natural polymers (collagen), synthetic or semi-synthetic polymers

(HPMC, PVA) and are degraded in the eye. Lacrisert® (Idis Limited, Weybridge, UK) is an example of commercial soluble ophthalmic drug insert. This product is used against dry eye. After its placement in the periocular space, the polymer soaked of lachrymal fluid from the tears and the conjunctiva and dissolved slowly.

Bioerodible inserts are made of biodegradable polymers (polyorthoester, polyorthocarbonate) and they do not require removal at the end of use. The polymer is gradually eroded or disintegrated, and the drug is slowly released from the hydrophilic matrix. Recently, inserts of diclofenac sodium were developed using HPMC both for the drug reservoir and for the rate controlling membrane and dibutylphtalate as plasticizer [61]. Formulation made with 3% of HPMC in drug reservoir and 3% of HPMC in rate controlling membrane increased residence time and reduced the frequency of administration. HPMC was also used in association with cyclodextrins and PVA to make ocular insert of lidocaine for topical ocular anesthesia [62]. The results revealed that lidocaine with β-cyclodextrin (βCD), 4% of HPMC and 2% of PVA have appropriate flexibility, good characteristics and the addition of β-cyclodextrins increase the drug content in the aqueous humor.

Insoluble inserts, also called ocusert, are composed of different types: osmotic systems, diffusion systems and hydrophilic contact lenses [60]. This form needs to be removed from the eye after use. The drug can be dissolved or dispersed in a reservoir. This reservoir is liquid, semi-solid, solid or can contained nanocarriers (nanoparticles). Osmotic inserts are constituted of two parts; a central part with one or two compartments surrounded by a peripheral part. Drug release occurs by the solubilization of the constituents. They generate a hydrostatic pressure against the polymer matrix that allows the release of the drug [63]. Dispersible systems are composed of semi-permeable or microporous membrane (polycarbonate, polyvinylchloride) and a central reservoir (glycerin, ethylene glycol, propylene glycol). The lachrymal fluid controls the drug release and the membrane of the system controls the rate of drug release [64].

3.6. Contact Lenses

Contact lenses are circulated shaped system. It is a thin, curve, round piece of transparent plastic placed directly on the surface of the eye. They are used to increase the residence time of the drug in the eye [65] and allow treating anterior eye disorders. The incorporation of the drug is achieved with methods like imprinting, simple soaking and colloidal nanoparticles [66]. Important settings of the lenses development are the preservation of the oxygen permeability and the transparency of the form. They have many advantages as the exempt of preservative and the control of the size and the shape. Although contact lenses are an alternative and promising ophthalmic drug delivery system, they are an expensive form which needs handling and cleaning. Some limitations of this form are the oxygen permeability of the lenses and it potential issue, the possibility of premature drug release or the limitation of some methodology to develop therapeutic contact lenses.

The first contact lenses were made of glass, but the use of polymethylmethacrylate allowed the development of rigid lens improving the comfort of the patient which did not let oxygen pass. Since the last three decades, contact lenses were made most of the time with silicone hydrogel [67]. They are traditionally used to improve vision defects, for cosmetic effects (change the appearance of the eye like the color) or more recently for therapeutic reasons. There are two types of therapeutic contact lenses: the scleral rigid gas permeable (RGP) lenses and the soft lenses. Scleral lenses are large, thin lenses, having a diameter from 18 mm to 24 mm. They are used in several indications [68] such as several ocular conditions [69], the correction of refractive disorders [70], provide relief on corneal irregularity [71–73], protection of the cornea for ocular chronic disease [74] and treatment of different ocular conditions such as glaucoma, chronic dry eye, allergies and infections [75].

3.7. Intraocular Injections

Intraocular injections are performed for posterior segment diseases. This technique is used in specific pathologies and requires the presence of trained and competent personnel. The surface of the eye is anesthetized during all the procedure. This technique needs a clean room, sterile materials and takes 15 to 30 min. Only solution or suspension of drug can be injected. Medications are injected through the corneal barrier, in the vitreous. Clear solutions contain antibiotic, antifungal, anticancer agent or antiviral. Avastin® (Roche, Bazel, Swizerland) or Lucentis® (Norvatis, Bazel, Swizerland) are commonly used in the treatment of the age-related macular degeneration. Other diseases such as the endophthalmitis, the uveitis, the diabetic retinopathy and the retinal vein occlusion are treated with intraocular injections.

3.8. Innovative Forms

For many years, researchers explored and discovered different forms for ocular administration. Among them, colloidal dispersions such as microemulsions, nanoemulsions, micro- or nanoparticles and liposomes were mainly described as innovative systems for ophthalmic delivery during last decades. They are able to penetrate the eye by the anterior or the posterior segment. These structures are presented in Figure 2.

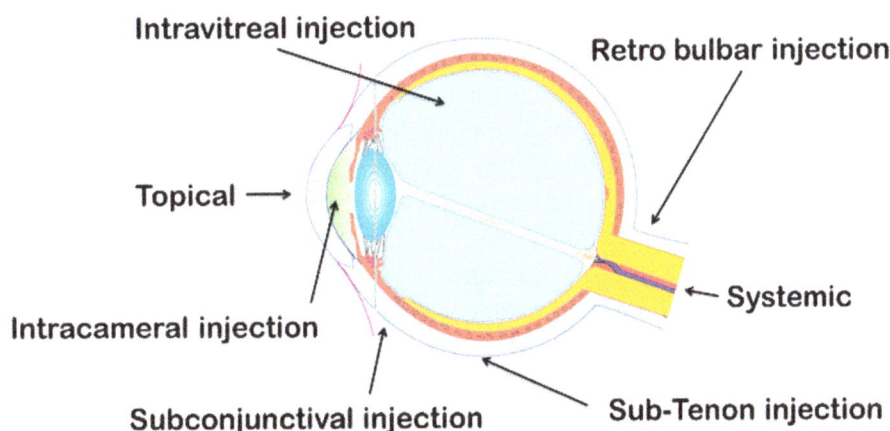

Figure 2. Routes of ocular administration.

Microemulsions are clear, transparent and thermodynamically stable systems of two immiscible fluids. This system is a dispersion of oil in water stabilized by a surfactant and sometimes a co-surfactant. Microemulsions allow the improvement of drug solubilization (hydrophilic and lipophilic) and dissolution efficiency of poorly water-soluble drugs. Its long shelf life, easy preparation (spontaneous formation) and improvement of bioavailability make it a potential ocular drug delivery system [52,53].

In ocular administration, nanoemulsion is privileged due to their small size; below 1 μm. Nanoemulsions are structured as follow: an aqueous phase, a lipophilic phase and a surfactant phase. A co-surfactant may be required in some cases. In some case, this dispersed system as the advantages of not required much energy because of its spontaneously formation [54]. This carrier has natural biodegradability; his small size allows an easy sterilization by filtration.

Nanoparticles are a nanotechnology defined as solid particles with at least one dimension less than 1 μm. These carriers have the capacity to entrapped drugs in different ways. According to the composition of the particles, there are two types of nanoparticles composed of natural or synthetic polymers, metals, lipids and phospholipids; the nanospheres and the nanocapsules [76]. Nanospheres are nanovesicles of polymeric matrix where the drug can be entrapped or attached to the surface of the particles. Nanocapsules are composed of a hydrophilic or lipophilic core surrounded by a polymeric coating. Active substances are dissolved and encapsulated in the core. Nanocarriers present many advantages; the small size and the large surface characteristic of the particles and their potential to be easily incorporated into topical formulations for ophthalmic administration with topical forms, the controlled and sustained release profiles of drugs, the spontaneous entrapment of active substance, the improvement of drug therapy and the decrease of side effects and the potential specific-site targeting [77,78]. In addition, there are some limitations; the potential particles aggregation due to their small size and their large surface area, the physical handling may be difficult in liquid and dry forms and the small size may limited the entrapment of the drug [77,79]. Moreover, due to their physical characteristics, some potential systemic toxicity can occur [80]; the systemic toxicity of nanoparticles refers to the ability of particles to adversely affect the normal physiology. From a biomedical perspective, nanoparticles toxicology reveals an interaction between the physicochemical characteristics of particles and their biological effects. The cytotoxicity of the nanoparticles can be related to the oxidative stress with the generation of reactive oxygen species or pro-inflammatory gene activation. Type of the particles (metallic substances or not), nanoparticle characteristics (morphology, size and surface) or route of administration are parameters that can induce some toxicity. Due to their small sizes, when used in intraocular way, nanoparticles could pass across ophthalmic barriers such as the trabecular meshwork leading to a systemic drug diffusion [81]. Used for topical application, nanoparticles usually do not cross corneal epithelium; Mun et al. have showed that even nanoparticles small as 21 nm do not cross neither intact cornea nor denatured cornea [82].

Introduced in 1965 as drug delivery carriers [83], liposomes are biodegradable and biocompatible vesicular systems composed of phospholipid bilayers surrounding aqueous compartments. According to their size and their structure liposomes are in: small unilamellar vesicles (SUV) with a size ranged from 20 nm to 200 nm; large unilamellar vesicles (LUV) from 200 to 3000 nm and multilamellar vesicles (MLV) higher than 1 μm. Unilamellar vesicles are composed of one layer of lipids and multilamellar are composed of various layers of lipids. Lipophilic drugs and hydrophilic drugs are entrapped in the phospholipid bilayer and the aqueous core respectively. In ocular drug delivery, liposomes offer the advantages of a nanocarrier system with a higher biocompatibility and tolerance, and can treat both anterior and posterior segment eye diseases after topical, subconjunctival or intravitreal administration [84,85]. The surface of the vesicle can be negatively, neutral or positively charged, depending of its composition. Because of the negatively charge of the ocular mucus, the positively charged liposomes seem to be the most efficient for a prolonged adhesion to the corneal surface [86].

Niosomes are non-ionic surfactant vesicles and specific type of liposomes. With a ranged size from 10 to 1000 nm, they are biodegradable, bilayered structures stable and have low toxicity due to its non-ionic nature. Sorbitan monooleate (Span), polysorbate (Tween®) and cholesterol are popularly used as surfactant [87,88].

Dendrimers are "tree-like", nanostructured polymers. This system is a potential carrier for ocular drug delivery due to its nanosize dimensions (1–100 nm) and its low polydispersity. They are structured as a three-dimensional globular shape (Figure 3). The core is in the center of the structure, it can be an atom or a functional molecule. The branching units are covalently bound and there are a large number of branging points regrouped in a series of radically concentric layer called generation. The terminal groups are located at the surface of the dendrimer and are functional molecules [89]. Dendrimers have lipophilic properties. New generation of dendrimers is cationic charged and potentially toxic for an ocular delivery. The old generation of anionic and neutral charged dendrimer have a higher biocompatibility of the ocular delivery [90]. Vandamme et al. formulate dendrimer with amine, carboxylate and hydroxyl surface group to increase residence time in the eye. Albino rabbit were used as an in vivo model to determine the residence time of the dendrimer in the eye and the ocular tolerance of the solution. After an instillation of 25 μL, the residence time increase with carboxylic and hydroxyl surface group. Moreover, when the dendrimer concentration increases, there is not a prolongation of the residence time, but this parameter depends of the size and the molecular weight of the dendrimer [91].

4. Recent Advances for Ocular Antibiotics Administration

4.1. Antibiotics and Ophthalmic Delivery

The first antibiotic industrially developed was penicillin, discovered by Fleming [92], which saved millions of lives and revolutionized therapies. Antibiotics are chemical substances produced naturally by microorganisms or chemically synthetized. They are used to treat or prevent infection caused by germs (bacteria or other parasites). They work by preventing bacteria from reproducing and spreading (bacteriostatic) or by killing them (bactericidal). Bacteria are unicellular microorganisms with a circular double-stranded DNA and a cell wall except for mycoplasma genus. They may be cylindric (bacilli), spherical (cocci) or spiral (spirochetes). *Streptococcus pneumoniae*, *Haemophilus* influenzae are example of bacteria that have a capsule and this encapsulation increases its virulence. Aerobic bacteria need oxygen to produce energy and growths in culture and the other bacteria are either anaerobic or facultative (can growth with or without oxygen).

The classification of the antibiotics can be done in different ways; mechanisms of action, spectrum and mechanism of action. Mechanisms of action are different from an antibiotic to another [93]; they can work on cell wall synthesis as beta-lactam (penicillin, cephalosporin), fosfomycine and glyco-, lipo- and peptides. Bacteria cells are composed of peptidoglycan and their growth is preventing by inhibiting the synthesis of this macromolecule. Aminoside, macrolide/lincosamide, chloramphenicol and tetracycline are active on protein synthesis from the bacteria. They inhibit the 30S ribosome subunit (aminoside and tetracycline) or the 50S ribosome subunit (macrolide/lincosamide, chloramphenicol), responsible for the binding of the tRNA to the receptor site on mRNA. Other antibiotics inhibit folate synthesis as sulfamides, and dihydrofolate reductase inhibitor. They block nucleotides, lipids and amino acid synthesis from bacteria cell. Finally, fluoroquinolone, sulfamide and rifampicin are working on DNA and RNA synthesis. Antibiotics can also be classified by their spectrum; broad spectrum antibiotics affect numerous infections, including gram-negative and gram-positive bacteria, and narrow spectrum antibiotics are active against a selective type of bacteria. Among broad spectrums antibiotics we can find amoxicillin (beta-lactam), tetracycline, cephalosporin, chloramphenicol, and erythromycin (macrolide). Short spectrum antibiotics group are composed of penicillin-G, vancomycine (glycopeptide).

Antibiotics can be bacteriostatic as tetracycline, chloramphenicol, and erythromycin. Cephalosporin, erythromycin and penicillin are examples of bactericidal antibiotics. Bacteriostatic antibiotics do not work if a bactericidal antibiotic is given concurrently. To avoid interaction between these drugs, they have to be alternatively administrated and not in combination [94].

Eye infections must be treated by appropriate and safe use of antibiotics. Antibiotics can be administrated by several routes (oral, parenteral, local) and the most appropriate administration depends on the area of the eye to be treated. The anterior segment (cornea, conjunctiva) is frequently treated with local administration. Topical administration is used for eye drops, ointments or gels; each form presents a main advantage like an immediate action for eye drops, a decrease of the administration frequency for gels or an increase of the drug biodisponibility for ointments. The intraocular (intravitreal, intracameral) administrations lead to a greater intraocular concentration of antibiotics than any other administration. Intravitreal injections are used as prophylaxis or curative treatments of endophthalmitis with combination of vancomycin and ceftazidimeb for example [95]. Subconjunctival and retrobulbar administrations are periorbital administration. Subconjunctival is used to achieve high concentration of drugs and large size molecules or the administration of drug with low bioavailability by the topical way. Retrobulbar injections are usually used for the treatment of optic neuritis. Generally, subconjunctival route allows achieving equal or higher drug concentration than retrobulbar injections [96].

Because of the ocular barriers, the targeting of the posterior segment (retina, choroid, and sclera) always requires systemic administration (oral, parenteral). Oral administration is easy to develop and to deliver to the patient, but this way of administration is limited by the antibiotics bioavailability;

only low molecular weight and lipophilic drugs can cross the blood barriers and the ocular barriers. Systemic toxicity and safety have to be considered for an oral administration with an ocular response [14]. Parenteral administration is used for preseptal cellulitis, orbital cellulitis, dacryocystitis, or in adjunction to others treatments in the ocular adnexa, orbital and periorbital tissues [97]. However, parenteral route is not the most common administration way for the treatment of ocular diseases.

Antibiotics usually have a short half-life and need repeated administrations. Using antibiotics requires knowledge of the pharmacokinetic and the toxicity of the drug for the different routes of administration. Due to their low solubility, molecules such as penicillins, cephalosporins and aminoglycosides penetrate the eye with great difficulty. In dermal application, penicillin is highly allergic and causes skin rashes and allergic sensitivity. Via oral route, tetracyclines present major side effects toward intestinal microflora. Modern betalactams and aminoglycosides have to be injected because of their low bioavailability by oral route. All of these side effects favor the ophthalmic administration to increase the tolerance of the active substance.

4.2. Recent Advances in Ocular Delivery of Antibiotics

4.2.1. Improvement of Drug Dissolution and Stability Using Cyclodextrins

Cyclodextrins (CD) were discovered in the 1900 and more recently used in ocular drug delivery. They are cyclic oligosaccharides with an inner lipophilic cavity and a hydrophilic outer surface. They are used as solubilizer, drug stabilizer, permeation enhancers, separation agent in HPLC or catalyst and additives. These excipients increase solubility and stability of drugs, prevent side effects as irritation and discomfort [98]. Cyclodextrins should be non-irritating, non-toxic, well tolerated, inert and enhance permeability of the drug through the corneal mucosa. CD can be used in particles (nanosphere, microsphere, liposome) [99].

Hydroxylpropyl-β-cyclodextrin (HPβCD) was used to create a complex with ciprofloxacin in order to formulate eye drops. The inclusion complex showed a better stability, an ocular tolerance and a higher biological activity in comparison to marketed eye drops and simple aqueous solutions [100]. The same combination increased the solubility of ciprofloxacin from 3-fold at pH 5.5 and 2-fold at pH 7.4. The authors noticed that the complex at pH 5.5 had a higher stability after two months of storage than the complex at pH 7.4. The stability of the drug increased with the HPβCD and the complex improved the in vitro release of the drug [101].

Novel βCD polymers are incorporated at complexes with rifampicine, novobycin or vancomycin into a hydrogel showed a slower release of the drug compared to the dextrose-based gels. The study demonstrated that the larger and more hydrophilic drugs had release profiles less altered than small hydrophobic drugs [102].

4.2.2. Contact Lens for Antibiotic Delivery

Contact lenses were used as drug reservoir or support for the active ingredient in antibiotic ocular delivery. Initially, they are used as ophthalmic system to correct vision. The scleral RPG (Rigid Gaz Permeable)) lenses trap a tear reservoir, which can be used as a drug container. It prevents tear evaporation or adhesion from mucus filament in the cornea, has a potential cornea healing or hydrates the cornea in severe case of dry eye disease [103]. It prevents eyes of the patient from exposure to their irregular cornea and the reservoir can contain some artificial tears needed to lubricate the surface of the eye. In the toxic epidermal necrosis and Steven-Johnson syndrome, wearing scleral lens improves the relieving symptoms. The liquid reservoir of this lens can contain some drug as topical corticosteroids and cyclosporine [104]. More recently, a study describes the in vivo release of ofloxacin from a scleral lens in rabbit with keratitis. This preclinical study assesses local tolerance and intraocular diffusion of the antibiotic administered by a contact lens. The authors found a higher level of drug in aqueous humor and cornea than those reported with other administration route [105].

Soft contact lenses are often composed of hydrogels, like hydroxyethyl polymetacrylate hydrogel [106]. More recently the use of silicone hydrogel was described offering more oxygen transmission than the standard hydrogel lenses. The most common preparation technique of contact lenses for controlled drug delivery is the "soaking" technique. Briefly, lenses are immersed in an antibiotic solution. The uptake and release of antibiotics were explored to compare the ability of different commercial lenses to release fluoroquinolone; 1-Day Acuvue® (Johnson & Johnson, New Brunswick, NJ, USA) Medalist® (Bausch & Lomb, Rochester, NY, USA) and 14UV. There were soaked in fluoroquinolone solutions during different times. In conclusion, the higher uptake of drug was for the 1-Day Acuvue® lens and the release rates were slower for the 1-Day and the Medallist® than for the 14UV, but the most practicable system was the 1-Day Acuvue® [107]. These conclusions were previously exposed by Hehl et al. [108]. Fluoroquinolone and aminoglycosides loaded contact lenses (gentamycin, kanamycin, tobramycin, ciprofloxacin, ofloxacin) were studied to improve the ocular penetration of topically applied drugs. They used Acuvue® contact lenses, soaked in the different antibiotic solutions. In conclusion, kanamycin was not able to cross the corneal barrier and only gentamicin, ciprofloxacin and ofloxacin produced bacteriostatic concentrations in the aqueous humor.

Derivate from the soaking technique, the supercritical CO_2 impregnation/dispersion method is also explored due to its non-toxicity, its low surface tension of the polymer and its high diffusivity [109]. This technique permits to prepare commercial soft contact lenses such as FocusDailies® (Novartis, Basel, Switzerland), Proclear® Compatibles (CooperVision, Lake Forest, CA, USA), Frequency® 55 (CooperVision, Lake Forest, CA, USA) and SofLens® 59 Comfort (Bausch & Lomb, Rochester, NY, USA). The study concludes that this drug delivery system obtained with the supercritical solvent impregnation can be viable, safe and efficient such as the impregnated lens obtained with the soaked method [110]. The molecular imprinting technology during the lens manufacturing forms, in the contact lens, structures like pockets, which are memorizing the spatial feature and the bonding preferences of the drug [111]. A norfloxacin (quinolone) delivery system with imprinting method was described using different ratios of drug and acrylic acid. With the most efficient ratio (1:4), they demonstrated that the high affinity binding point allows to make lenses able to control drug delivery release from several hours to days [112]. The development of drug-soft contact lenses with polymyxin B and vancomycin against *Pseudomonas aeruginosa* demonstrated a good biocompatibility of the two hydrogels but imprinting effect only exhibited with polymyxin B [113].

4.2.3. Ocular Inserts for Antibiotic Delivery

Ocular insert is solid or semi-solid preparation placed in the cul-de-sac to deliver a controlled flow of drug. The use of ocular insert for antibiotic delivery was also described in the literature. In 1980, some researchers studied the in vitro and the in vivo release of antibiotics such as erythromycin and erythromycin estolate from matricial ocular inserts. They discovered that when the water content of the hydrogel insert is more than 30%, the elution rate of a low aqueous solubility drug is constant [114]. In the same time, drug-inserts with copolymers of *N*-vinylpyrrolidone tested completely suppressed the chlamydia trachomatis infection in the monkey eyes [115]. In a study, macrolide antibiotics (erythromycin) and penicillin were evaluated as a potential ocular drug delivery system in an antibiotic-impregnated collagen insert. The system with the erythromycin and the soluble collagen produced the most interesting system due to his sustained drug delivery [116]. To treat external ophthalmic infections, a combination of the aminoglycoside, gentamicin sulfate, and dexamethasone phosphate in a soluble insert was developed. The matricial insert was composed of HPMC, ethylcellulose and carbomer. This new form prolonged the release of gentamycin above the minimum inhibitory concentration value (MIC) of $4\mu g \cdot mL^{-1}$ for nearly 50 h. The dexamethasone side effects caused by repeated instillation were avoided and the compliance improved [117].

Many fluoroquinolones were used as drug for ocular controlled delivery in an insert. For example, ofloxacin was studied in erodible insert with poly(ethylene oxide) (PEO). After application of the insert (6 mm of diameter and 20 mg of weight), a gel formed. The aqueous maximum concentration was higher than the commercial eye drops. Bioavailability improved due to the mucoadhesion of PEO and tear fluid viscosity [118]. This gelling system was explored with different molecular weight of PEO (from 200 to 2000 kDa). The molecular weight of PEO had huge influence on the erosion time consequently on the transcorneal absorption, the gel residence time, the drug release, the drug residence time in the aqueous humor at concentration higher than MIC. The optimal mucoadhesion was for the 400 kDa PEO. The 400 kDa PEO and 900 kDa PEO have some potential for a topical treatment in endophthalmitis [119]. The in vitro release and the ocular delivery of ofloxacin in chitosan microspheres and insert were explored by the same researchers. The microspheres were added to the insert formulation to evaluate their effects on drug release mechanism from the insert and the drug penetration into the aqueous humor of the rabbit eyes. This addition produced structural changes, accelerating the erosion of the insert and the release of the drug. In conclusion, chitosan microspheres enhanced the transcorneal permeability of the drug [120]. More recently, inserts with ofloxacin encapsulated in nanolipid carriers showed a preocular retention up to 24 h and a maximum concentration in aqueous humor increased six times in comparison with the commercial. Keratitis in rabbit's eyes were healed in 7 days [121].

Other fluoroquinolone-inserts, such as pefloxacin, were developed. They were used in bacterial conjunctivitis and were a reservoir type ocular insert. Eudragit® (Evonik, Essen, Deutschland) is copolymers derived from esters of acrylic and methacrylic acid. Different ratios of Eudragit® RS100 and RL100 (ethyl prop-2-enoate methyl 2-methylprop-2-enoate trimethyl-[2-(2-methylprop-2-enoyloxy)ethyl]azanium chloride) were studied. The ratio 4:1 (RS/RL) allowed a drug release from 90-98% within 48 to 120 h. This optimized formulation remained stable and intact at room temperature and provided the desired drug sustained release in vitro for 5 days [122]. Ciprofloxacin drug reservoir inserts were studied to achieve once a day administration. A hydrophilic polymer, gelatin, was used in drug reservoir and the rate controlling membrane was made by hydrophobic ethylcellulose. This form showed an increasing residence time in the eye, a sustained drug release, a decreasing frequency of administration and improved compliance of the patient [123]. These conclusions are supported by the in vitro and in vivo studies revealing the efficacy of the formulation [124].

In another study, Pawar et al. prepared an ocular insert of moxifloxacin and PVA by the film casting method. The soluble insert obtained (5.5 mm of diameter) was coated with different Eudragit® (S-100, RL-100, RS-100, E-100 or L-100) and cross-linked by $CaCl_2$. The mucoadhesion time and the drug content were found satisfactory. The coating and the cross linking extended drainage from insert and the formulation with Eudragit® RL100 showed maximum drug penetration [125].

Macrolides were also studied in ocular insert. Azithromycin ocular inserts were formulated and evaluated. The polymer HPMC was used as drug reservoir and the Eudragit® RL100 as rate controlled membrane. The concentration of 1.5% HPMC and 3% Eudragit® RL100 was found to be optimized formulation. It controlled release over a 12 h period, had a better ocular tolerability and improved ocular bioavailability in ocular infections [126].

4.2.4. In Situ Gelling Systems for Antibiotic Delivery

Some antibiotics were studied in different in situ gelling systems during the past two decades to improve patient compliance by: prolonging and controlling drug release, prolonging corneal contact time and enhancing ocular bioavailability. Different in situ gelling systems are used in ocular drug delivery as the thermosensitive, the ion-activated and the pH sensitive gelling system.

Different concentrations of active substance in the formulation allowed screening the efficiency on referential bacteria as *Staphylococcus aureus*, *Pseudomonas aeruginosa* or *Escherichia coli*. In a study, various concentrations of clarithromycin or levofloxacin in ophthalmic gels were tested. Two drops of each gel were administered four times per day during 4 days. The 0.25% clarithromycin ophthalmic gel had a better action again *Staphylococcus aureus* than the 0.1% clarithromycin ophthalmic gel [127].

Different excipients are used for the formulation of in situ gelling systems in order to control the mucoadhesion force and the viscosity of the formulation. HPMC is a viscosity enhancer commonly employed in gel formulation. The combination of alginate as ionic-induced gelation agent and HPMC with gatifloxacin demonstrated a higher efficacy than the alginate alone. The mixture could be used as an in situ gelling system to improve compliance of patient and increase ocular bioavailability [128]. These conclusions were confirmed by a recent study testing HPMC and sodium alginate in a pH induced gelation system developed for a ciprofloxacin ocular gel [46]. In some cases, the addition of HPMC and methylcellulose is used to increase the viscosity of the gel and decrease the concentration of carbomer in the formulation. This pH or ionic sol-in-gel transition system with ciprofloxacin, used in corneal ulcer and corneal infection, allowed prolonging the antimicrobial effect against bacteria for instance *Escherichia coli*, *Staphylococcus strains* and *Pseudomonas aeruginosa* [129].

Ciprofloxacin was also tested alone in poloxamer-based thermosensitive gel. The combination of poloxamer (407 and 188) and HPMC or HEC, as bioadhesive agents, allowed formulating an in situ gelling system with a gelation temperature between 28 and 34°C. The addition of poloxamer 407, HPMC and HEC improved the bioadhesion force, the viscosity of the formulation and decreases the in vitro drug release [130]. Moreover, the elastic properties of the ocular gelling systems allow the limitation of drug ocular drainage. Combination of poloxamer 401 and 188 with sodium alginate and xanthan gum were also explored with the moxifloxacin. The increase of the mucoadhesive polymer concentration decreased the rate of drug release. The thermoreversible mucoadhesive gels obtained have a pH of 6.8 to 7.4, were safe and sustained ocular delivery of moxifloxacin [42]. More recently, different polymers; polyox (pH sensitive agent), poloxamer (a temperature-sensitive gelling agent) and sodium alginate (an ion-sensitive gelling agent) were tested in combination with HPMC as viscosity enhancer. The in vivo assays showed sustained release of moxifloxacin hydrochloride over 8 h and the formulation were therapeutically efficient, stable and non-irritant [131]. The combination of sodium alginate and methylcellulose in an ion-sensitive gel confirmed this conclusion with a sustained release of sparfloxacin for a period up to 24 h with no ocular damage [132]. The bioavailability of pefloxacin was increased by the addition of carbomer and methylcellulose. This combination increased the gel strength. The 0.18% pefloxacin gel showed a drug level in the aqueous humor above the MIC-values over a period of 12 h compared to the 0.3% commercial eye drops indicating that the developed form is better considering this parameter. This mixture showed a better ability to retain the drug than the carbomer or methyl cellulose solutions alone [133].

An ion activated in situ gelling system of gatifloxacin showed a higher bioavailability and a longer residence time in the eye by microdialysis. Compared to conventional eye drops, this system could be viable as a potential ocular drug delivery [134].

In another study, a Gelrite® in situ ophthalmic gelling system was compared to Vigamox® (Alcon, Fort Worth, TX, USA) commercial eye drop for the local administration of moxifloxacin. They concluded that compared to the eye drop, higher amount of moxifloxacin was retained in the aqueous humor. Against the bacterial corneal inflammation, they had a major improvement after four days compared to seven days for the conventional eye drops [135].

4.2.5. Colloidal Systems for Antibiotic Delivery

Colloidal systems are popularly employed in the development of formulation for the treatment of ocular diseases (Table 2).

They have many advantages; prolonging the residence time of the drug on the surface of the eye, sustained release, increasing the bioavailability of the drug. The dosages' forms included microemulsions, nanoemulsions, nanoparticles, liposomes or niosomes (Figure 3) [5,136].

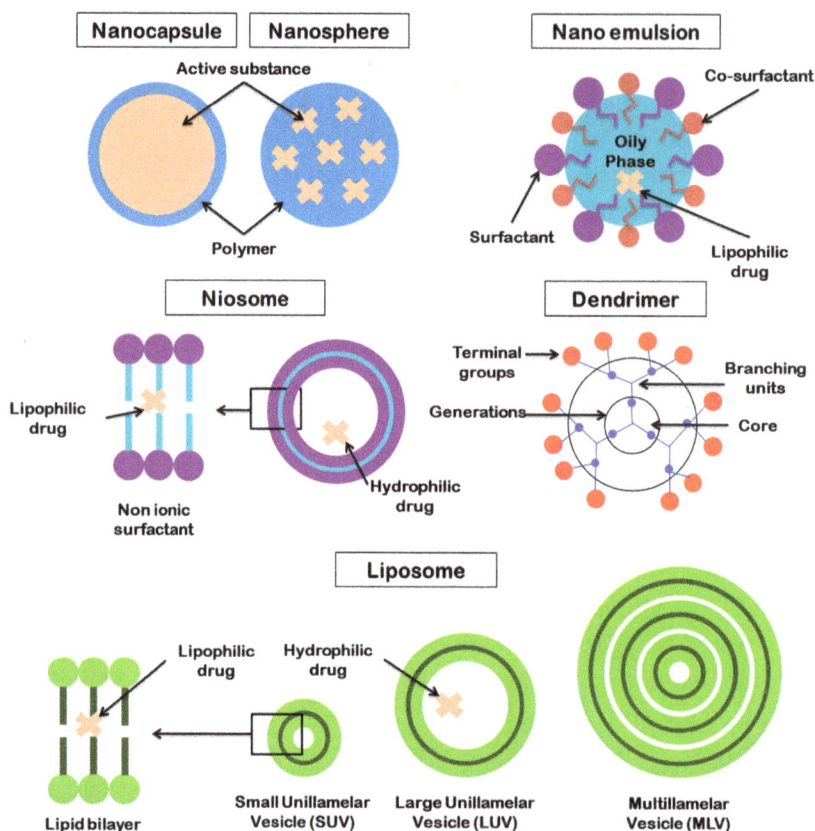

Figure 3. Schema of micro- and nanostructure intended for ocular drug delivery.

Microemulsions for Antibiotic Delivery

Microemulsions are colloidal systems kinetically stable. They are used for their ability to deliver both lipophilic and hydrophilic drugs and to increase the bioavailability of active substances. Tween® 80 (polyoxyethylene sorbitan monooleate) and Span® 20 (sorbitan monolaurate) are mainly used as a non-ionic surfactant and co-surfactant for microemulsion formulation. Tween® 80 is recognized as a practically non-irritating and non-toxic surfactant for ophthalmic use [137].

Lv et al. studied the stability of microemulsion containing 0.3% of chloramphenicol for the treatment of trachoma and keratitis. The organic phase is composed of butanol, isopropyl palmitate and isopropyl myristate and the aqueous phase is composed of water. They concluded with an improvement of the stability of the drug after three months compared to classical chloramphenicol eye drops. Chloramphenicol was in hydrophilic shells of microemulsion drops [138]. This improvement of stability was confirmed by another study using microemulsion for the ocular delivery of moxifloxacin for the treatment of bacterial keratitis. Droplet sizes were below 40 nm and exhibited a sustained drug release profile. The in vivo study showed a greater antimicrobial activity on bacterial keratitis in rabbit eyes than the commercial eye drops [139].

Üstündag-Okur et al. studied the addition of ethanol as co-surfactant, Tween® 80 as surfactant, oleic acid as oil phase and sodium chloride in water as aqueous phase as a promising strategy for ocular drug delivery. The preocular residence time was higher with the microemulsion than the solution. The authors studied the effect of the addition of 0.75% chitosan oligosaccharide lactate (COL) in microemulsion on ofloxacin ocular penetration compared to a simple microemulsion (without COL) and a solution of ofloxacin. They observed that the permeation rate was lower with COL microemulsion than the formulation without COL. However, the COL microemulsion had a slower release of ofloxacin and a higher antimicrobial activity than the simple microemulsion. The MIC values were the same for the two microemulsions [140]. The combination of Tween® 80 and the

Transcutol® P (diethylene glycol monoethyl ether) (Gattefossé, Saint-Priest, France) as a co-surfactant with 0.3% of gatifloxaxin formulated an oil-in-water microemulsion was explored for the intraocular drug delivery. Zeta potential ranged from +15 to +24 mV and the droplet size ranged from 51 to 74 nm. The optimized formulation, composed of 10% isopropyl miristate, 10% Tween® 80, 10% Transcutol® P and 70% deionized water, showed a better stability, adherence to corneal surface, permeation rate of gatifloxacin and tolerance than the commercial eye drops, Zigat® (FDC Limited, Maharashtra, India). However, the transcorneal permeation of gatifloxaxin using commercial eye drops was higher during the first hour than the microemulsion due to the un-ionized forms of the drug. Finally, the developed formulation increased intraocular penetration of the drug and was a promising alternative to the eye drops [141].

Nanoemulsions for Antibiotic Delivery

Many studies describe the use of nanoemulsion in ocular administration. Their small size and god tolerance by the patient are advantages for an effective treatment. Unfortunately, this form is sparsely described in the literature in association with antibiotics.

Researchers explored a mucoadhesive cationic nanoemulsion of dexamethasone and polymyxin B. The innovation was in the use of a positively charged drug and preservatives to achieve mucoadhesion of cationic emulsion. The lipid phase was composed of dexamethasone 0.5% (w/w), Lipoid® S100-Eutanol® G (30%:70%) (soy phosphatdylcholine-octyldodecanol) (BASF Corporation, Ludwigshafen, Deutschland)) and the aqueous phase contained polymyxin B 0.1% (w/w), cetylpiridium chloride 0.01% (w/w) and glycerol 2.6% (w/w). The pH of the formulation was 5.31, droplets size was below 200 nm, and zeta potential ranged from 11 to +9 mV and the emulsion was stable after six months at room temperature and +4°C. The in vitro study demonstrated the non-cytotoxicity of the nanoemulsion and its ocular potential application as viable alternative to commercial solutions [142].

Nanoparticles and Microparticles for Antibiotic Delivery

Nanoparticles were explored in many cases of eye diseases. With their ability to cross the ocular tissues [143] without any influence on cornea, iris or retina, they are promising technology for increasing the therapeutic efficacy of ophthalmic therapies [144].

Das et al. studied polymeric nanoparticles composed of Eudragit® RL100 and prepared by the nanoprecipitation method for ophthalmic delivery of amphotericin B against *Fusarium solani*. The particles had a size ranged from 130 to 300 nm, a positive zeta potential and encapsulation efficiency from 60% to 80%. They showed no signs of eye irritation and were stable for two months at +4°C and room temperature [145]. Other authors confirmed this conclusion. The combination of Eudragit® RL100 and Pluronic® F108 (BASF Corporation, Ludwigshafen, Deutschland) formulated small positive particles (below 500 nm) with no significant chemical interaction between the polymer and the drug. They noticed that changing the pH of the external phase of nanoparticle suspension increased the encapsulation efficiency of sulfacetamide [146].

Ibrahim et al., developed Eudragit® RL100 / RS100 nanoparticles of coated with hyaluronic acid as bioadhesive polymer, to extend the release of gatifloxacin and prednisolone (glucocorticoid) compared to the free drug and to improve the patient compliance. The authors demonstrated that the increase of drugs:polymers ratio improved the drug encapsulation efficiency and the increase of Eudragit® RS100 amount decreased the release efficiency values. The particles had a size ranged from 315 nm to 473 nm and showed better bioavailability of drugs in the aqueous humor and corneal tissue than the marketed eye drops [147]. In another study, a 50:50 (w/w) ratio of Eudragit® RS100 and RL100 was tested with Tween® 80 and poly(vinyl alcohol) (PVA) to improve the residence time of the gatifloxacin. The nanoparticles were prepared via the double emulsion technique or the nanoprecipitation method. The particle size was higher with the double emulsion technique and the Tween® 80. The optimized positive nanoparticles had a gatifloxacin encapsulation efficiency of 46%, a prolonged release rate of gatifloxacin and prolonged antimicrobial effects against *Escherichia coli*, *Staphylococcus aureus* and *Pseudomonas aeruginosa* [81].

Poly(lactic-*co*-glycolic acid) (PLGA) is a copolymer widely used in medical and pharmaceutical applications. It is a biodegradable excipient evaluated, for example, in a rifampicin microparticulate system for an intraocular injection in order to prevent endophthalmitis during cataract surgery. The in vitro release of rifampicin and its antibacterial assessment were explored. The PLGA microparticles showed a sustained release profile of rifampicin in vitro and bactericidal effect against *Staphyloccocus epidermidis* mainly involved in endophthalmitis [148]. Similar PLGA microparticles prepared by w/o/w emulsion-diffusion method were studied for the vancomycin delivery. Depending of formulation parameters, microparticles have a negative zeta potential and a size ranged from 1.6 to 11.8 μm. The release of the vancomycin in the first 24 h was around 90% [149].

Another study explored a sparfloxacin nanoparticle system with PLGA as polymer and PVA as stabilizant. The negatively charged particles had a size from 180 nm to 190 nm and showed non-irritant properties. In vivo study and gamma scintigraphy exploration suggested that there was no drug in systemic circulation, an increase of the precorneal residence time and of the sparfloxacin ocular penetration [150]. The PLGA gave the same size and zeta potential results and an entrapment efficiency of 85% in combination with levofloxacin. Images of scintigraphy showed a good spread and good retention of the drug on the cornea. Nanoparticles retained the drug for a longer time and allowed slowing down the drain out of the drug from the eye compared to the marketed formulation. Moreover, the in vitro release showed an initial burst followed by a slow drug release over a period of 24 h [151]. Another study confirmed this in vitro conclusion. Clarithromycin loaded PLGA nanoparticles were prepared via the nanoprecipitation method with different ratio of drug:polymer (1:1, 1:2, 1:3). The negative particles obtained had a size below 300 nm and an entrapment efficiency of clarithromycin from 57% to 80%. Under encapsulated form, he drug crystallinity was decreased and the authors demonstrated that a dosing at 1/8 concentration in the particles of the intact drug is more effective against *Staphylococcus aureus* than the free drug [152].

More recently, a study developed doxycycline hyclate loaded nanoparticles prepared via the emulsion cross-linking method to improve precorneal residence time and drug penetration. Gellan gum, Aerosol® OT (dioctyl sodium sulfosuccinate) (anionic surfactant) (Cytec Solvay Group, Woodland Park, NJ, USA) and PVA composed the particles. They had a size ranged from 331 nm to 850 nm and entrapment efficiency of doxycycline from 45% to 80%. *Ex-vivo* studies showed a higher sustained release from particles in both *Staphylococcus aureus* and *Escherichia coli* strains than the doxycycline hyclate aqueous solution. The authors noticed that formulations were non-irritating for the eye, inhibited bacterial growth and were a potential drug delivery system for ocular bacterial infections [153].

Chitosan is a natural mucoadhesive, biocompatible, positively charged polymer. In combination with sodium alginate and Pluronic® F127, nanoparticles demonstrated a prolonged topical ophthalmic delivery of gatifloxacin. They are positively charged (+18 to +48 mV) and had a size from 205 to 572 nm. The in vitro studies showed a fast release for the first hour and non-Fickian diffusion process for the gradual drug release during the next 24 h [154]. In addition, Silva et al. developed mucoadhesive chitosan, sodium tripolyphosphate particles for daptomycin ocular delivery prepared by the ionotropic gelation method. Particles exhibited small size (200 to 500 nm, polydispersity index from 0.1 to 0.2) and round-shape. They obtained a total release of the drug within 4 h and the incubation of the particles with lysozyme positively affected their mucoadhesive properties [155]. More recently, a study demonstrated that the combination of chitosan and sodium alginate as a mucoadhesive coating for nanoparticles (size from 380 to 420 nm, entrapment efficiency from 79% to 92%) allowed an epithelial retention of daptomycin compared to the solution of the free drug [156].

Solid lipid nanoparticles (SLN) were considered as promising carrier for ocular drug delivery strategies. There are characterized by a physiological lipid core surrounded by an aqueous phase and stabilized by surfactants. Hydrophilic and lipophilic drugs are entrapped in this particles presenting the advantages of a good safety; a large-scale industrial and sterilizable production feasibility [157]. SLN for example, were studied for the ocular administration of gatifloxacin, with stearic acid alone or a stearic acid/Compritol® (Glyceryl behenate) (Gattefossé, Saint-Priest, France) mixture and poloxamer 188 as surfactant. The authors concluded to a higher average size, entrapment efficiency and lower crystallinity for the lipid matrix SLN (composed of stearic acid/Compritol®) than for the stearic acid alone SLN. In addition, the formulations had a positive zeta potential and were physiologically tolerable by the eye [158]. A Box Behnken statistical design with 3 variables and 3 responses were used to optimize the development of a gatifloxacin SLN. The cationic carriers were composed of lipids (stearic acid and Compritol® or stearic acid and Gelucire® (Gattefossé, Saint-Priest, France), poloxamer 188 and sodium taurocholate and prepared by o/w-emulsion method. SLN size ranged from 250 nm to 305 nm had a zeta potential from +29 to +36 mV and gatifloxacin entrapment efficiencies from 47% to 79%. The authors studied the corneal permeation of drug on a freshly excised goat cornea and its effect on corneal hydration level compared to Gate® (gatifloxacin 0.3%) (Ajanta Pharma, Maharashtra, India) eye drops. They concluded to an increase of 3.37-fold for the bioavailability of the drug, 2.34-fold for the half-life and 1.09-fold of concentration of drug in the aqueous humor in favor of the SLN. The authors suggested that, with no signs of irritation, the formulations could prolong the residence time in the eye and enhance the bioavailability of the drug [159,160].

A Box Behnken experimental design with 3 variables (stearic acid, Tween® 80 and sodium taurocholate concentrations) and 2 responses was also performed to optimize the preparation of levofloxacin SLN. With a particles size of 238 nm and a entrapment efficiency of 79%, the optimized formulation showed a flux of 0.2493 μm/cm/h through excised goat cornea, a prolonged drug release and an equivalent antibacterial activity against *Staphylococcus aureus* and *Escherichia coli* compared to the marketed eye drops [161].

In another study, the double emulsion method was used to prepare vancomycin SLN and enhance the ocular penetration of the drug and its residence time in the eye. The molar ratio lipid:drug of 1:1 (glycerylpalmitate:vancomycin) with low molecular weight of PVA allowed nanoparticles of 278 nm, a zeta potential of −20 mV and an entrapment efficiency of 20%. The authors concluded that the encapsulation efficiency of the drug was not enough due to the high water solubility of the drug, clinical application are consequently not possible [162].

Finally, intraocular delivery of tobramycin with stearic acid SLN was studied for targeting the posterior segment and the inner parts of the eye against *Pseudomonas aeruginosa*. The vesicles had a size of 80 nm, a polydispersity index of 0.15 and a zeta potential of −26 mV. They demonstrated a higher concentration of drug in the ocular tissue with a topical administration compared to the commercial Tobral® (Alcon, Fort Worth, TX, USA) eyedrops and a slow and constant release of tobramycin [163].

Liposomes for Antibiotic Delivery

Phosphatidylcholine (egg and soy) (PC) and cholesterol (CH) are lipids popularly used in liposomes preparation. To provide long-term drug delivery without avoiding systemic drug exposure, a study explored a ciprofloxacin hydrochloride liposomal system. Different molar concentrations of CH were studied, and it appeared that this parameter influenced the particle size, the drug entrapment efficiency and its release. The sizes of the particles ranged from 2.5 to 7.2 μm. Ciprofloxacin had a fast release profile during the first hours, then the drug release followed the Higuchi diffusion model. The authors showed that the drug release was controlled by the drug concentration during the first 10 h and, after 10 h, by the concentration of CH [164]. More recently, Chetoni et al. compared the efficacy of distamycin a liposomes to a simple solution, for Herpes simplex virus treatment. The combination of PC and CH was used. Using PC/CH liposomes, the authors showed that the ocular tissue toxicity was reduced with this formulation and that the ocular bioavailability and retention into the cornea were increased [165].

Another study investigated the influence of different molecular weights and concentrations of chitosan for the coating of ciprofloxacin liposomes. Despite a lower encapsulation efficiency of the drug, coated liposomes improved ocular penetration and antimicrobial activity of ciprofloxacin. In vitro studies showed that the formulation inhibited the growth of *Pseudomonas aeruginosa* in rabbit's eyes for 24 h. In addition, a higher concentration and molecular weight of chitosan increased the mucoadhesion properties of the liposomes [166]. More recently, a study with the combination of chitosan, liposomes and ciprofloxacin hydrochloride concluded to the improvement of the bioavailability of the drug. The liposomes were composed of PC, CH at different ratio and stearylamine. Optimized formulation obtained with a ratio PC:CH of 10:0 showed the better entrapment efficiency of ciprofloxacin of 39% and an in vitro release after 8 h of 79% [167].

To increase the contact time between the drug and the surface of the eye, the liposomal gels showed great potential. MLV were formulated with lecithin and PC in a bioadhesive poyl(vinyl alcohol) and polymethacrylic acid gel. This formulation aimed to minimize the dilution effect of tear in the conjunctival sac and ensured a steady and prolonged drug release. The liposomal encapsulation of the ciprofloxacin extended the in vitro release of the antibiotic [168]. Hosny et al. developed a hydrogel of liposomal suspension for the ophthalmic delivery of ofloxacin. The use of an ophthalmic solution requires a frequently instillation in the eyes and due to its pH dependent solubility ofloxacin tends to deposit on the eye surface. MLV and reverse-phase evaporation vesicle (REV) are formulated. MLV have better entrapment efficiency and the liposomal hydrogel enhanced the transcorneal permeation 7-fold more than the aqueous solution. Authors also demonstrated that a thermosensitive prolonged release liposomal hydrogel provided in vitro ocular bioavailability through albino rabbit cornea. This formulation allowed minimizing the frequency of administration and decreased ocular side effects of ofloxacin [169].

Gatifloxacin and ciprofloxacin were studied with the same liposomal hydrogel to enhance transcorneal permeation. Liposomes are composed of phosphatidylcholine and CH, stearylamine or dicetyl phosphate, both used to respectively provide to liposomes either a positive charge or a negative charge. Liposomes were dispersed in a Carbopol® 940 (carbomer) hydrogel. Optimal entrapment efficiency was obtained for the ratio 5:3 (PC:CH) and the best release of hydrogel and transcorneal penetration was obtained for the ratio 5:3:1 (PC:CH:stearylamine). In addition, the increase of CH content above this limit decreased the entrapment efficiency and the positively charged liposomes entrapped more drug than the negatively charged liposomes. They concluded that the hydrogel ensured steady prolonged transcorneal permeation and improved the ocular bioavailability of the antibiotics [170,171].

Intravitreal injections are mainly used as conventional therapy for bacterial endophthalmitis. To improve these treatments and prolong intravitreal therapeutic concentrations of antibiotics, these drugs were entrapped in liposomes. For example, Zeng et al. encapsulated amikacin into liposomes with an entrapment efficiency of 91%. The half-time release of the drug from liposomes in PBS was 84.8 h. This formulation prolonged half-life of the drug in the vitreous and the pharmacokinetic analysis suggested that in severe case of endophthalmitis, liposomes should be preferred to conventional formulations [172]. These conclusions were confirmed by another study, with a ciprofloxacin liposomal system. The authors demonstrated that the liposomes improved the intraocular bioavailability of the drug. MLV showed a concentration of drug in vitreous higher than the MIC90 value after three days of the intravitreal injection, and after 14 days, they found no drug in the vitreous [173].

In a recent study, minocycline-liposomes were developed for a subconjunctival injection and compared to free minocycline injection. They obtained SUV (Small Unilamellar Vesicles) with an average particle size of 80 nm $\pm$ 20 nm. The authors concluded on a higher release of drug than free minocycline in the retina with loaded liposomes [174].

Niosomes for Antibiotic Delivery

Antiglaucoma therapy requires a continuous and chronic administration of antibiotics. To improve the low corneal penetration and bioavailability of drugs in conventional ocular forms, azetazolamide-niosomes were tested as ocular drug delivery vesicles. Span® 40 or 60 and CH were used in different molar ratios. The results showed that the ratio 7:6 (Span® 60:CH) made MLV and had the higher entrapment efficiency. The formulation showed a high retention of drug with 75% of active substance in the vesicles after 3 months at +4°C. The intraocular pressure (IOP) was measured to establish the treatment efficacy due to the antimicrobial activity of acetazolamide. There was a better decrease of IOP with the niosomes compared to the free drug solution. The most effective molar ratio was 7:4 (Span® 60:CH) with a prolonged decrease of IOP. In addition a reversible irritation in the rabbit's eyes was noted with no major change in ocular tissues [175].

Another study explored acetazolamide-niosomes coated with Carbopol® (bioadhesive effect) for a glaucoma treatment. The low solubility (0.7mg/mL) and low permeability coefficient of the drug require frequent administration. They compared the coated niosome with an aqueous suspension with 1% w/v of Tween® 80 as dispersing agent. They demonstrated a concentration of acetazolamide in the aqueous humor (determined by a microdialys method) two fold higher with niosomes than using aqueous suspension and a longer effect; 6 h for the niosomes against 3 h for the aqueous suspension [176].

Gentamicin is a water-soluble antibiotic which was studied in a niosomal system with Tween® (60 or 80) or Brij 35, CH and dicetylphosphate. With in vitro drug release, the study demonstrated a higher drug concentration inside the vesicles and slower drug release compared to the aqueous solution. They observed that the size of vesicles depended of amount of cholesterol and surfactant type. The molar ratio of 1:1:0.1 (Tween® 60:CH:dicetylphosphate) had the higher entrapment efficiency (92%) and the higher release rate of drug 8 h after administration (66%) with no sign of ocular irritation [177].

More recently, a study confirmed this conclusion. Ciprofloxacin-niosomes were developed with different concentrations of Span®, Tween® and CH to treat conjunctiva and corneal ulcer. They obtained a ranged size from 8.6 to 61.3 μm and an entrapment efficiency of 74% and demonstrated that the MIC values with niosomes were 2-fold higher compared to the free ciprofloxacin. In addition, the authors concluded of the higher release of drug for the combination of Span® and Tween® [178].

Table 2. Example of colloidal system for ocular drug delivery of antibiotics.

Formulation	Antibiotic	Anterior (AS) or Posterior (PS) Segment	Disease Targeted	References
Microemulsion	Chloramphenicol	AS	Trachoma Keratitis	[138]
	Moxifloxacin	AS	Bacterial keratitis	[139]
Nanoemulsion	Polymixin B	AS	Ophthalmic infection	[142]
Nanoparticles	Tobramycin	AS + PS	Bacterial infection *Pseudomonas aeruginosa*	[163]
	Levofloxacin	AS	Bacterial infection *S. aureus* and *E. coli*	[161]
Liposomes	Ciprofloxacin	PS	Bacterial endophthalmitis	[173]
	Distamycin A	AS	Herpes simplex virus	[165]
Niosomes	Acetazolamide	AS	Glaucoma	[175]
	Ciprofloxacin	AS	Conjunctiva + corneal ulcer	[178]

5. Conclusions

Topical eye drops represent 90% of all ocular dosage forms. In recent years, medical and pharmaceutical researchers have made major advances in the field of ophthalmic administration and in ocular drug delivery systems. New ocular drug delivery systems have great potential to improve drug bioavailability in the eye. Limitations of the ocular barriers are major issues to solve for an optimal formulation. Active substance limitations are decreased with the choice of an adaptable form and composition. Patient compliance improves with a tolerable and non-irritating formulation; this parameter is primary for an acceptable administration.

This review showed various development studies of ocular delivery forms. Many studies explored the possibility to decrease the side effects of ocular barrier to prolong ophthalmic residence of the drugs in the eyes, to improve the bioavailability of the active substances and to enhance ocular penetration. Various antibiotics with different characteristics were tested with different delivery systems in order to improve their ophthalmic bioavailability. Antibiotic administration required optimal antimicrobial efficacy. These drugs are used in eye surgeries, anterior segment and posterior segment diseases. Some improvements to limit the impact of the antibiotic's disadvantages on the eye are under study and under development. Existing forms and new shapes make it possible to increase the ocular therapy efficacy. In the next few years, drug development allowing local action without the need for systemic passage will decrease the frequency of administration, dosage of the drug and improve patient compliance.

Author Contributions: Marion Dubald was the primary author of this paper. She wrote the article and designed figures and tables. Sandrine Bourgeois, Véronique Andrieux and Hatem Fessi conceived the design of the review with Marion Dubald and supervised its writing and the submission process.

References

1. Gan, L.; Wang, J.; Jiang, M.; Bartlett, H.; Ouyang, D.; Eperjesi, F.; Liu, J.; Gan, Y. Recent advances in topical ophthalmic drug delivery with lipid-based nanocarriers. *Drug Discov. Today* **2013**, *18*, 290–297. [CrossRef] [PubMed]

2. Le Bourlais, C.; Acar, L.; Zia, H.; Sado, P.A.; Needham, T.; Leverge, R. Ophthalmic drug delivery systems—Recent advances. *Prog. Retin. Eye Res.* **1998**, *17*, 33–58. [CrossRef]

3. Achouri, D.; Alhanout, K.; Piccerelle, P.; Andrieu, V. Recent advances in ocular drug delivery. *Drug Dev. Ind. Pharm.* **2013**, *39*, 1599–1617. [CrossRef] [PubMed]

4. Yellepeddi, V.K.; Palakurthi, S. Recent advances in topical ocular drug delivery. *J. Ocul. Pharmacol. Ther. Off. J. Assoc. Ocul. Pharmacol. Ther.* **2016**, *32*, 67–82. [CrossRef] [PubMed]

5. Kalhapure, R.S.; Suleman, N.; Mocktar, C.; Seedat, N.; Govender, T. Nanoengineered drug delivery systems for enhancing antibiotic therapy. *J. Pharm. Sci.* **2015**, *104*, 872–905. [CrossRef] [PubMed]

6. Sharma, S. Antibiotic resistance in ocular bacterial pathogens. *Indian J. Med. Microbiol.* **2011**, *29*, 218–222. [CrossRef] [PubMed]

7. Remington, L.A. *Clinical anatomy and physiology of the visual system*, 3rd ed.; Elsevier/Butterworth Heinemann: St. Louis, MO, USA, 2012; ISBN 978-1-4377-1926-0.

8. Rathbone, M.J.; Hadgraft, J.; Roberts, M.S.; Lane, M.E. *Modified-release drug delivery technology (Drugs and the pharmaceutical sciences)*, 2nd ed.; Informa Healthcare: New York, NY, USA, 2008; Volume 2, ISBN 978-1-4200-4435-5.

9. Goel, M.; Picciani, R.G.; Lee, R.K.; Bhattacharya, S.K. Aqueous humor dynamics: A review. *Open Ophthalmol. J.* **2010**, *4*, 52–59. [CrossRef] [PubMed]

10. Cholkar, K.; Dasari, S.R.; Pal, D.; Mitra, A.K. Eye: anatomy, physiology and barriers to drug delivery. In *Ocular Transporters and Receptors*; Mitra, A.K., Ed.; Woodhead Publishing: Cambridge, UK, 2013; pp. 1–36. ISBN 978-1-907568-86-2.

11. Occhiutto, M.L.; Freitas, F.R.; Maranhao, R.C.; Costa, V.P. Breakdown of the Blood-Ocular Barrier as a Strategy for the Systemic Use of Nanosystems. *Pharmaceutics* **2012**, *4*, 252–275. [CrossRef] [PubMed]

12. Cunha-Vaz, J. The blood-ocular barriers. *Surv. Ophthalmol.* **1979**, *23*, 279–296. [CrossRef]

13. Chen, M.-S.; Hou, P.-K.; Tai, T.-Y.; Lin, B.J. Blood-ocular barriers. *Tzu Chi Med. J.* **2008**, *20*, 25–34. [CrossRef]

14. Gaudana, R.; Ananthula, H.K.; Parenky, A.; Mitra, A.K. Ocular drug delivery. *AAPS J.* **2010**, *12*, 348–360. [CrossRef] [PubMed]

15. Patel, A. Ocular drug delivery systems: An overview. *World J. Pharmacol.* **2013**, *2*, 47. [CrossRef] [PubMed]

16. Pisella, P.J.; Fillacier, K.; Elena, P.P.; Debbasch, C.; Baudouin, C. Comparison of the effects of preserved and unpreserved formulations of timolol on the ocular surface of albino rabbits. *Ophthalmic Res.* **2000**, *32*, 3–8. [CrossRef] [PubMed]

17. Van der Bijl, P.; van Eyk, A.D.; Meyer, D. Effects of three penetration enhancers on transcorneal permeation of cyclosporine. *Cornea* **2001**, *20*, 505–508. [CrossRef] [PubMed]

18. Bartlett, J.D.; Jaanus, S.D. *Clinical ocular pharmacology*; Butterworth-Heinemann: Oxford, United Kingdom, 1989; ISBN 0-409-90058-3.

19. Bakkour, Y.; Vermeersch, G.; Morcellet, M.; Boschin, F.; Martel, B.; Azaroual, N. Formation of cyclodextrin inclusion complexes with doxycyclin-hyclate: NMR investigation of their characterisation and stability. *J. Incl. Phenom. Macrocycl. Chem.* **2006**, *54*, 109–114. [CrossRef]

20. Sigurdsson, H.H.; Stefánsson, E.; Gudmundsdóttir, E.; Eysteinsson, T.; Thorsteinsdóttir, M.; Loftsson, T. Cyclodextrin formulation of dorzolamide and its distribution in the eye after topical administration. *J. Controlled Release* **2005**, *102*, 255–262. [CrossRef] [PubMed]

21. Loftsson, T.; Järvinen, T. Cyclodextrins in ophthalmic drug delivery. *Adv. Drug Deliv. Rev.* **1999**, *36*, 59–79. [CrossRef]

22. Al-Ghabeish, M.; Xu, X.; Krishnaiah, Y.S.R.; Rahman, Z.; Yang, Y.; Khan, M.A. Influence of drug loading and type of ointment base on the in vitro performance of acyclovir ophthalmic ointment. *Int. J. Pharm.* **2015**, *495*, 783–791. [CrossRef] [PubMed]

23. Kirchhof, S.; Goepferich, A.M.; Brandl, F.P. Hydrogels in ophthalmic applications. *Eur. J. Pharm. Biopharm.* **2015**, *95*, 227–238. [CrossRef] [PubMed]

24. Khare, A.; Grover, K.; Pawar, P.; Singh, I. Mucoadhesive polymers for enhancing retention in ocular drug delivery: A critical review. *Rev. Adhes. Adhes.* **2014**, *2*, 467–502. [CrossRef]

25. Roy, S.; Pal, K.; Anis, A.; Pramanik, K.; Prabhakar, B. Polymers in mucoadhesive drug-delivery systems: A brief note. *Des. Monomers Polym.* **2009**, *12*, 483–495. [CrossRef]

26. Bora, M.; Mundargi, R.C.; Chee, Y.; Wong, T.T.L.; Venkatraman, S.S. 5-Flurouracil microencapsulation and impregnation in hyaluronic acid hydrogel as composite drug delivery system for ocular fibrosis. *Cogent Med.* **2016**, *3*. [CrossRef]

27. Lai, J.-Y.; Ma, D.H.-K.; Cheng, H.-Y.; Sun, C.-C.; Huang, S.-J.; Li, Y.-T.; Hsiue, G.-H. Ocular biocompatibility of Carbodiimide cross-linked hyaluronic acid hydrogels for cell sheet delivery carriers. *J. Biomater. Sci. Polym. Ed.* **2010**, *21*, 359–376. [CrossRef] [PubMed]

28. Widjaja, L.K.; Bora, M.; Chan, P.N.P.H.; Lipik, V.; Wong, T.T.L.; Venkatraman, S.S. Hyaluronic acid-based nanocomposite hydrogels for ocular drug delivery applications: Ha-based nanocomposite hydrogels. *J. Biomed. Mater. Res. A* **2014**, *102*, 3056–3065. [CrossRef] [PubMed]

29. Rajoria, G.; Gupta, A. In situ Gelling System: A novel approach for ocular drug delivery. *Am. J. PharmTech Res.* **2012**, *2*, 25–53.

30. Cao, Y.; Zhang, C.; Shen, W.; Cheng, Z.; Yu, L.; Ping, Q. Poly(N-isopropylacrylamide)–chitosan as thermosensitive in situ gel-forming system for ocular drug delivery. *J. Controlled Release* **2007**, *120*, 186–194. [CrossRef] [PubMed]

31. Al Khateb, K.; Ozhmukhametova, E.K.; Mussin, M.N.; Seilkhanov, S.K.; Rakhypbekov, T.K.; Lau, W.M.; Khutoryanskiy, V.V. In situ gelling systems based on Pluronic F127/Pluronic F68 formulations for ocular drug delivery. *Int. J. Pharm.* **2016**, *502*, 70–79. [CrossRef] [PubMed]

32. Almeida, H.; Amaral, M.H.; Lobão, P.; Lobo, J.M.S. In situ gelling systems: a strategy to improve the bioavailability of ophthalmic pharmaceutical formulations. *Drug Discov. Today* **2014**, *19*, 400–412. [CrossRef] [PubMed]

33. Mane, K.; Dhole, S. In situ gelling system - A novel approach for ocular drug delivery. *World J. Pharm. Pharm. Sci.* **2014**, *3*, 317–333.

34. Gonjari, I.D.; Karmarkar, A.B.; Khade, T.S.; Hosmani, A.H.; Navale, R.B. Use of factorial design in formulation and evaluation of ophthalmic gels of gatifloxacin: Comparison of different mucoadhesive polymers. *Drug Discov. Ther.* **2010**, *4*, 423–434. [PubMed]

35. Buchan, B.; Kay, G.; Heneghan, A.; Matthews, K.H.; Cairns, D. Gel formulations for treatment of the ophthalmic complications in cystinosis. *Int. J. Pharm.* **2010**, *392*, 192–197. [CrossRef] [PubMed]

36. Peppas, N.A.; Bures, P.; Leobandung, W.; Ichikawa, H. Hydrogels in pharmaceutical formulations. *Eur. J. Pharm. Biopharm. Off. J. Arbeitsgemeinschaft Pharm. Verfahrenstechnik EV* **2000**, *50*, 27–46. [CrossRef]

37. Jeong, B.; Kim, S.W.; Bae, Y.H. Thermosensitive sol–gel reversible hydrogels. *Adv. Drug Deliv. Rev.* **2002**, *54*, 37–51. [CrossRef]

38. Almeida, H.; Amaral, M.H.; Lobão, P.; Sousa Lobo, J.M. Applications of poloxamers in ophthalmic pharmaceutical formulations: An overview. *Expert Opin. Drug Deliv.* **2013**, *10*, 1223–1237. [CrossRef] [PubMed]

39. He, Z.; Wang, Z.; Zhang, H.; Pan, X.; Su, W.; Liang, D.; Wu, C. Doxycycline and hydroxypropyl-β-cyclodextrin complex in poloxamer thermal sensitive hydrogel for ophthalmic delivery. *Acta Pharm. Sin. B* **2011**, *1*, 254–260. [CrossRef]

40. Cho, K. Release of ciprofloxacin from poloxamer-graft-hyaluronic acid hydrogels in vitro. *Int. J. Pharm.* **2003**, *260*, 83–91. [CrossRef]

41. Mayol, L.; Quaglia, F.; Borzacchiello, A.; Ambrosio, L.; Rotonda, M. A novel poloxamers/hyaluronic acid in situ forming hydrogel for drug delivery: Rheological, mucoadhesive and in vitro release properties. *Eur. J. Pharm. Biopharm.* **2008**, *70*, 199–206. [CrossRef] [PubMed]

42. Shastri, D.H.; Prajapati, S.T.; Patel, L.D. Studies on poloxamer based mucoadhesive insitu ophthalmic hydrogel of moxifloxacin HCL. *Curr. Drug Deliv.* **2010**, *3*, 238–243. [CrossRef]

43. Gratieri, T.; Gelfuso, G.M.; Rocha, E.M.; Sarmento, V.H.; de Freitas, O.; Lopez, R.F.V. A poloxamer/chitosan in situ forming gel with prolonged retention time for ocular delivery. *Eur. J. Pharm. Biopharm.* **2010**, *75*, 186–193. [CrossRef] [PubMed]

44. Srividya, B.; Cardoza, R.M.; Amin, P. Sustained ophthalmic delivery of ofloxacin from a pH triggered in situ gelling system. *J. Controlled Release* **2001**, *73*, 205–211. [CrossRef]

45. Patil, S.; Kadam, A.; Bandgar, S.; Patil, S. Formulation and evaluation of an in situ gel for ocular drug delivery of anticonjunctival drug. *Cellulose Chem. Technol.* **2015**, *49*, 35–40.

46. Makwana, S.B.; Patel, V.A.; Parmar, S.J. Development and characterization of in situ gel for ophthalmic formulation containing ciprofloxacin hydrochloride. *Results Pharma Sci.* **2016**, *6*, 1–6. [CrossRef] [PubMed]

47. Mandal, S.; Prabhushankar, G.; Thimmasetty, M.; Geetha, M. Formulation and evaluation of an in situ gel-forming ophthalmic formulation of moxifloxacin hydrochloride. *Int. J. Pharm. Investig.* **2012**, *2*, 78. [CrossRef] [PubMed]

48. Carlfors, J.; Edsman, K.; Petersson, R.; Jörnving, K. Rheological evaluation of Gelrite® in situ gels for ophthalmic use. *Eur. J. Pharm. Sci.* **1998**, *6*, 113–119. [CrossRef]

49. Sultana, Y.; Aqil, M.; Ali, A. Ion-Activated, Gelrite®-Based in Situ Ophthalmic Gels of Pefloxacin Mesylate: Comparison with Conventional Eye Drops. *Drug Deliv.* **2006**, *13*, 215–219. [CrossRef] [PubMed]

50. Joshi, A.; Ding, S.; Himmelstein, K.J. Reversible Gelation Compositions and Methods of Use. U.S. Patent 5252318 A, 15 June 1990.

51. Liu, Y.; Liu, J.; Zhang, X.; Zhang, R.; Huang, Y.; Wu, C. In situ gelling gelrite/alginate formulations as vehicles for ophthalmic drug delivery. *AAPS PharmSciTech* **2010**, *11*, 610–620. [CrossRef] [PubMed]

52. Fanun, M. Microemulsions as delivery systems. *Curr. Opin. Colloid Interface Sci.* **2012**, *17*, 306–313. [CrossRef]

53. Ghosh, P.K.; Murthy, R.S.R. Microemulsions: A potential drug delivery system. *Curr. Drug Deliv.* **2006**, *3*, 167–180. [CrossRef] [PubMed]

54. Vandamme, T.F. Microemulsions as ocular drug delivery systems: Recent developments and future challenges. *Prog. Retin. Eye Res.* **2002**, *21*, 15–34. [CrossRef]

55. Tamilvanan, S.; Benita, S. The potential of lipid emulsion for ocular delivery of lipophilic drugs. *Eur. J. Pharm. Biopharm.* **2004**, *58*, 357–368. [CrossRef] [PubMed]

56. Lallemand, F.; Daull, P.; Benita, S.; Buggage, R.; Garrigue, J.-S. Successfully improving ocular drug delivery using the cationic nanoemulsion, Novasorb. *J. Drug Deliv.* **2012**, *2012*, 604204. [CrossRef] [PubMed]

57. Van, A. Eye irritation: studies relating to responses in man and laboratory animals. *J. Soc. Cosmet. Chem. Jpn.* **1973**, *24*, 685–692.

58. Yin, J.; Xiang, C.; Lu, G. Cationic lipid emulsions as potential bioadhesive carriers for ophthalmic delivery of palmatine. *J. Microencapsul.* **2016**, *33*, 718–724. [CrossRef] [PubMed]

59. Higuchi, T. Ocular Insert. U.S. Patent 3,630,200 A, 28 December 1971.

60. Kumari, A.; Sharma, P.; Garg, V.; Garg, G. Ocular inserts—Advancement in therapy of eye diseases. *J. Adv. Pharm. Technol. Res.* **2010**, *1*, 291. [CrossRef] [PubMed]

61. Ara, T.; Sharma, S.; Bhat, S.A.; Bhandari, A.; Deva, A.S.; Rathore, M.S.; Khan, R.A.; Bhatia, N. Preparation and evaluation of ocular inserts of diclofenac sodium for controlled drug delivery. *Int. J. Sci. Res. Publ.* **2015**, *5*, 93–99.

62. Shukr, M. Formulation, in vitro and in vivo evaluation of lidocaine HCl ocular inserts for topical ocular anesthesia. *Arch. Pharm. Res.* **2014**, *37*, 882–889. [CrossRef] [PubMed]

63. Sampath Kumar, K.P.; Bhowmik, D.; Harish, G.; Duraivel, S.; Pragathi Kumar, B. Ocular inserts: A novel controlled drug delivery system. *The Pharm. Innov.* **2012**, *1*, 1–16.

64. Gurtler, F.; Gurny, R. Patent literature review of ophthalmic inserts. *Drug Dev. Ind. Pharm.* **1995**, *21*, 1–18. [CrossRef]

65. Baranowski, P.; Karolewicz, B.; Gajda, M.; Pluta, J. Ophthalmic drug dosage forms: Characterisation and research methods. *Sci. World J.* **2014**, *2014*, 1–14. [CrossRef] [PubMed]

66. Guzman-Aranguez, A.; Colligris, B.; Pintor, J. Contact lenses: promising devices for ocular drug delivery. *J. Ocul. Pharmacol. Ther. Off. J. Assoc. Ocul. Pharmacol. Ther.* **2013**, *29*, 189–199. [CrossRef] [PubMed]

67. Stapleton, F.; Stretton, S.; Papas, E.; Skotnitsky, C.; Sweeney, D.F. Silicone hydrogel contact lenses and the ocular surface. *Ocul. Surf.* **2006**, *4*, 24–43. [CrossRef]

68. Van der Worp, E.; Bornman, D.; Ferreira, D.L.; Faria-Ribeiro, M.; Garcia-Porta, N.; González-Meijome, J.M. Modern scleral contact lenses: A review. *Contact Lens Anterior Eye J. Br. Contact Lens Assoc.* **2014**, *37*, 240–250. [CrossRef] [PubMed]

69. Harthan, J.S. Therapeutic use of mini-scleral lenses in a patient with Graves' ophthalmopathy. *J. Optom.* **2014**, *7*, 62–66. [CrossRef] [PubMed]

70. Rathi, V.M.; Dumpati, S.; Mandathara, P.S.; Taneja, M.M.; Sangwan, V.S. Scleral contact lenses in the management of pellucid marginal degeneration. *Contact Lens Anterior Eye* **2016**, *39*, 217–220. [CrossRef] [PubMed]

71. Severinsky, B.; Behrman, S.; Frucht-Pery, J.; Solomon, A. Scleral contact lenses for visual rehabilitation after penetrating keratoplasty: Long term outcomes. *Contact Lens Anterior Eye* **2014**, *37*, 196–202. [CrossRef] [PubMed]

72. Romero-Rangel, T.; Stavrou, P.; Cotter, J.; Rosenthal, P.; Baltatzis, S.; Foster, C.S. Gas-permeable scleral contact lens therapy in ocular surface disease. *Am. J. Ophthalmol.* **2000**, *130*, 25–32. [CrossRef]

73. Kramer, E.G.; Boshnick, E.L. Scleral lenses in the treatment of post-LASIK ectasia and superficial neovascularization of intrastromal corneal ring segments. *Contact Lens Anterior Eye* **2015**, *38*, 298–303. [CrossRef] [PubMed]

74. Inamoto, Y.; Sun, Y.-C.; Flowers, M.E.D.; Carpenter, P.A.; Martin, P.J.; Li, P.; Wang, R.; Chai, X.; Storer, B.E.; Shen, T.T.; et al. Bandage soft contact lenses for ocular graft-versus-host disease. *Biol. Blood Marrow Transplant.* **2015**, *21*, 2002–2007. [CrossRef] [PubMed]

75. Glisoni, R.J.; García-Fernández, M.J.; Pino, M.; Gutkind, G.; Moglioni, A.G.; Alvarez-Lorenzo, C.; Concheiro, A.; Sosnik, A. β-Cyclodextrin hydrogels for the ocular release of antibacterial thiosemicarbazones. *Carbohydr. Polym.* **2013**, *93*, 449–457. [CrossRef] [PubMed]

76. Teixeira, M.; Alonso, M.J.; Pinto, M.M.M.; Barbosa, C.M. Development and characterization of PLGA nanospheres and nanocapsules containing xanthone and 3-methoxyxanthone. *Eur. J. Pharm. Biopharm.* **2005**, *59*, 491–500. [CrossRef] [PubMed]

77. Diebold, Y.; Calonge, M. Applications of nanoparticles in ophthalmology. *Prog. Retin. Eye Res.* **2010**, *29*, 596–609. [CrossRef] [PubMed]

78. Xu, Q.; Kambhampati, S.P.; Kannan, R.M. Nanotechnology approaches for ocular drug delivery. *Middle East Afr. J. Ophthalmol.* **2013**, *20*, 26–37. [CrossRef] [PubMed]

79. Mohanraj, V.J.; Chen, Y. Nanoparticles—A review. *Trop. J. Pharm. Res.* **2006**, *5*, 561–573. [CrossRef]

80. Yildirimer, L.; Thanh, N.T.K.; Loizidou, M.; Seifalian, A.M. Toxicology and clinical potential of nanoparticles. *Nano Today* **2011**, *6*, 585–607. [CrossRef] [PubMed]

81. Duxfield, L.; Sultana, R.; Wang, R.; Englebretsen, V.; Deo, S.; Swift, S.; Rupenthal, I.; Al-Kassas, R. Development of gatifloxacin-loaded cationic polymeric nanoparticles for ocular drug delivery. *Pharm. Dev. Technol.* **2016**, *21*, 172–179. [CrossRef] [PubMed]

82. Mun, E.A.; Morrison, P.W.J.; Williams, A.C.; Khutoryanskiy, V.V. On the barrier properties of the cornea: A microscopy study of the penetration of fluorescently labeled nanoparticles, polymers, and sodium fluorescein. *Mol. Pharm.* **2014**, *11*, 3556–3564. [CrossRef] [PubMed]

83. Bangham, A.D.; Standish, M.M.; Watkins, J.C. Diffusion of univalent ions across the lamellae of swollen phospholipids. *J. Mol. Biol.* **1965**, *13*, 238–252. [CrossRef]

84. Meisner, D.; Mezei, M. Liposome ocular delivery systems. *Adv. Drug Deliv. Rev.* **1995**, *16*, 75–93. [CrossRef]

85. Mishra, G.P.; Bagui, M.; Tamboli, V.; Mitra, A.K. Recent applications of liposomes in ophthalmic drug delivery. *J. Drug Deliv.* **2011**, *2011*, e863734. [CrossRef] [PubMed]

86. Hathout, R.M.; Mansour, S.; Mortada, N.D.; Guinedi, A.S. Liposomes as an ocular delivery system for acetazolamide: in vitro and in vivo studies. *AAPS PharmSciTech* **2007**, *8*, 1. [CrossRef] [PubMed]

87. Khanam, N.; Alam, M.I.; Sachan, A.K.; Sharma, R. Recent trends in drug delivery by niosomes: A review. *Research Gate* **2013**, *1*, 115–122.

88. Pham, T.T.; Jaafar-Maalej, C.; Charcosset, C.; Fessi, H. Liposome and niosome preparation using a membrane contactor for scale-up. *Colloids Surf. B* **2012**, *94*, 15–21. [CrossRef] [PubMed]

89. Kalomiraki, M.; Thermos, K.; Chaniotakis, N.A. Dendrimers as tunable vectors of drug delivery systems and biomedical and ocular applications. *Int. J. Nanomedicine* **2015**, *11*, 1–12. [CrossRef] [PubMed]

90. Burçin, Y.; Bozdag Pehlivan, S.; Ünlü, S. Dendrimeric systems and their applications in ocular drug delivery. *Sci. World J.* **2013**, *2013*. [CrossRef]

91. Vandamme, T.F.; Brobeck, L. Poly(amidoamine) dendrimers as ophthalmic vehicles for ocular delivery of pilocarpine nitrate and tropicamide. *J. Controlled Release* **2005**, *102*, 23–38. [CrossRef] [PubMed]

92. Fleming, A. On the antibacterial action of cultures of a penicillium, with special reference to their use in the isolation of B. influenzæ. *Br. J. Exp. Pathol.* **1929**, *10*, 226–236. [CrossRef]

93. Gualerzi, C.O.; Brandi, L.; Fabbretti, A.; Pon, C.L. (Eds.) *Antibiotics: Targets, Mechanisms and Resistance*; Wiley-VCH Verlag GmbH & Co. KGaA: Weinheim, Germany, 2013; ISBN 978-3-527-65968-5.

94. Kapoor, A.; Malhotra, R.; Grover, V.; Grover, D. Systemic antibiotic therapy in periodontics. *Dent. Res. J.* **2012**, *9*, 505–515. [CrossRef]

95. Cornut, P.-L.; Chiquet, C. Intravitreal injection of antibiotics in endophthalmitis. *J. Fr. Ophtalmol.* **2008**, *31*, 815–823. [CrossRef]

96. Barza, M. Factors affecting the intraocular penetration of antibiotics. The influence of route, inflammation, animal species and tissue pigmentation. *Scand. J. Infect. Dis. Suppl.* **1978**, 151–159.

97. Snyder, R.W.; Glasser, D.B. Antibiotic therapy for ocular infection. *West. J. Med.* **1994**, *161*, 579–584. [PubMed]

98. Shimpi, S.; Chauhan, B.; Shimpi, P. Cyclodextrins: application in different routes of drug administration. *Acta Pharm. Zagreb Croat.* **2005**, *55*, 139–156.

99. Tiwari, G.; Tiwari, R.; Rai, A.K. Cyclodextrins in delivery systems: Applications. *J. Pharm. Bioallied Sci.* **2010**, *2*, 72. [CrossRef] [PubMed]

100. Nijhawan, R.; Agarwal, S.P. Development of an ophthalmic formulation containing ciprofloxacin-hydroxypropyl-b-cyclodextrin complex. *Boll. Chim. Farm.* **2003**, *142*, 214–219. [PubMed]

101. Bozkir, A.; Denli, Z.F.; Basaran, B. Effect of hydroxypropyl-beta-cyclodextrin on the solubility, stability and in-vitro release of ciprofloxacin for ocular drug delivery. *Acta Pol. Pharm.* **2012**, *69*, 719–724. [PubMed]

102. Thatiparti, T.R.; von Recum, H.A. Cyclodextrin complexation for affinity-based antibiotic delivery. *Macromol. Biosci.* **2010**, *10*, 82–90. [CrossRef] [PubMed]

103. Pullum, K.W. The unique role of scleral lenses in contact lens practice. *Contact Lens Anterior Eye* **1999**, *22*, S26–S34. [CrossRef]

104. Tougeron-Brousseau, B.; Delcampe, A.; Gueudry, J.; Vera, L.; Doan, S.; Hoang-Xuan, T.; Muraine, M. Vision-related function after scleral lens fitting in ocular complications of stevens-johnson syndrome and toxic epidermal necrolysis. *Am. J. Ophthalmol.* **2009**, *148*, 852–859.e2. [CrossRef] [PubMed]

105. Laballe, R.; Vigne, J.; Denion, E.; Lemaitre, F.; Goux, D.; Pisella, P.-J. Preclinical assessment of scleral lens as a reservoir-based ocular therapeutic system. *Contact Lens Anterior Eye J. Br. Contact Lens Assoc.* **2016**, *39*, 394–396. [CrossRef] [PubMed]

106. Hu, X.; Tan, H.; Hao, L. Functional hydrogel contact lens for drug delivery in the application of oculopathy therapy. *J. Mech. Behav. Biomed. Mater.* **2016**, *64*, 43–52. [CrossRef] [PubMed]

107. Tian, X.; Iwatsu, M.; Sado, K.; Kanai, A. Studies on the uptake and release of fluoroquinolones by disposable contact lenses. *CLAO J. Off. Publ. Contact Lens Assoc. Ophthalmol. Inc.* **2001**, *27*, 216–220.

108. Hehl, E.M.; Beck, R.; Luthard, K.; Guthoff, R.; Drewelow, B. Improved penetration of aminoglycosides and fluorozuinolones into the aqueous humour of patients by means of Acuvue contact lenses. *Eur. J. Clin. Pharmacol.* **1999**, *55*, 317–323. [CrossRef] [PubMed]

109. Yokozaki, Y.; Sakabe, J.; Shimoyama, Y. Enhanced impregnation of hydrogel contact lenses with salicylic acid by addition of water in supercritical carbon dioxide. *Chem. Eng. Res. Des.* **2015**, *104*, 203–207. [CrossRef]

110. Costa, V.P.; Braga, M.E.M.; Guerra, J.P.; Duarte, A.R.C.; Duarte, C.M.M.; Leite, E.O.B.; Gil, M.H.; de Sousa, H.C. Development of therapeutic contact lenses using a supercritical solvent impregnation method. *J. Supercrit. Fluids* **2010**, *52*, 306–316. [CrossRef]

111. Alvarez-Lorenzo, C.; Yañez, F.; Concheiro, A. Ocular drug delivery from molecularly-imprinted contact lenses. *J. Drug Deliv. Sci. Technol.* **2010**, *20*, 237–248. [CrossRef]

112. Alvarez-Lorenzo, C.; Yañez, F.; Barreiro-Iglesias, R.; Concheiro, A. Imprinted soft contact lenses as norfloxacin delivery systems. *J. Controlled Release* **2006**, *113*, 236–244. [CrossRef] [PubMed]

113. Malakooti, N.; Alexander, C.; Alvarez-Lorenzo, C. Imprinted contact lenses for sustained release of polymyxin B and related antimicrobial peptides. *J. Pharm. Sci.* **2015**, *104*, 3386–3394. [CrossRef] [PubMed]

114. Ozawa, H.; Hosaka, S.; Kunitomo, T.; Tanzawa, H. Ocular inserts for controlled release of antibiotics. *Biomaterials* **1983**, *4*, 170–174. [CrossRef]

115. Hosaka, S.; Ozawa, H.; Tanzawa, H.; Kinitomo, T.; Nichols, R.L. In vivo evaluation of ocular inserts of hydrogel impregnated with antibiotics for trachoma therapy. *Biomaterials* **1983**, *4*, 243–248. [CrossRef]

116. Punch, P.I.; Costa, N.D.; Edwards, M.E.; Wilcox, G.E. The release of insoluble antibiotics from collagen ocular inserts in vitro and their insertion into the conjunctival sac of cattle. *J. Vet. Pharmacol. Ther.* **1987**, *10*, 37–42. [CrossRef] [PubMed]

117. Baeyens, V.; Kaltsatos, V.; Boisramé, B.; Varesio, E.; Veuthey, J.-L.; Fathi, M.; Balant, L.P.; Gex-Fabry, M.; Gurny, R. Optimized release of dexamethasone and gentamicin from a soluble ocular insert for the treatment of external ophthalmic infections. *J. Controlled Release* **1998**, *52*, 215–220. [CrossRef]

118. Di Colo, G.; Burgalassi, S.; Chetoni, P.; Fiaschi, M.P.; Zambito, Y.; Saettone, M.F. Gel-forming erodible inserts for ocular controlled delivery of ofloxacin. *Int. J. Pharm.* **2001**, *215*, 101–111. [CrossRef]

119. Di Colo, G.; Burgalassi, S.; Chetoni, P.; Fiaschi, M.P.; Zambito, Y.; Saettone, M.F. Relevance of polymer molecular weight to the in vitro/in vivo performances of ocular inserts based on poly(ethylene oxide). *Int. J. Pharm.* **2001**, *220*, 169–177. [CrossRef]

120. Di Colo, G.; Zambito, Y.; Burgalassi, S.; Serafini, A.; Saettone, M.F. Effect of chitosan on in vitro release and ocular delivery of ofloxacin from erodible inserts based on poly(ethylene oxide). *Int. J. Pharm.* **2002**, *248*, 115–122. [CrossRef]

121. Üstündağ-Okur, N.; Gökçe, E.H.; Bozbıyık, D.İ.; Eğrilmez, S.; Ertan, G.; Özer, Ö. Novel nanostructured lipid carrier-based inserts for controlled ocular drug delivery: Evaluation of corneal bioavailability and treatment efficacy in bacterial keratitis. *Expert Opin. Drug Deliv.* **2015**, *12*, 1791–1807. [CrossRef] [PubMed]

122. Sultana, Y.; Aqil, M.; Ali, A. Ocular inserts for controlled delivery of pefloxacin mesylate: Preparation and evaluation. *Acta Pharm. Zagreb Croat.* **2005**, *55*, 305–314.

123. Mundada, A.S.; Shrikhande, B.K. Design and evaluation of soluble ocular drug insert for controlled release of ciprofloxacin hydrochloride. *Drug Dev. Ind. Pharm.* **2006**, *32*, 443–448. [CrossRef] [PubMed]

124. Mundada, A.S.; Shrikhande, B.K. Formulation and evaluation of ciprofloxacin hydrochloride soluble ocular drug insert. *Curr. Eye Res.* **2008**, *33*, 469–475. [CrossRef] [PubMed]

125. Pawar, P.K.; Katara, R.; Majumdar, D.K. Design and evaluation of moxifloxacin hydrochloride ocular inserts. *Acta Pharm. Zagreb Croat.* **2012**, *62*, 93–104. [CrossRef] [PubMed]

126. Thakur, R.; Swami, G.; Rahman, M. Development and optimization of controlled release bioerodable anti infective ophthalmic insert. *Curr. Drug Deliv.* **2014**, *11*, 2–10. [CrossRef] [PubMed]

127. Wang, J.; Li, X.; Xiong, L.; Sun, N. Different concentrations of clarithromycin ophthalmic gel for rabbits corneal ulcers induced by Staphylococcus aureus. *Yan Ke Xue Bao* **2008**, *24*, 18–22. [PubMed]

128. Liu, Z.; Li, J.; Nie, S.; Liu, H.; Ding, P.; Pan, W. Study of an alginate/HPMC-based in situ gelling ophthalmic delivery system for gatifloxacin. *Int. J. Pharm.* **2006**, *315*, 12–17. [CrossRef] [PubMed]

129. Al-Kassas, R.S.; El-Khatib, M.M. Ophthalmic controlled release in situ gelling systems for ciprofloxacin based on polymeric carriers. *Drug Deliv.* **2009**, *16*, 145–152. [CrossRef] [PubMed]

130. Mansour, M.; Mansour, S.; Mortada, N.D.; Abd Elhady, S.S. Ocular poloxamer-based ciprofloxacin hydrochloride in situ forming gels. *Drug Dev. Ind. Pharm.* **2008**, *34*, 744–752. [CrossRef] [PubMed]

131. Nanjwade, B.K.; Deshmukh, R.V.; Gaikwad, K.R.; Parikh, K.A.; Manvi, F.V. Formulation and evaluation of micro hydrogel of Moxifloxacin hydrochloride. *Eur. J. Drug Metab. Pharmacokinet.* **2012**, *37*, 117–123. [CrossRef] [PubMed]

132. Khan, N.; Aqil, M.; Imam, S.S.; Ali, A. Development and evaluation of a novel in situ gel of sparfloxacin for sustained ocular drug delivery: In vitro and ex vivo characterization. *Pharm. Dev. Technol.* **2015**, *20*, 662–669. [CrossRef] [PubMed]

133. Sultana, Y.; Aqil, M.; Ali, A.; Zafar, S. Evaluation of carbopol-methyl cellulose-based sustained-release ocular delivery system for pefloxacin mesylate using rabbit eye model. *Pharm. Dev. Technol.* **2006**, *11*, 313–319. [CrossRef] [PubMed]

134. Liu, Z.; Yang, X.-G.; Li, X.; Pan, W.; Li, J. Study on the ocular pharmacokinetics of ion-activated in situ gelling ophthalmic delivery system for gatifloxacin by microdialysis. *Drug Dev. Ind. Pharm.* **2007**, *33*, 1327–1331. [CrossRef] [PubMed]

135. El-Laithy, H.M.; Nesseem, D.I.; El-Adly, A.A.; Shoukry, M. Moxifloxacin-Gelrite in situ ophthalmic gelling system against photodynamic therapy for treatment of bacterial corneal inflammation. *Arch. Pharm. Res.* **2011**, *34*, 1663–1678. [CrossRef] [PubMed]

136. Ameeduzzafar; Ali, J.; Fazil, M.; Qumbar, M.; Khan, N.; Ali, A. Colloidal drug delivery system: Amplify the ocular delivery. *Drug Deliv.* **2014**, *23*, 700–716. [CrossRef]

137. Ammar, H.O.; Salama, H.A.; Ghorab, M.; Mahmoud, A.A. Nanoemulsion as a Potential Ophthalmic Delivery System for Dorzolamide Hydrochloride. *AAPS PharmSciTech* **2009**, *10*, 808–817. [CrossRef] [PubMed]

138. Lv, F.-F.; Zheng, L.-Q.; Tung, C.-H. Phase behavior of the microemulsions and the stability of the chloramphenicol in the microemulsion-based ocular drug delivery system. *Int. J. Pharm.* **2005**, *301*, 237–246. [CrossRef] [PubMed]

139. Bharti, S.K.; Kesavan, K. Phase-transition W/O Microemulsions for ocular delivery: Evaluation of antibacterial activity in the treatment of bacterial keratitis. *Ocul. Immunol. Inflamm.* **2016**, 1–12. [CrossRef] [PubMed]

140. Üstündag-Okur, N.; Gökçe, E.H.; Eğrilmez, S.; Özer, Ö.; Ertan, G. Novel ofloxacin-loaded microemulsion formulations for ocular delivery. *J. Ocul. Pharmacol. Ther. Off. J. Assoc. Ocul. Pharmacol. Ther.* **2014**, *30*, 319–332. [CrossRef] [PubMed]

141. Kalam, M.A.; Alshamsan, A.; Aljuffali, I.A.; Mishra, A.K.; Sultana, Y. Delivery of gatifloxacin using microemulsion as vehicle: Formulation, evaluation, transcorneal permeation and aqueous humor drug determination. *Drug Deliv.* **2016**, *23*, 896–907. [CrossRef] [PubMed]

142. Li, X.; Müller, R.H.; Keck, C.M.; Bou-Chacra, N.A. Mucoadhesive dexamethasone acetate-polymyxin B sulfate cationic ocular nanoemulsion–novel combinatorial formulation concept. *Int. J. Pharm. Sci.* **2016**, *71*, 327–333. [CrossRef]

143. Almeida, H.; Amaral, M.H.; Lobao, P.; Frigerio, C.; Sousa Lobo, J.M. Nanoparticles in Ocular Drug Delivery Systems for Topical Administration: Promises and Challenges. *Curr. Pharm. Des.* **2015**, *21*, 5212–5224. [CrossRef] [PubMed]

144. Zhou, H.-Y.; Hao, J.-L.; Wang, S.; Zheng, Y.; Zhang, W.-S. Nanoparticles in the ocular drug delivery. *Int. J. Ophthalmol.* **2013**, *6*, 390–396. [CrossRef] [PubMed]

145. Das, S.; Suresh, P.K.; Desmukh, R. Design of Eudragit RL 100 nanoparticles by nanoprecipitation method for ocular drug delivery. *Nanomedicine Nanotechnol. Biol. Med.* **2010**, *6*, 318–323. [CrossRef] [PubMed]

146. Mandal, B.; Alexander, K.S.; Riga, A.T. Sulfacetamide loaded Eudragit® RL100 nanosuspension with potential for ocular delivery. *J. Pharm. Pharm. Sci. Publ. Can. Soc. Pharm. Sci. Soc. Can. Sci. Pharm.* **2010**, *13*, 510–523.

147. Ibrahim, H.K.; El-Leithy, I.S.; Makky, A.A. Mucoadhesive nanoparticles as carrier systems for prolonged ocular delivery of gatifloxacin/prednisolone bitherapy. *Mol. Pharm.* **2010**, *7*, 576–585. [CrossRef] [PubMed]

148. Lee, M.Y.; Bourgeois, S.; Almouazen, E.; Pelletier, J.; Renaud, F.; Fessi, H.; Kodjikian, L. Microencapsulation of rifampicin for the prevention of endophthalmitis: In vitro release studies and antibacterial assessment. *Int. J. Pharm.* **2016**, *505*, 262–270. [CrossRef] [PubMed]

149. Hachicha, W.; Kodjikian, L.; Fessi, H. Preparation of vancomycin microparticles: Importance of preparation parameters. *Int. J. Pharm.* **2006**, *324*, 176–184. [CrossRef] [PubMed]

150. Gupta, H.; Aqil, M.; Khar, R.K.; Ali, A.; Bhatnagar, A.; Mittal, G. Sparfloxacin-loaded PLGA nanoparticles for sustained ocular drug delivery. *Nanomedicine Nanotechnol. Biol. Med.* **2010**, *6*, 324–333. [CrossRef] [PubMed]

151. Gupta, H.; Aqil, M.; Khar, R.K.; Ali, A.; Bhatnagar, A.; Mittal, G. Biodegradable levofloxacin nanoparticles for sustained ocular drug delivery. *J. Drug Target.* **2011**, *19*, 409–417. [CrossRef] [PubMed]

152. Mohammadi, G.; Nokhodchi, A.; Barzegar-Jalali, M.; Lotfipour, F.; Adibkia, K.; Ehyaei, N.; Valizadeh, H. Physicochemical and anti-bacterial performance characterization of clarithromycin nanoparticles as colloidal drug delivery system. *Colloids Surf. B Biointerfaces* **2011**, *88*, 39–44. [CrossRef] [PubMed]

153. Pokharkar, V.; Patil, V.; Mandpe, L. Engineering of polymer-surfactant nanoparticles of doxycycline hydrochloride for ocular drug delivery. *Drug Deliv.* **2015**, *22*, 955–968. [CrossRef] [PubMed]

154. Motwani, S.K.; Chopra, S.; Talegaonkar, S.; Kohli, K.; Ahmad, F.J.; Khar, R.K. Chitosan-sodium alginate nanoparticles as submicroscopic reservoirs for ocular delivery: Formulation, optimisation and in vitro characterisation. *Eur. J. Pharm. Biopharm. Off. J. Arbeitsgemeinschaft Pharm. Verfahrenstechnik EV* **2008**, *68*, 513–525. [CrossRef] [PubMed]

155. Silva, N.C.; Silva, S.; Sarmento, B.; Pintado, M. Chitosan nanoparticles for daptomycin delivery in ocular treatment of bacterial endophthalmitis. *Drug Deliv.* **2015**, *22*, 885–893. [CrossRef] [PubMed]

156. Costa, J.R.; Silva, N.C.; Sarmento, B.; Pintado, M. Potential chitosan-coated alginate nanoparticles for ocular delivery of daptomycin. *Eur. J. Clin. Microbiol. Infect. Dis. Off. Publ. Eur. Soc. Clin. Microbiol.* **2015**, *34*, 1255–1262. [CrossRef] [PubMed]

157. Sánchez-López, E.; Espina, M.; Doktorovova, S.; Souto, E.B.; García, M.L. Lipid nanoparticles (SLN, NLC): Overcoming the anatomical and physiological barriers of the eye–Part II—Ocular drug-loaded lipid nanoparticles. *Eur. J. Pharm. Biopharm.* **2017**, *110*, 58–69. [CrossRef] [PubMed]

158. Kalam, M.A.; Sultana, Y.; Ali, A.; Aqil, M.; Mishra, A.K.; Chuttani, K. Preparation, characterization, and evaluation of gatifloxacin loaded solid lipid nanoparticles as colloidal ocular drug delivery system. *J. Drug Target.* **2010**, *18*, 191–204. [CrossRef] [PubMed]

159. Abul Kalam, M.; Sultana, Y.; Ali, A.; Aqil, M.; Mishra, A.K.; Aljuffali, I.A.; Alshamsan, A. Part I: Development and optimization of solid-lipid nanoparticles using Box-Behnken statistical design for ocular delivery of gatifloxacin. *J. Biomed. Mater. Res. A* **2013**, *101*, 1813–1827. [CrossRef] [PubMed]

160. Abul Kalam, M.; Sultana, Y.; Ali, A.; Aqil, M.; Mishra, A.K.; Chuttani, K.; Aljuffali, I.A.; Alshamsan, A. Part II: Enhancement of transcorneal delivery of gatifloxacin by solid lipid nanoparticles in comparison to commercial aqueous eye drops. *J. Biomed. Mater. Res. A* **2013**, *101*, 1828–1836. [CrossRef] [PubMed]

161. Baig, M.S.; Ahad, A.; Aslam, M.; Imam, S.S.; Aqil, M.; Ali, A. Application of Box-Behnken design for preparation of levofloxacin-loaded stearic acid solid lipid nanoparticles for ocular delivery: Optimization, in vitro release, ocular tolerance, and antibacterial activity. *Int. J. Biol. Macromol.* **2016**, *85*, 258–270. [CrossRef] [PubMed]

162. Yousry, C.; Fahmy, R.H.; Essam, T.; El-Laithy, H.M.; Elkheshen, S.A. Nanoparticles as tool for enhanced ophthalmic delivery of vancomycin: A multidistrict-based microbiological study, solid lipid nanoparticles formulation and evaluation. *Drug Dev. Ind. Pharm.* **2016**, *42*, 1752–1762. [CrossRef] [PubMed]

163. Chetoni, P.; Burgalassi, S.; Monti, D.; Tampucci, S.; Tullio, V.; Cuffini, A.M.; Muntoni, E.; Spagnolo, R.; Zara, G.P.; Cavalli, R. Solid lipid nanoparticles as promising tool for intraocular tobramycin delivery: Pharmacokinetic studies on rabbits. *Eur. J. Pharm. Biopharm. Off. J. Arbeitsgemeinschaft Pharm. Verfahrenstechnik EV* **2016**, *109*, 214–223. [CrossRef] [PubMed]

164. Mehanna, M.M.; Elmaradny, H.A.; Samaha, M.W. Ciprofloxacin liposomes as vesicular reservoirs for ocular delivery: Formulation, optimization, and in vitro characterization. *Drug Dev. Ind. Pharm.* **2009**, *35*, 583–593. [CrossRef] [PubMed]

165. Chetoni, P.; Monti, D.; Tampucci, S.; Matteoli, B.; Ceccherini-Nelli, L.; Subissi, A.; Burgalassi, S. Liposomes as a potential ocular delivery system of distamycin A. *Int. J. Pharm.* **2015**, *492*, 120–126. [CrossRef] [PubMed]

166. Mehanna, M.M.; Elmaradny, H.A.; Samaha, M.W. Mucoadhesive liposomes as ocular delivery system: Physical, microbiological, and in vivo assessment. *Drug Dev. Ind. Pharm.* **2010**, *36*, 108–118. [CrossRef] [PubMed]

167. Abdelbary, G. Ocular ciprofloxacin hydrochloride mucoadhesive chitosan-coated liposomes. *Pharm. Dev. Technol.* **2011**, *16*, 44–56. [CrossRef] [PubMed]

168. Budai, L.; Hajdú, M.; Budai, M.; Gróf, P.; Béni, S.; Noszál, B.; Klebovich, I.; Antal, I. Gels and liposomes in optimized ocular drug delivery: Studies on ciprofloxacin formulations. *Int. J. Pharm.* **2007**, *343*, 34–40. [CrossRef] [PubMed]

169. Hosny, K.M. Preparation and evaluation of thermosensitive liposomal hydrogel for enhanced transcorneal permeation of ofloxacin. *AAPS PharmSciTech* **2009**, *10*, 1336–1342. [CrossRef] [PubMed]

170. Hosny, K.M. Ciprofloxacin as ocular liposomal hydrogel. *AAPS Pharm. Sci. Tech.* **2010**, *11*, 241–246. [CrossRef] [PubMed]

171. Hosny, K.M. Optimization of gatifloxacin liposomal hydrogel for enhanced transcorneal permeation. *J. Liposome Res.* **2010**, *20*, 31–37. [CrossRef] [PubMed]

172. Zeng, S.; Hu, C.; Wei, H.; Lu, Y.; Zhang, Y.; Yang, J.; Yun, G.; Zou, W.; Song, B. Intravitreal pharmacokinetics of liposome-encapsulated amikacin in a rabbit model. *Ophthalmology* **1993**, *100*, 1640–1644. [CrossRef]

173. Wiechens, B.; Krausse, R.; Grammer, J.B.; Neumann, D.; Pleyer, U.; Duncker, G.I. Clearance of liposome-incorporated ciprofloxacin after intravitreal injection in rabbit eyes. *Klin. Monatsbl. Augenheilkd.* **1998**, *213*, 284–292. [CrossRef] [PubMed]

174. Kaiser, J.M.; Imai, H.; Haakenson, J.K.; Brucklacher, R.M.; Fox, T.E.; Shanmugavelandy, S.S.; Unrath, K.A.; Pedersen, M.M.; Dai, P.; Freeman, W.M.; et al. Nanoliposomal minocycline for ocular drug delivery. *Nanomedicine Nanotechnol. Biol. Med.* **2013**, *9*, 130–140. [CrossRef] [PubMed]

175. Guinedi, A.S.; Mortada, N.D.; Mansour, S.; Hathout, R.M. Preparation and evaluation of reverse-phase evaporation and multilamellar niosomes as ophthalmic carriers of acetazolamide. *Int. J. Pharm.* **2005**, *306*, 71–82. [CrossRef] [PubMed]

176. Aggarwal, D.; Pal, D.; Mitra, A.K.; Kaur, I.P. Study of the extent of ocular absorption of acetazolamide from a developed niosomal formulation, by microdialysis sampling of aqueous humor. *Int. J. Pharm.* **2007**, *338*, 21–26. [CrossRef] [PubMed]

177. Abdelbary, G.; El-Gendy, N. Niosome-encapsulated gentamicin for ophthalmic controlled delivery. *AAPS PharmSciTech* **2008**, *9*, 740–747. [CrossRef] [PubMed]

178. Akbari, V.; Abedi, D.; Pardakhty, A.; Sadeghi-Aliabadi, H. Release studies on ciprofloxacin loaded non-ionic surfactant vesicles. *Avicenna J. Med. Biotechnol.* **2015**, *7*, 69–75. [PubMed]

12

Hydrogels for Atopic Dermatitis and Wound Management: A Superior Drug Delivery Vehicle

Ian P. Harrison and Fabrizio Spada * (iD)

Department of Research and Development, Ego Pharmaceuticals Pty Ltd., 21-31 Malcolm Road, Braeside, VIC 3195, Australia; ian.harrison@egopharm.com
* Correspondence: fabrizio.spada@egopharm.com

Abstract: Wound management, in addition to presenting a significant burden to patients and their families, also contributes significantly to a country's healthcare costs. Treatment strategies are numerous, but in most cases not ideal. Hydrogels, three-dimensional polymeric materials that can withstand a great degree of swelling without losing structural integrity, are drawing great attention for their use as topical wound management solutions in the form of films and as vehicles for drug delivery, due to their unique properties of high water content, biocompatibility, and flexibility. Hydrogels, both naturally and synthetically derived, can be tuned to respond to specific stimuli such as pH, temperature and light and they are ideally suited as drug delivery vehicles. Here we provide a brief overview of the history and characteristics of hydrogels, assess their uses in wound management and drug delivery, and compare them with other types of common drug delivery vehicle.

Keywords: hydrogels; skin; wound healing; drug delivery

1. Introduction

The intricate structure of the human skin both repels environmental insults to the barrier and protects the body's internal organs, two mechanisms crucial to survival. The skin is subjected to an almost constant barrage of potential injuries, from environmental injury due to exposure to the likes of UV radiation, to physical wounds where one or more layers of the skin are cut, broken, or otherwise damaged. Wounds to the skin, if not properly treated, can become infected, further increasing local tissue damage and potentially leading to systemic inflammation and life-threatening immunological responses, such as sepsis in the worst cases [1]. As a result, the process of wound healing is a crucial component of ensuring the host's continuing health [2].

Wound healing is a rapid, dynamic, and complex process, encompassing multiple, distinct, and overlapping processes, including haemostasis, inflammation, cellular proliferation, and granulation tissue formation and maturation [3]. While members of other species such as fish [3] and amphibians [4] have demonstrated the ability to perfectly regenerate skin, mammals, including humans, experience great difficulty in completely regenerating damaged tissue, especially if the damage is significant. Human wound repair leads to scarring and the loss of skin appendages, such as hair follicles that contribute to normal skin functions (e.g., sensation) [5]. While most cases of wound healing are successful in a basic sense, in that the process completes and the dermal layers are repaired (thus restoring the skins fundamental role of keeping pathogens out and moisture in), some instances of wound healing may become disrupted, leading to chronic wounds, such as pressure ulcers [6], diabetic leg and foot ulcers, and infected wounds [7]. Chronic wounds, or wounds that have not progressed through the ordered healing process [8], exist in a self-perpetuating inflammatory stage [9], prolonging the burden on the patient and their families and on society as a whole, with an estimated AUD$2.85 billion spent annually on chromic wound management in Australia [10].

Numerous regimens are employed for treating wounds, from dressings, bandages, and surgery to targeted drug delivery via optimized vehicles (for a recent review on methods employed for the treatment of wounds, see [11]). Of these optimized vehicles, hydrogels in particular are garnering a lot of interest from the medical and pharmaceutical wound care market, because of their unique characteristics of biocompatibility, high water content, and flexibility. This review aims to provide a brief overview of hydrogels, their applications in drug delivery and wound management, and their benefits over other commonly-used drug delivery vehicles.

2. A Brief Research History of Hydrogels

Hydrogels are hydrophilic, three-dimensional polymeric matrices that are able to absorb and swell with water without dissolving [12,13]. Though a proto-hydrogel concept of a three-dimensional network of hydrophilic natural polymers and gums existed as early as 1894 [14], the first mention of hydrogels that defined them in terms of properties—such as biocompatibility and high water affinity—was in 1960 by Wichterle and Lim [15]. From here on, the focus on hydrogels in research steadily increased until the 1990s. Since then, there has been a near exponential growth in the number of publications on hydrogels [14,16]. This explosion in interest in hydrogels can be ascribed to their evolution over time into the highly versatile products available today. Buwalda and colleagues suggest three distinct phases of hydrogel development [17]. The first phase encompassed the basic concept of Wichterle and Lim, which aimed to develop a relatively simple material with good swelling and mechanical properties. The second stage, beginning in the 1970s, included a more complex type of hydrogel that was able to respond to specific stimuli, such as pH and temperature, and elicit specific responses to these stimuli. The third stage of hydrogel development comprises supramolecular inclusion complexes with excellent biocompatibility and versatility. For example, a complex between Polyethylene Glycol (PEG) and α-cyclodextrins can produce a supramolecular hydrogel that can be tailored to respond to numerous specific stimuli [18], from temperature and pH to electrical fields. This third stage of hydrogel development gave rise to the development of so-called "smart hydrogels": these are hydrogels with a vast array of tunable properties and possible applications [16], such as drug delivery (Figure 1).

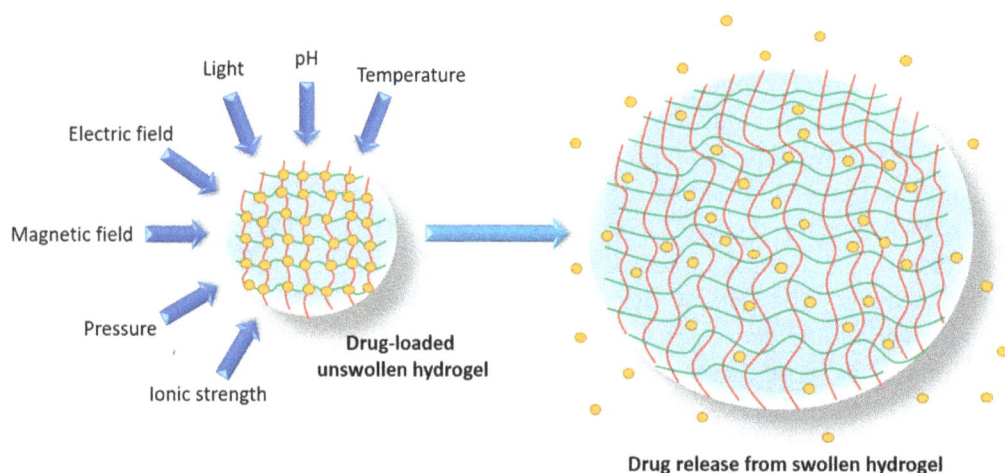

Figure 1. Swelling of a drug delivery hydrogel in response to various chemical and physical stimuli. Red and yellow lines indicate the interwoven matrix structure of a hydrogel, with the yellow dots representing drug molecules.

3. Hydrogel Classification

Hydrogels can be classified according to various characteristics: their origin (natural, synthetic, or a combination of both), their properties (mechanical or physical), the nature of their polymer side groups (ionic or non-ionic), the type of cross-link (chemical or physical), and their response to various chemical and physical stimuli, to name a few [19] (Figure 2). In the following two sections, we will focus briefly on the categories of hydrogels and their physical and mechanical properties.

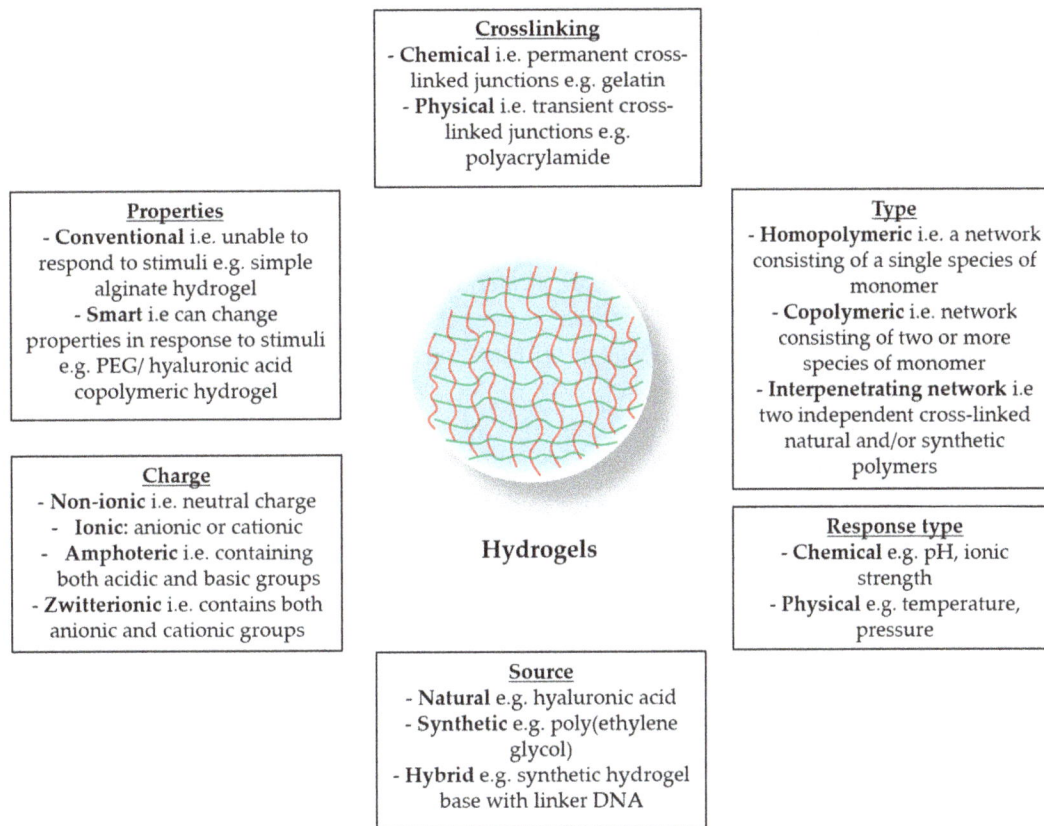

Crosslinking
- **Chemical** i.e. permanent cross-linked junctions e.g. gelatin
- **Physical** i.e. transient cross-linked junctions e.g. polyacrylamide

Properties
- **Conventional** i.e. unable to respond to stimuli e.g. simple alginate hydrogel
- **Smart** i.e can change properties in response to stimuli e.g. PEG/ hyaluronic acid copolymeric hydrogel

Type
- **Homopolymeric** i.e. a network consisting of a single species of monomer
- **Copolymeric** i.e. network consisting of two or more species of monomer
- **Interpenetrating network** i.e two independent cross-linked natural and/or synthetic polymers

Charge
- **Non-ionic** i.e. neutral charge
- **Ionic**: anionic or cationic
- **Amphoteric** i.e. containing both acidic and basic groups
- **Zwitterionic** i.e. contains both anionic and cationic groups

Hydrogels

Response type
- **Chemical** e.g. pH, ionic strength
- **Physical** e.g. temperature, pressure

Source
- **Natural** e.g. hyaluronic acid
- **Synthetic** e.g. poly(ethylene glycol)
- **Hybrid** e.g. synthetic hydrogel base with linker DNA

Figure 2. The various parameters by which hydrogels are classified.

Three distinct categories of hydrogels exist: the natural hydrogels that are often composed of polysaccharide chains, such as chitosan [20], cellulose [21] and hyaluronic acid [22], or protein chains such as collagen [23]; the synthetic hydrogels that consist of polymers, such as poly (ethylene glycol) [24] and poly (acrylamide) [25]; and a third group, the hybrid hydrogels, which are composed of a combination of natural and synthetic polymers. Natural and synthetic hydrogels both have their advantages and disadvantages.

3.1. Natural Hydrogels

Natural hydrogels offer the greatest biocompatibility, as they are natural components of the Extracellular Matrix (ECM) [16]. Examples include Matrigel™, a basement-membrane extract from Engelbrecht–Holm–Swarm (EHS) mouse sarcoma cells, and gels made from fibrin and hyaluronic acid. Matrigel™ is an oft-used natural hydrogel matrix, and its composition of type IV collagen, laminin, and nidogen make it a very close fit to the in vivo basement membrane [26]. Fibrin gels, made from fibrinogen and thrombin (the key proteins in blood clotting), are well-characterised hydrogels used in the promotion of wound healing [27]. Hydrogels made from hyaluronic acid have numerous applications in the fields of tissue engineering and regenerative medicine through their ability to be tuned by various chemical, mechanical, and spatial cues [22]. Despite the biocompatibility of natural hydrogels, they are limited by the fact that their natural origin means that there will be inherent variability between batches, variables difficult to control between experiments.

Additionally, the translational potential of natural hydrogels is limited by the source of the hydrogel to begin with [16,25].

3.2. Synthetic Hydrogels

An alternative to natural hydrogels are the synthetic hydrogels, engineered matrices that, by being synthetic, are not susceptible to the limits imposed on natural hydrogels. Examples include Poly (Ethylene Glycol), or PEG, one of the most widely-used synthetic hydrogel materials, owing to its bio-inertness and its effectiveness in suppressing bacterial adhesion, protein adsorption, and cell adhesion [28,29]. Synthetic hydrogels are more reproducible, tend to provide more flexibility for tuning their chemical or mechanical properties [16], and have structures that can be more tightly controlled. The mechanical structure of synthetic hydrogels also tends to be more robust; a hydrogel containing slide-ring polymers for example can stretch to more than ten times its initial length [30]. Given their non-natural origin however, synthetic hydrogels cannot offer the same biocompatibility as that of a natural hydrogel: they will often lack the self-healing abilities of biological tissues, even though they are engineered to mimic them.

3.3. Hybrid Hydrogels

The third category of hydrogels, the hybrid hydrogels, use both natural and synthetic polymers to harness the potential of both types [31]. This synergy between the two types of hydrogels can provide the mechanical strength of a synthetic non-natural hydrogel with the biocompatibility and recoverability of natural hydrogels [32]. For example, natural collagen or extracellular matrix-based hydrogels can be strengthened by cross-linking with multi-armed PEG stars containing esters on the termini that react with amine residues on the protein, creating a hybrid hydrogel with a robust synthetic backbone but the same biochemical cues as the natural hydrogel, due to the inertness of PEG [33,34].

4. The Properties of Hydrogels

4.1. Physical Properties

Given the fact that hydrogels are polymeric matrices swollen with water, the characteristics of the water within a hydrogel will naturally be an important determinant of how a hydrogel functions. When water is first taken in by a dry hydrogel, it is the most polar hydrophilic groups that will interact first with the water molecules and become hydrated, leading to what is termed 'primary bound water' [16]. Once these groups are hydrated, the hydrophobic groups are in turn exposed and interact with water molecules, leading to 'secondary bound water' [16]. The combination of primary and secondary bound water is known as 'total bound water'. Osmotic forces will take in additional water, but any additional swelling in the structure will be opposed by the covalent or physical crosslinks so that the swelling level of the hydrogel reaches equilibrium [16]. This excess, or 'free', water is assumed to fill the center of larger pores or the space between network chains [16].

4.2. Mechanical Properties

The appeal of hydrogels in numerous and varied applications is in large part due to the fact that their mechanical properties can vary considerably depending on requirements. For instance, the rigidity of the structure can be lessened by heating it, while it can be made more rigid by increasing the degree of crosslink within its structure. The pores within a hydrogel structure that are thought to absorb free water when the structure reaches swelling equilibrium can also increase or decrease in size by varying the degree of crosslink within the hydrogel matrix. The structure of conventional hydrogels tends to be more fragile when swollen, but recent studies show that the ability of hydrogels to swell with great amounts of water need not be at the expense of durability [35,36]. It is due to this considerable flexibility in mechanical properties that hydrogels have become a subject of great interest in the fields of wound healing and drug delivery.

5. Hydrogels and Wound Healing

As stated previously, wounds, and especially chronic wounds, present a significant burden to the sufferer, their families and the economy. Numerous wound treatment interventions exist in the form of topical pharmacological formulations and wound dressings. The characteristics of the ideal dressing as outlined by Jones and colleagues [37] include the maintenance of high humidity at the wound site, the removal of excess exudate, freedom from particles and toxic contaminants, the ability to be removed without causing further trauma, impermeability to bacteria, comfortability, the allowance of gaseous exchange, and infrequent changes. Though many wound treatment strategies exist, they all invariably lack one or more properties that prevent them from being the optimal strategy. Bandages and dressings, for example, can protect a wound from bacteria, but they need frequent changing and cannot remove excess exudate, maintain a moist environment, nor be removed without causing at least some trauma to the wound.

Hydrogel-based products, on the other hand, present a more attractive wound management solution. The hydrophilic nature of hydrogels ensures that they are able to retain large amounts of water at the wound site, while their mechanical structure prevents the dissolution of the polymer. The closely woven nature of the hydrogel matrix allows the passage of bioactive molecules, such as antimicrobials and pharmaceutical agents to the wound while preventing bacteria from getting in [38,39]. Additionally, hydrogels do not readily bind to highly hydrophilic surfaces like wounds, so the potential for harm caused by dressing changes is drastically reduced when compared to bandages, gauze, or non-hydrogel films, all of which are either at least low-adherent or not amenable to a constantly moist environment, causing the covering to stick to the wound. Finally, in what is perhaps their most remarkable property, hydrogels can reversibly absorb and release water in response to changes in environmental stimuli such as temperature and light [40].

In a mouse model of diabetic ulcers, Chen et al. found that a biocompatible, multifunctional crosslinker-based temperature-sensitive hydrogel with Bone Marrow-derived Mesenchymal stem Cells (BSMC) inhibited pro-inflammatory M1 macrophage expression at the site and significantly improved wound contraction and healing, compared with control [41]. Histology and immunohistochemistry confirmed that this was due to the BSMC-laden hydrogel, promoting granulation tissue formation, angiogenesis, re-epithelialization, extracellular matrix secretion, and wound contraction. Similarly, Xiao et al. demonstrated that a chitosan-collagen hydrogel with an angiopoietin-1-derived integrin-binding prosurvival peptide significantly accelerated and enhanced wound healing, compared with a clinically-approved collagen wound dressing control in a mouse model of diabetic ulcers [42]. A poly (vinyl alcohol)/chitosan hydrogel containing bee venom has been shown to accelerate healing of diabetic wounds in rats, with an anti-inflammatory effect similar to that of diclofenac gel, the standard nonsteroidal anti-inflammatory drug treatment [43]. Kanokpanont and colleagues reported that a bi-layered wound dressing consisting of a non-adhesive wax-coated silk fibroin fabric layer and a glutaraldehyde-crosslinked silk fibroin/gelatin bioactive layer increased epithelialization and collagen formation and decreased wound size to a greater degree than a clinically-used wound dressing in a model of full-thickness wounds [44]. Seow et al. showed that a cysteine-containing ultrashort peptide hydrogel accelerated re-epithelialization of full-thickness excision wounds in mice compared with controls [45]. In a rat model of wound infection, Zhao et al. found that a thermosensitive hydrogel with a sustained curcumin-releasing profile closed wounds at a quicker rate than gauze and led to improved histological outcomes [46]. In vitro analysis indicated that the hydrogel had distinct antimicrobial, anti-oxidative, and anti-nuclear factor-κB activity. Similarly, Gong and colleagues showed that a curcumin-loaded thermosensitive hydrogel had better tissue adhesiveness than a control dressing and could release curcumin over an extended period [47]. At the wound site, the curcumin-loaded hydrogel group also exhibited greater collagen content, greater wound maturity, better granulation, a decrease in superoxide dismutase, and an increase in catalase. Henderson et al. reported that a sustained delivery of the angiogenic chemokine stromal-derived factor-1 via an alginate hydrogel vehicle significantly decreased the observed wound area on the dorsum of mice and significantly increased endothelial cell invasion into the wound bed, compared with a saline-loaded control [48]. Yasasvini et al. showed that poly (vinyl alcohol) hydrogels loaded with Simvastatin-chitosin microparticles at an optimum low dose significantly improved wound healing in Wistar rats, compared with low-dose ointment and untreated controls [49].

The versatility of hydrogels also make them ideal delivery materials for antibiotics in the treatment of infected wounds. The broad-spectrum antibiotic silver has been used for centuries in the treatment of infections, yet the high reactivity of the silver cation means that its incorporation into delivery vehicles is often quite challenging. Pinto et al. found that a silver-loaded soft agar hydrogel had good antibacterial efficacy at the wound site in a model of skin and soft tissue infections [50], while providing an easier, more stable, and acceptable material to work with. Similarly, a chloramphenicol-loaded 2,3-dialdehyde cellulose hydrogel prepared by Laçin was found to have prolonged antibacterial effects and greater fibroblast adhesion and proliferation than a cellulose control [51]. The author concludes that this hydrogel is ideally suited to wound healing, due to its biodegradability, biocompatibility, and antimicrobial effectiveness.

Hydrogels as synthetic skins in the treatment of wounds have been a subject of study for at least two decades [52]. Kao et al. was able to construct a three-dimensional dermis, using fibroblasts mixed with a biocompatible peptide hydrogel scaffold, which, when combined with keratinocytes, formed a synthetic skin with three to five keratinocyte layers. These layers were found to contain human type 1 collagen, which indicated expression of basement membrane proteins, functional expression around fibroblasts in the dermis, and keratinocyte differentiation in the epidermis [53]. Similarly, Lee et al. found that optimized hydrogel semi-interpenetrating polymer networks of PEG diacrylate and hyaluronic acid were able to support both long-term survival of encapsulated fibroblasts and cell migration [54], results that would have potential in the therapeutic transplantation of cells for wound healing.

The potential of hydrogels in wound healing is not only limited to efficacy: the cost and ease of use of hydrogels as a delivery system can help overcome the limitations of other systems. Murphy et al. found that a hyaluronic acid-based hydrogel containing solubilized amnion membrane not only accelerated wound closure, it also provided an easy-to-use delivery system that overcame the significant cost and handling limitations presented by the placing of thin sheets of living cellularized tissue that had been the preferred treatment strategy [55].

6. Hydrogels in Drug Delivery

Hydrogels have become increasingly attractive as vehicles for drug delivery, due to their unique properties. Their highly porous nature allows the loading and releasing of drugs, a property that can be easily tuned by altering the density of cross-links in their matrix structure. Sustained delivery of a drug is a particular advantage offered by hydrogels through the tuning of mechanisms such as diffusion and swelling and by programming responses to environmental stimuli, such as pH or temperature. The versatility of hydrogels also makes them ideal vehicles for proteins and peptides that normally have very short duration of action; conjugation of a drug to PEG for instance can retard kidney filtration and as a result increase plasma half-life of the drug considerably [56]. Previously, hydrogels had been limited to carrying only hydrophilic drugs, due to the limited homogeneity of hydrophobic drugs loaded in hydrogel matrices [57], but recent studies have utilized hydrogels composed of networks of small micelles (around 200 nm) [58] that have a hydrophobic core and hydrophilic shell, allowing the delivery of both hydrophobic and hydrophilic compounds [57,59]. Polo Fonseca and colleagues found in an oral administration simulation that a polyurethane hydrogel was able to deliver the hydrophobic acidic NSAID sodium diclofenac in a sustained fashion for up to 40 h in a neutral solution and to achieve 80% of cumulative release [60]. Pillai et al. developed a folic acid-conjugated cross-linked pH sensitive hydrogel for site-specific delivery of the hydrophobic compound curcumin [61]. This cross-linked conjugated hydrogel showed higher cellular uptake of curcumin than a non-conjugated form. Similarly,

Deepa et al. showed in an in vitro study pH-sensitive sustained release of curcumin from a cross-linked hydrogel prepared via inverse emulsion polymerization [62].

A number of studies have examined hydrogel-based products for the transdermal delivery of drugs, a route of administration of obvious importance in the field of wound healing. Carafa et al. found in an in vitro study that a hydrogel composed of two polysaccharides, locust bean gum and xanthan, showed a protective effect on the integrity of drug-loaded niosomes (non-ionic surfactant vesicular structures) for topical application, leading to slower sustained release of the drug-loaded niosomes from the hydrogel system [63]. Transdermal diclofenac transport over 24 h from a solid hydrogel has been shown to be greater than any other known diclofenac formulation [64], with temperature-dependent sustained release of diclofenac, made possible through the entrapment of temperature-responsive nanogels within the solid hydrogel structure. Sun et al. developed composite membranes that cast a linear poly (2-Hydroxyethyl Methacrylate) (pHEMA) solution onto polyester non-woven supports that, depending on the preparation conditions, could be tailored to provide a permeation flux in the range of 4 to 68 $\mu g/cm^2$ per hour of nitroglycerin [65]. Gayet et al. found that high water content (>96%) hydrogels created from a copolymerization of Bovine Serum Albumin (BSA) and PEG allowed the release of soluble and hydrophobic substances from a 2.4 mm-thick hydrogel disk [66]. The authors also showed that the greater the molecular weight of PEG, the more porous the hydrogel. Gabriel et al. showed that a methoxy PEG hexyl substituted poly (lactic acid) composite hydrogel delivered the poorly-solubilised psoriasis drug tacrolimus to the skin of mice with imiquimod-induced psoriasis at a rate twice that of the Protopic™ control, a commercially-available tacrolimus ointment [67]. A hydrogel-thickened microemulsion system for the delivery of the corticosteroid betamethasone diproprionate, which normally has poor permeability through the skin, was found to inhibit inflammation by 72.11% compared with a 43.96% inhibition by a marketed gel in a psoriasis model of rat hind paw edema [68]. Hydrogels as delivery vehicles have also been shown to help improve cosmetic considerations of the skin. Kwankaew et al. reported that a chitosan hydrogel patch incorporating the poorly-solubilized *Artocarpus altilis* heartwood extract (that contains the melanogenesis inhibitor artocarpin) significantly improved hyperpigmentation of the skin via both rapid and slow release of the extract [69].

7. Comparing Hydrogels with Other Drug-Delivery Vehicles

The properties of the vehicle used for topical medications can have a significant influence on parameters such as drug delivery, tolerance, and efficacy. In addition, the aesthetic acceptability of these vehicles plays a major role in patient compliance; a vehicle preparation that is difficult to apply or uncomfortable once applied is understandably unappealing to most. Creams and lotions are less greasy than occlusive vehicles and therefore tend to be more appealing to patients, leading to better compliance. They are also easily removed from the skin and allow surface evaporation, which can provide a cooling effect. However, they can cause the formation of mucilaginous slime on the wound surface and require chemical preservatives that may impede wound repair. Surface evaporation also means that they tend to provide less epidermal hydration than occlusive vehicles. Ointments tend to be paraffin-based and form an occlusive barrier over the wound, which can increase both skin hydration and percutaneous drug absorption. Their occlusive, water-free nature protects the skin from aqueous irritants, reduces the risk of sensitization through the lack of preservatives, and provides a longer contact time than creams or lotions. Ointments tend to be greasy and difficult to remove however, which may impact patient compliance, and they lack the ability to provide a cooling effect through surface evaporation, potentially exacerbating discomfort. They also prevent excessive exudate from escaping from a wound, which may cause maceration of healthy skin [70].

Hydrogels on the other hand can offer the advantages of creams, lotions and ointments while accounting for their shortcomings (Table 1). In a small split-body, double-blind randomized assessment of the effects of a cream vehicle versus a hydrogel vehicle in 80 men, women, and children with contact dermatitis [71], Draelos found that both investigators and subjects reported that the hydrogel product resulted in a significant improvement in the symptoms of contact dermatitis, compared with the cream-based product. Sabale et al. concluded that a microemulsion-based hydrogel improved the solubility and skin permeability of the broad spectrum antifungal bifonazole, with comparable skin irritancy and antifungal activity to a marketed bifonazole cream [72]. A participant preference study by Trookman et al. reported that the use of a hydrogel formulation containing desonide was found by atopic dermatitis sufferers to be easy to use, comfortable and soothing, disappeared quickly, and was not drying, greasy, or shiny on the skin [73]. The same author reported more recently that desonide hydrogel 0.05% is as effective at reducing the symptoms of mild-to-moderate eczema as a desonide ointment 0.05% preparation, but was rated by patients as significantly better than the ointment for absorbability and lack of greasiness [74]. Similarly, Yentzer et al. found that a hydrogel preparation was consistently rated higher than other vehicles in all categories in a four-week study of desonide treatment for 41 subjects with mild-to-moderate atopic dermatitis [75]. They also found the hydrogel formulation to be efficacious in a shorter timeframe than other vehicles and that patients were more judicious in their adherence to the treatment regimen. The authors conclude that these results may suggest that the reliance on ointments as a first choice in the treatment of atopic dermatitis may actually be counterproductive. A small, single-center, randomized split-body exploratory study of 20 participants with mild-to-moderate atopic dermatitis reported that a hydrogel formulation significantly improved skin hydration at baseline when compared with a moisturizing lotion [76]. The hydrogel also had no significant effect on Transepidermal Water Loss (TEWL), whereas the lotion was found to actually increase TEWL.

We have previously reported that a hydrogel formulation containing 0.1% mometasone furoate is bioequivalent to a 0.1% mometasone furoate lotion, but also provides better moisturisation [77]. Application of the hydrogel resulted in a significant decrease of 43% in TEWL after 2 h, which remained significant (29%) after 24 h. Skin hydration was also significant after 24 h, at 38% above baseline. Based on the similarity of this mometasone furoate hydrogel with a desonide hydrogel, we expected there to be improved patient adherence to the hydrogel application regimen based on previous preference studies with a desonide hydrogel [73,75,78,79]. As desonide is a low-potency topical corticosteroid indicated for use in the treatment of conditions such as atopic dermatitis, it stands to reason that these studies showing patient preference for hydrogels would also apply for similar low-potency topical corticosteroid hydrogel formulations. Recently, we have developed a 1% hydrocortisone hydrogel based on the well-established DermAid™ range. According to the Australian Regulatory Guide for Over-the-Counter Medicines, hydrocortisone is formulation-independent in terms of efficacy and safety, so long as the level of the active ingredient is the same. Comparative diffusion testing using Franz Cell methodology showed that DermAid™ 1% Hydrogel is comparable with other 1% hydrocortisone formulations. As to be expected with different formulations, the results of this Franz Cell testing showed substantial differences in the permeation of hydrocortisone through synthetic membranes of currently registered 1% hydrocortisone products. However, the physiochemical properties that vary the release rates of different hydrocortisone formulations do not necessarily affect bioequivalence or therapeutic equivalence. The stratum corneum has been shown to act as a reservoir and retain topically-applied hydrocortisone [80], and the rate-controlling step is generally the diffusion of the drug from this reservoir, which is relatively slow, rather than the comparatively fast release of the drug from the dosage form. Based on these results, the plethora of efficacy data available on hydrocortisone and the bioequivalence of DermAid™ 1% Hydrogel with other 1% hydrocortisone formulations, DermAid™ 1% Hydrogel offers a more versatile, patient-friendly option for the treatment of mild atopic dermatitis and associated conditions.

Table 1. Advantages and disadvantages of hydrogels compared with the most common drug-delivery vehicles.

Vehicle	Advantages	Disadvantages
Creams and lotions	• Not as greasy as occlusive agents, therefore they may have better skin feel and improved patient compliance • Water base allows evaporation from the surface of the skin, leading to a cooling effect • Easily washed from the skin and clothes	• Non-occlusive nature usually leads to less epidermal hydration • Non-occlusive nature also means decreased percutaneous drug absorption • Water base necessitates the use of preservatives, which may lead to sensitization • May cause the formation of mucilaginous slime on the surface of wounds
Ointments	• Occlusive base leads to better retention of moisture in the epidermis • Water-proof, and thus has a long contact time with the skin • Long contact time ensures better percutaneous drug absorption than creams • Can protect the skin from aqueous irritants • Usually a preservative-free system, thereby reducing the risk of sensitisation	• Tend to be very greasy and may have a comparably poor skin feel, which may reduce patient compliance • Occlusive nature prevents any cooling effect on the skin • Can be difficult to remove from the skin or clothing • Oil base tends to prevent exudate from escaping a wound • Some oils such as lanolin may lead to sensitisation
Hydrogels	• High water content ensures that they are not greasy • Better skin feel may improve patient compliance • Surface evaporation can lead to a cooling effect on the skin • Improves skin hydration and reduces transepidermal water loss • Improved drug absorption as contact time tends to be longer than creams or lotions • Easily removed from the skin or clothing • Natural hydrogels tend to be extremely biocompatible • Synthetic hydrogels are hugely tunable, with the ability to respond to many stimuli • Tunable drug delivery capabilities mean that drugs can be delivered to the area when needed	• Conventional hydrogels tend to be fragile • Can be expensive, especially tunable smart hydrogels • Synthetic hydrogels are not as biocompatible as natural hydrogels

8. Conclusions

In this review, we provide a brief overview of hydrogels and their applications in wound management and drug delivery for atopic dermatitis. We also briefly outline the pros of hydrogel vehicles compared with the common drug delivery vehicles of creams, lotions, and ointments. Hydrogels show great potential as tools in wound management, as they overcome most of the limitations associated with more traditional forms of wound management solutions like bandages and dressings. Additionally, the biocompatibility, ease-of-use, and incredible versatility and programmability of hydrogels make them ideally suited as vehicles for drug delivery. As alternatives to other drug delivery vehicles, hydrogels have been shown to have at least bioequivalence, and in many cases are more efficacious. They are also consistently rated higher for acceptability by users and may present as the preferred drug delivery vehicle for patient compliance alone. These reasons, and the constant progress being made in hydrogel research, point to hydrogels as the first-choice platform for wound management and drug delivery.

Funding: This research received no external funding

References

1. Church, D.; Elsayed, S.; Reid, O.; Winston, B.; Lindsay, R. Burn wound infections. *Clin. Microbiol. Rev.* **2006**, *19*, 403–434. [CrossRef] [PubMed]

2. Wilkins, R.G.; Unverdorben, M. Wound cleaning and wound healing: A concise review. *Adv. Skin Wound Care* **2013**, *26*, 160–163. [CrossRef] [PubMed]

3. Richardson, R.; Slanchev, K.; Kraus, C.; Knyphausen, P.; Eming, S.; Hammerschmidt, M. Adult zebrafish as a model system for cutaneous wound-healing research. *J. Investig. Dermatol.* **2013**, *133*, 1655–1665. [CrossRef] [PubMed]

4. Seifert, A.W.; Monaghan, J.R.; Voss, S.R.; Maden, M. Skin regeneration in adult axolotls: A blueprint for scar-free healing in vertebrates. *PLoS ONE* **2012**, *7*, e32875. [CrossRef] [PubMed]

5. Li, L.; Rutlin, M.; Abraira, V.E.; Cassidy, C.; Kus, L.; Gong, S.; Jankowski, M.P.; Luo, W.; Heintz, N.; Koerber, H.R.; et al. The functional organization of cutaneous low-threshold mechanosensory neurons. *Cell* **2011**, *147*, 1615–1627. [CrossRef] [PubMed]

6. Stansby, G.; Avital, L.; Jones, K.; Marsden, G.; Guideline Development Group. Prevention and management of pressure ulcers in primary and secondary care: Summary of NICE guidance. *BMJ* **2014**, *348*, g2592. [CrossRef] [PubMed]

7. Mattera, E.; Iovene, M.R.; Rispoli, C.; Falco, G.; Rocco, N.; Accurso, A. Assessment of bacterial infection in chronic wounds in the elderly: Biopsy versus VERSAJET. *Int. J. Surg.* **2014**, *12* (Suppl. 2), S50–S55. [CrossRef] [PubMed]

8. Tricco, A.C.; Antony, J.; Vafaei, A.; Khan, P.A.; Harrington, A.; Cogo, E.; Wilson, C.; Perrier, L.; Hui, W.; Straus, S.E. Seeking effective interventions to treat complex wounds: An overview of systematic reviews. *BMC Med.* **2015**, *13*, 89. [CrossRef] [PubMed]

9. Zhao, R.; Liang, H.; Clarke, E.; Jackson, C.; Xue, M. Inflammation in Chronic Wounds. *Int. J. Mol. Sci.* **2016**, *17*, 2085. [CrossRef]

10. Graves, N.; Zheng, H. Modelling the direct health care costs of chronic wounds in Australia. *Wound Pract. Res. J. Aust. Wound Manag. Assoc.* **2014**, *22*, 20–33.

11. Han, G.; Ceilley, R. Chronic Wound Healing: A Review of Current Management and Treatments. *Adv. Ther.* **2017**, *34*, 599–610. [CrossRef] [PubMed]

12. Kopecek, J. Polymer chemistry: Swell gels. *Nature* **2002**, *417*, 388–391. [CrossRef] [PubMed]

13. Ahmed, E.M. Hydrogel: Preparation, characterization, and applications: A review. *J. Adv. Res.* **2015**, *6*, 105–121. [CrossRef] [PubMed]

14. Lee, S.C.; Kwon, I.K.; Park, K. Hydrogels for Delivery of Bioactive Agents: A Historical Perspective. *Adv. Drug Deliv. Rev.* **2013**, *65*, 17–20. [CrossRef] [PubMed]

15. Wichterle, O.; Lím, D. Hydrophilic Gels for Biological Use. *Nature* **1960**, *185*, 117–118. [CrossRef]

16. Yahia, L.; Chirani, N.; Gritsch, L.; Motta, F.L.; SoumiaChirani; Fare, S. History and Applications of Hydrogels. *J. Biomed. Sci.* **2015**, *4*, 13. [CrossRef]

17. Buwalda, S.J.; Boere, K.W.M.; Dijkstra, P.J.; Feijen, J.; Vermonden, T.; Hennink, W.E. Hydrogels in a historical perspective: From simple networks to smart materials. *J. Control. Release* **2014**, *190*, 254–273. [CrossRef] [PubMed]

18. Zhang, J.; Ma, P.X. Cyclodextrin-based supramolecular systems for drug delivery: Recent progress and future perspective. *Adv. Drug Deliv. Rev.* **2013**, *65*, 1215–1233. [CrossRef] [PubMed]

19. Sharpe, L.A.; Daily, A.M.; Horava, S.D.; Peppas, N.A. Therapeutic applications of hydrogels in oral drug delivery. *Expert Opin. Drug Deliv.* **2014**, *11*, 901–915. [CrossRef] [PubMed]

20. Lajud, S.A.; Nagda, D.A.; Qiao, P.; Tanaka, N.; Civantos, A.; Gu, R.; Cheng, Z.; Tsourkas, A.; O'Malley, B.W., Jr.; Li, D. A novel chitosan-hydrogel-based nanoparticle delivery system for local inner ear application. *Otol. Neurotol.* **2015**, *36*, 341–347. [CrossRef] [PubMed]

21. Qiu, X.; Hu, S. "Smart" Materials Based on Cellulose: A Review of the Preparations, Properties, and Applications. *Materials* **2013**, *6*, 738–781. [CrossRef] [PubMed]

22. Lam, J.; Truong, N.F.; Segura, T. Design of Cell-Matrix Interactions in Hyaluronic Acid Hydrogel Scaffolds. *Acta Biomater.* **2014**, *10*, 1571–1580. [CrossRef] [PubMed]

23. Antoine, E.E.; Vlachos, P.P.; Rylander, M.N. Review of collagen I hydrogels for bioengineered tissue microenvironments: Characterization of mechanics, structure, and transport. *Tissue Eng. Part B Rev.* **2014**, *20*, 683–696. [CrossRef] [PubMed]

24. Zhu, J. Bioactive modification of poly(ethylene glycol) hydrogels for tissue engineering. *Biomaterials* **2010**, *31*, 4639–4656. [CrossRef] [PubMed]

25. Cruz-Acuña, R.; García, A.J. Synthetic Hydrogels Mimicking Basement Membrane Matrices to Promote Cell-Matrix Interactions. *Matrix Biol.* **2017**, *57–58*, 324–333. [CrossRef] [PubMed]

26. Hughes, C.S.; Postovit, L.M.; Lajoie, G.A. Matrigel: A complex protein mixture required for optimal growth of cell culture. *Proteomics* **2010**, *10*, 1886–1890. [CrossRef] [PubMed]

27. Janmey, P.A.; Winer, J.P.; Weisel, J.W. Fibrin gels and their clinical and bioengineering applications. *J. R. Soc. Interface* **2009**, *6*, 1–10. [CrossRef] [PubMed]

28. Zhang, M.; Desai, T.; Ferrari, M. Proteins and cells on PEG immobilized silicon surfaces. *Biomaterials* **1998**, *19*, 953–960. [CrossRef]

29. Krsko, P.; Kaplan, J.B.; Libera, M. Spatially controlled bacterial adhesion using surface-patterned poly(ethylene glycol) hydrogels. *Acta Biomater.* **2009**, *5*, 589–596. [CrossRef] [PubMed]

30. Okumura, Y.; Ito, K. The Polyrotaxane Gel: A Topological Gel by Figure-of-Eight Cross-links. *Adv. Mater.* **2001**, *13*, 485–487. [CrossRef]

31. Chu, T.-W.; Feng, J.; Yang, J.; Kopeček, J. Hybrid Polymeric Hydrogels via Peptide Nucleic Acid (PNA)/DNA Complexation. *J. Control. Release* **2015**, *220*, 608–616. [CrossRef] [PubMed]

32. Haraguchi, K.; Takehisa, T. Nanocomposite Hydrogels: A Unique Organic–Inorganic Network Structure with Extraordinary Mechanical, Optical, and Swelling/De-swelling Properties. *Adv. Mater.* **2002**, *14*, 1120–1124. [CrossRef]

33. Sargeant, T.D.; Desai, A.P.; Banerjee, S.; Agawu, A.; Stopek, J.B. An in situ forming collagen-PEG hydrogel for tissue regeneration. *Acta Biomater.* **2012**, *8*, 124–132. [CrossRef] [PubMed]

34. Grover, G.N.; Rao, N.; Christman, K.L. Myocardial Matrix-Polyethylene Glycol Hybrid Hydrogels for Tissue Engineering. *Nanotechnology* **2014**, *25*, 014011. [CrossRef] [PubMed]

35. Sun, J.-Y.; Zhao, X.; Illeperuma, W.R.K.; Chaudhuri, O.; Oh, K.H.; Mooney, D.J.; Vlassak, J.J.; Suo, Z. Highly stretchable and tough hydrogels. *Nature* **2012**, *489*, 133–136. [CrossRef] [PubMed]

36. Zhang, Y.; An, D.; Pardo, Y.; Chiu, A.; Song, W.; Liu, Q.; Zhou, F.; McDonough, S.P.; Ma, M. High-water-content and resilient PEG-containing hydrogels with low fibrotic response. *Acta Biomater.* **2017**, *53*, 100–108. [CrossRef] [PubMed]

37. Jones, V.; Grey, J.E.; Harding, K.G. Wound dressings. *BMJ* **2006**, *332*, 777–780. [CrossRef] [PubMed]

38. Song, A.; Rane, A.A.; Christman, K.L. Antibacterial and Cell-adhesive Polypeptide and Poly(ethylene glycol) Hydrogel as a Potential Scaffold for Wound Healing. *Acta Biomater.* **2012**, *8*, 41–50. [CrossRef] [PubMed]

39. Roy, D.C.; Tomblyn, S.; Burmeister, D.M.; Wrice, N.L.; Becerra, S.C.; Burnett, L.R.; Saul, J.M.; Christy, R.J. Ciprofloxacin-Loaded Keratin Hydrogels Prevent Pseudomonas aeruginosa Infection and Support Healing in a Porcine Full-Thickness Excisional Wound. *Adv. Wound Care (New Rochelle)* **2015**, *4*, 457–468. [CrossRef] [PubMed]

40. Strong, L.E.; West, J.L. Hydrogel-Coated Near Infrared Absorbing Nanoshells as Light-Responsive Drug Delivery Vehicles. *ACS Biomater. Sci. Eng.* **2015**, *1*, 685–692. [CrossRef] [PubMed]

41. Chen, S.; Shi, J.; Zhang, M.; Chen, Y.; Wang, X.; Zhang, L.; Tian, Z.; Yan, Y.; Li, Q.; Zhong, W.; et al. Mesenchymal stem cell-laden anti-inflammatory hydrogel enhances diabetic wound healing. *Sci. Rep.* **2015**, *5*, 18104. [CrossRef] [PubMed]

42. Xiao, Y.; Reis, L.A.; Feric, N.; Knee, E.J.; Gu, J.; Cao, S.; Laschinger, C.; Londono, C.; Antolovich, J.; McGuigan, A.P.; et al. Diabetic wound regeneration using peptide-modified hydrogels to target re-epithelialization. *Proc. Natl. Acad. Sci. USA* **2016**, *113*, E5792–E5801. [CrossRef] [PubMed]

43. Amin, M.A.; Abdel-Raheem, I.T. Accelerated wound healing and anti-inflammatory effects of physically cross linked polyvinyl alcohol-chitosan hydrogel containing honey bee venom in diabetic rats. *Arch. Pharm. Res.* **2014**, *37*, 1016–1031. [CrossRef] [PubMed]

44. Kanokpanont, S.; Damrongsakkul, S.; Ratanavaraporn, J.; Aramwit, P. An innovative bi-layered wound dressing made of silk and gelatin for accelerated wound healing. *Int. J. Pharm.* **2012**, *436*, 141–153. [CrossRef] [PubMed]

45. Seow, W.Y.; Salgado, G.; Lane, E.B.; Hauser, C.A.E. Transparent crosslinked ultrashort peptide hydrogel dressing with high shape-fidelity accelerates healing of full-thickness excision wounds. *Sci. Rep.* **2016**, *6*, 32670. [CrossRef] [PubMed]

46. Zhao, Y.; Liu, J.-G.; Chen, W.-M.; Yu, A.-X. Efficacy of thermosensitive chitosan/β-glycerophosphate hydrogel loaded with β-cyclodextrin-curcumin for the treatment of cutaneous wound infection in rats. *Exp. Ther. Med.* **2018**, *15*, 1304–1313. [CrossRef] [PubMed]

47. Gong, C.; Wu, Q.; Wang, Y.; Zhang, D.; Luo, F.; Zhao, X.; Wei, Y.; Qian, Z. A biodegradable hydrogel system containing curcumin encapsulated in micelles for cutaneous wound healing. *Biomaterials* **2013**, *34*, 6377–6387. [CrossRef] [PubMed]

48. Henderson, P.W.; Singh, S.P.; Krijgh, D.D.; Yamamoto, M.; Rafii, D.C.; Sung, J.J.; Rafii, S.; Rabbany, S.Y.; Spector, J.A. Stromal-derived factor-1 delivered via hydrogel drug-delivery vehicle accelerates wound healing in vivo. *Wound Repair Regen.* **2011**, *19*, 420–425. [CrossRef] [PubMed]

49. Yasasvini, S.; Anusa, R.S.; VedhaHari, B.N.; Prabhu, P.C.; RamyaDevi, D. Topical hydrogel matrix loaded with Simvastatin microparticles for enhanced wound healing activity. *Mater. Sci. Eng. C Mater. Biol. Appl.* **2017**, *72*, 160–167. [CrossRef] [PubMed]

50. Pinto, M.N.; Martinez-Gonzalez, J.; Chakraborty, I.; Mascharak, P.K. Incorporation of a Theranostic "Two-Tone" Luminescent Silver Complex into Biocompatible Agar Hydrogel Composite for the Eradication of ESKAPE Pathogens in a Skin and Soft Tissue Infection Model. *Inorg. Chem.* **2018**, *57*, 6692–6701. [CrossRef] [PubMed]

51. Laçin, N.T. Development of biodegradable antibacterial cellulose-based hydrogel membranes for wound healing. *Int. J. Biol. Macromol.* **2014**, *67*, 22–27. [CrossRef] [PubMed]

52. Yannas, I.V.; Lee, E.; Orgill, D.P.; Skrabut, E.M.; Murphy, G.F. Synthesis and characterization of a model extracellular matrix that induces partial regeneration of adult mammalian skin. *Proc. Natl. Acad. Sci. USA* **1989**, *86*, 933–937. [CrossRef] [PubMed]

53. Kao, B.; Kadomatsu, K.; Hosaka, Y. Construction of synthetic dermis and skin based on a self-assembled peptide hydrogel scaffold. *Tissue Eng. Part A* **2009**, *15*, 2385–2396. [CrossRef] [PubMed]

54. Lee, H.-J.; Sen, A.; Bae, S.; Lee, J.S.; Webb, K. Poly(ethylene glycol) diacrylate/hyaluronic acid semi-interpenetrating network compositions for 3-D cell spreading and migration. *Acta Biomater.* **2015**, *14*, 43–52. [CrossRef] [PubMed]

55. Murphy, S.V.; Skardal, A.; Song, L.; Sutton, K.; Haug, R.; Mack, D.L.; Jackson, J.; Soker, S.; Atala, A. Solubilized Amnion Membrane Hyaluronic Acid Hydrogel Accelerates Full-Thickness Wound Healing. *Stem Cells Transl. Med.* **2017**, *6*, 2020–2032. [CrossRef] [PubMed]

56. Ashley, G.W.; Henise, J.; Reid, R.; Santi, D.V. Hydrogel drug delivery system with predictable and tunable drug release and degradation rates. *Proc. Natl. Acad. Sci. USA* **2013**, *110*, 2318–2323. [CrossRef] [PubMed]

57. McKenzie, M.; Betts, D.; Suh, A.; Bui, K.; Kim, L.D.; Cho, H. Hydrogel-Based Drug Delivery Systems for Poorly Water-Soluble Drugs. *Molecules* **2015**, *20*, 20397–20408. [CrossRef] [PubMed]

58. Stocke, N.A.; Arnold, S.M.; Hilt, J.Z. Responsive Hydrogel Nanoparticles for Pulmonary Delivery. *J. Drug Deliv. Sci. Technol.* **2015**, *29*, 143–151. [CrossRef] [PubMed]

59. Simões, S.; Figueiras, A.; Veiga, F. Modular Hydrogels for Drug Delivery. *J. Biomater. Nanobiotechnol.* **2012**, *3*, 185–199. [CrossRef]

60. Polo Fonseca, L.; Trinca, R.B.; Felisberti, M.I. Amphiphilic polyurethane hydrogels as smart carriers for acidic hydrophobic drugs. *Int. J. Pharm.* **2018**, *546*, 106–114. [CrossRef] [PubMed]

61. Pillai, J.J.; Thulasidasan, A.K.T.; Anto, R.J.; Chithralekha, D.N.; Narayanan, A.; Kumar, G.S.V. Folic acid conjugated cross-linked acrylic polymer (FA-CLAP) hydrogel for site specific delivery of hydrophobic drugs to cancer cells. *J. Nanobiotechnol.* **2014**, *12*, 25. [CrossRef] [PubMed]

62. Deepa, G.; Thulasidasan, A.K.T.; Anto, R.J.; Pillai, J.J.; Kumar, G.S.V. Cross-linked acrylic hydrogel for the controlled delivery of hydrophobic drugs in cancer therapy. *Int. J. Nanomed.* **2012**, *7*, 4077–4088.

63. Carafa, M.; Marianecci, C.; Di Marzio, L.; Rinaldi, F.; Meo, C.; Matricardi, P.; Alhaique, F.; Coviello, T. A new vesicle-loaded hydrogel system suitable for topical applications: Preparation and characterization. *J. Pharm. Pharm. Sci.* **2011**, *14*, 336–346. [CrossRef] [PubMed]

64. Carmona-Moran, C.A.; Zavgorodnya, O.; Penman, A.D.; Kharlampieva, E.; Bridges, S.L.; Hergenrother, R.W.; Singh, J.A.; Wick, T.M. Development of gellan gum containing formulations for transdermal drug delivery: Component evaluation and controlled drug release using temperature responsive nanogels. *Int. J. Pharm.* **2016**, *509*, 465–476. [CrossRef] [PubMed]

65. Sun, Y.M.; Huang, J.J.; Lin, F.C.; Lai, J.Y. Composite poly(2-hydroxyethyl methacrylate) membranes as rate-controlling barriers for transdermal applications. *Biomaterials* **1997**, *18*, 527–533. [CrossRef]

66. Gayet, J.C.; Fortier, G. Drug release from new bioartificial hydrogel. *Artif. Cells Blood Substit. Immobil. Biotechnol.* **1995**, *23*, 605–611. [CrossRef] [PubMed]

67. Gabriel, D.; Mugnier, T.; Courthion, H.; Kranidioti, K.; Karagianni, N.; Denis, M.C.; Lapteva, M.; Kalia, Y.; Möller, M.; Gurny, R. Improved topical delivery of tacrolimus: A novel composite hydrogel formulation for the treatment of psoriasis. *J. Control. Release* **2016**, *242*, 16–24. [CrossRef] [PubMed]

68. Baboota, S.; Alam, M.S.; Sharma, S.; Sahni, J.K.; Kumar, A.; Ali, J. Nanocarrier-based hydrogel of betamethasone dipropionate and salicylic acid for treatment of psoriasis. *Int. J. Pharm. Investig.* **2011**, *1*, 139–147. [CrossRef] [PubMed]

69. Kwankaew, J.; Phimnuan, P.; Wanauppathamkul, S.; Viyoch, J. Formulation of chitosan patch incorporating Artocarpus altilis heartwood extract for improving hyperpigmentation. *J. Cosmet. Sci.* **2017**, *68*, 257–269. [PubMed]

70. Cutting, K.F.; White, R.J. Maceration of the skin and wound bed 1: Its nature and causes. *J. Wound Care* **2002**, *11*, 275–278. [CrossRef] [PubMed]

71. Draelos, Z.D. Hydrogel barrier/repair creams and contact dermatitis. *Am. J. Contact Dermat.* **2000**, *11*, 222–225. [CrossRef] [PubMed]

72. Sabale, V.; Vora, S. Formulation and evaluation of microemulsion-based hydrogel for topical delivery. *Int. J. Pharm. Investig.* **2012**, *2*, 140–149. [CrossRef] [PubMed]

73. Trookman, N.; Rizer, R.; Ford, R.; Gotz, V. The importance of vehicle properties to atopic dermatitis patients: A preference study with a novel desonide hydrogel treatment. *J. Am. Acad. Dermatol.* **2008**, *58*, AB52. [CrossRef]

74. Trookman, N.S.; Rizer, R.L. Randomized Controlled Trial of Desonlde Hydrogel 0.05% versus Desonide Ointment 0.05% in the Treatment of Mild-to-moderate Atopic Dermatitis. *J. Clin. Aesthet. Dermatol.* **2011**, *4*, 34–38. [PubMed]

75. Yentzer, B.; Camacho, F.; Young, T.; Fountain, J.; Clark, A.; Feldman, S. Good adherence and early efficacy using desonide hydrogel for atopic dermatitis: Results from a program addressing patient compliance. *J. Drugs Dermatol.* **2010**, *9*, 324–329. [PubMed]

76. Kircik, L. Transepidermal Water Loss (TEWL) and Corneometry with Hydrogel Vehicle in the Treatment of Atopic Dermatitis: A Randomized, Investigator-Blind Pilot Study. *J. Drugs Dermatol.* **2012**, *11*, 181–184.

77. Greive, K.A.; Barnes, T.M. Bioequivalence of 0.1% mometasone furoate lotion to 0.1% mometasone furoate hydrogel. *Australas. J. Dermatol.* **2016**, *57*, e39–e45. [CrossRef] [PubMed]

78. Kircik, L.; Del Rosso, J. A novel hydrogel vehicle formulated for the treatment of atopic dermatitis. *J. Drugs Dermatol.* **2007**, *6*, 718–722. [PubMed]

79. Kerney, D.L.; Ford, R.O.; Gotz, V. Self-reported participant experience with desonide hydrogel in the treatment of mild to moderate atopic dermatitis. *Cutis* **2011**, *88*, 18–24. [PubMed]

80. Turpeinen, M. Absorption of hydrocortisone from the skin reservoir in atopic dermatitis. *Br. J. Dermatol.* **1991**, *124*, 358–360. [CrossRef] [PubMed]

13

Anticancer Activity of Bacterial Proteins and Peptides

Tomasz M. Karpiński [1,*] 🆔 and Artur Adamczak [2] 🆔

[1] Department of Genetics and Pharmaceutical Microbiology, Poznań University of Medical Sciences, Święcickiego 4, 60-781 Poznań, Poland
[2] Department of Botany, Breeding and Agricultural Technology of Medicinal Plants, Institute of Natural Fibres and Medicinal Plants, Kolejowa 2, 62-064 Plewiska, Poland; artur.adamczak@iwnirz.pl
* Correspondence: tkarpin@ump.edu.pl or tkarpin@interia.pl

Abstract: Despite much progress in the diagnosis and treatment of cancer, tumour diseases constitute one of the main reasons of deaths worldwide. The side effects of chemotherapy and drug resistance of some cancer types belong to the significant current therapeutic problems. Hence, searching for new anticancer substances and medicines are very important. Among them, bacterial proteins and peptides are a promising group of bioactive compounds and potential anticancer drugs. Some of them, including anticancer antibiotics (actinomycin D, bleomycin, doxorubicin, mitomycin C) and diphtheria toxin, are already used in the cancer treatment, while other substances are in clinical trials (e.g., p28, arginine deiminase ADI) or tested in in vitro research. This review shows the current literature data regarding the anticancer activity of proteins and peptides originated from bacteria: antibiotics, bacteriocins, enzymes, nonribosomal peptides (NRPs), toxins and others such as azurin, p28, Entap and Pep27anal2. The special attention was paid to the still poorly understood active substances obtained from the marine sediment bacteria. In total, 37 chemical compounds or groups of compounds with antitumor properties have been described in the present article.

Keywords: anticancer; bacteria; proteins; anticancer antibiotics; anticancer enzymes; nonribosomal peptides; bacteriocins; bacterial toxins

1. Introduction

Cancer belongs to the main reasons of morbidity and mortality in the world. In the year 2012, approximately 14 million new cancer cases were detected [1]. In 2015, cancer was responsible for 8.8 million deaths. Lung, liver, colorectal, stomach and breast cancers were the most common causes of death [2,3]. To reduce premature mortality from cancer, the resolution: 'Cancer Prevention and Control in the Context of an Integrated Approach' (WHA70.12) was passed in 2017 by the World Health Assembly [4].

Cancerous cells are altered host cells without the natural mechanisms controlling their normal growth. Oncogenesis can be caused by environmentally induced or inherited genetic mutations. It leads to inhibition of cell reaction to the control mechanisms of normal growth and gives rise to the rapid development of cell clones producing neoplasm [5]. Treatment of cancer involves apoptosis induction and tumour-cell proliferation inhibition [6].

According to Hanahan and Weinberg [7], cancer cells exhibit six important changes in their own physiology: (1) self-sufficiency in signals of growth, (2) insensitivity to signals inhibiting growth, (3) resistance to apoptosis, (4) unlimited proliferative potential, (5) sustained angiogenesis and (6) metastasis. One of the available treatments for cancer is chemotherapy, which very often belongs to the main choice of treatment. Unfortunately, chemotherapy can lead to damage of healthy cells and tissues or development of drug resistance [8].

The most known examples of usage of bacteria and their metabolites for the cancer treatment are investigations made by William Coley [9], who utilized *Streptococcus pyogenes* and *Serratia marcescens* supernatants in the treatment of patients with unresectable tumours. This mixture, called today as 'Coley's toxins', was used in approximately 1200 patients with malignancy. Cancer regression in 52 cases, including complete cure of 30 patients, was observed. Mechanism of this reaction has now been partially recognized. Microbial infections can activate macrophages and lymphocytes and induce the cytotoxic substance production, particularly tumour necrosis factor α (TNF-α) [10]. Currently, bacterial proteins and peptides are important as antiproliferative agents. Some of these are already used in cancer treatment, others are in human clinical trials or studied in vitro. In this paper, main anticancer proteins and peptides of bacterial origin are presented. Suggested division of the described proteins and peptides is shown in Figure 1.

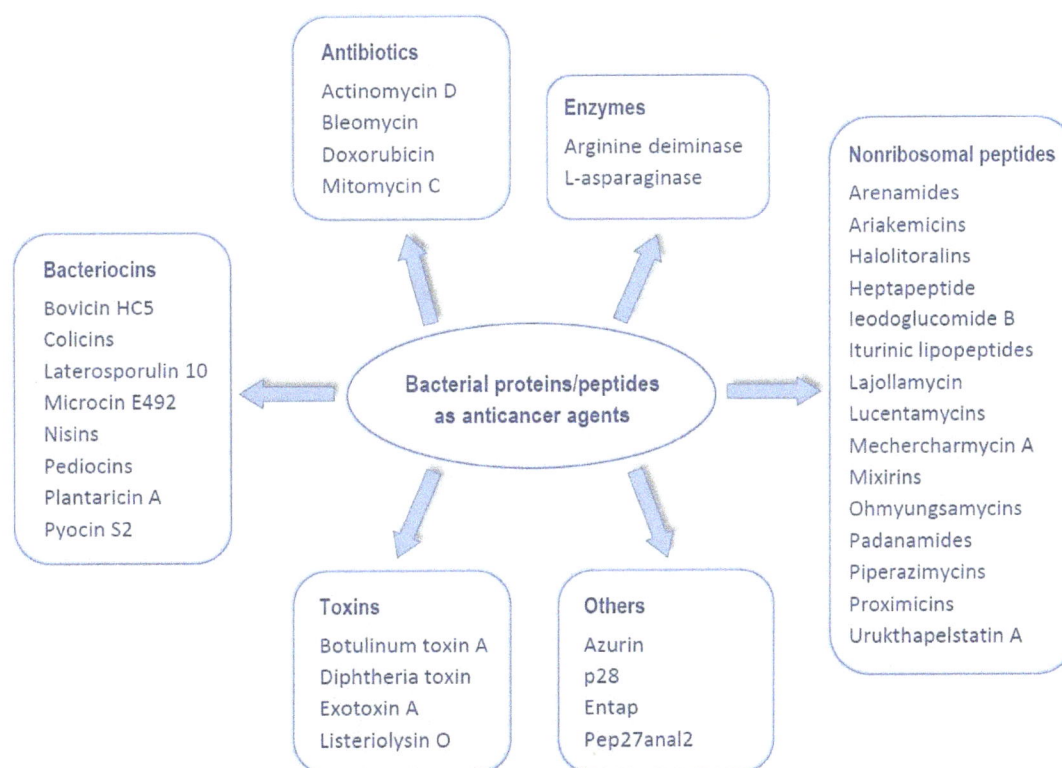

Figure 1. Division of the described anticancer proteins and peptides.

2. Antibiotics

According to *Encyclopaedia Britannica* [11], antibiotics are the chemical compounds produced mostly by the microorganisms and injurious to other organisms from this group. It has been observed that some of the antibiotics also have anticancer activity and recently they have been used mainly as antitumor drugs. The origin and biological target of four antibiotics already utilized in medicine as chemotherapeutic drugs are presented in Table 1 and their chemical structures in Figure 2.

Table 1. The origin and biological activity of anticancer antibiotics.

No.	Protein/Peptide	Source	Biological Target: Human Cancer Cells	IC_{50}	References
1	Actinomycin D	*Actinomyces antibioticus*	Wilms cancer, Ewing sarcoma, neuroblastomas, trophoblastic tumours	from 0.4 nM to 0.42 µM	[12–15]
2	Bleomycin	*Streptomyces verticillus*	head and neck squamous cell carcinomas, Hodgkin's disease, non-Hodgkin's lymphoma, testicular carcinomas, ovarian cancer, malignant pleural effusion	from 25.2 nM to 2.93 mM	[12,16–19]
3	Doxorubicin	*Streptomyces peucetius* var. *caesius*	acute lymphoblastic leukaemia, acute myeloblastic leukaemia, Wilms' tumour, neuroblastoma, soft tissue and bone sarcomas, breast carcinoma, ovarian carcinoma, transitional cell bladder carcinoma, thyroid carcinoma, gastric carcinoma, Hodgkin's disease, malignant lymphoma, bronchogenic carcinoma, oral squamous carcinoma	from 548.2 nM to 44.7 µM	[12,20–23]
4	Mitomycin C	*Streptomyces caespitosus*	cancers of the head and neck, lungs, breast, cervix, bladder, colorectal and anal carcinomas, hepatic cell carcinoma, melanoma, stomach and pancreatic carcinomas	from 9.48 nM to 249 µM	[12,24–26]

IC_{50}—half maximal inhibitory concentration.

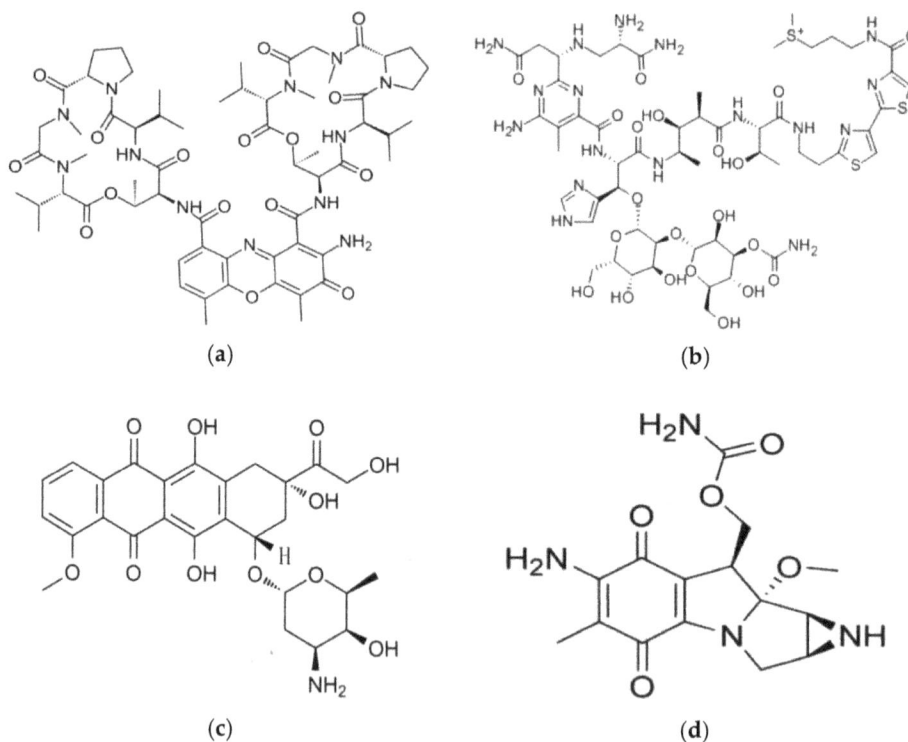

Figure 2. Chemical structures of anticancer antibiotics: (**a**) Actinomycin D; (**b**) Bleomycin A2; (**c**) Doxorubicin; (**d**) Mitomycin C.

2.1. Actinomycin D

Actinomycin D (dactinomycin) is a well-known antibiotic produced by *Actinomyces antibioticus* that exhibits antibacterial and antitumor activity. This drug has a chemical formula of $C_{62}H_{86}N_{12}O_{16}$ and a molecular weight of 1.26 kDa [15]. Actinomycin D has several mechanisms of its cytotoxic and antitumor action: intercalation to DNA and the stabilization of cleavable complexes of topoisomerases I and II with DNA, photodynamic activity and free radical formation [27]. Presented drug blocks both

DNA and RNA expression and as a consequence protein synthesis. Therefore, it induces cellular p53-independent apoptosis [28]. Actinomycin D is effective in the treatment of Wilms cancer, Ewing sarcoma, neuroblastomas and trophoblastic tumours, primarily in children. It is also used as a tool in the study of many cellular processes, such as the biosynthesis of cell macromolecules, RNA transport or viral replication [15,29]. Following drugs containing actinomycin D: Actinomycin D, Cosmegen and Lyovac are available, among others, on the market [30].

2.2. Bleomycin

Bleomycin (BLM) is a mixture of glycopeptide antibiotics with cytotoxic properties, obtained from *Streptomyces verticillus*. Bleomycin A2 has a chemical formula of $C_{55}H_{84}N_{17}O_{21}S_3$ and a molecular mass of 1.42 kDa, while in the case of bleomycin B2 it is $C_{55}H_{84}N_{20}O_{21}S_2$ and 1.43 kDa [31]. Bleomycin induces oxygen- and metal ion-dependent cleaving of DNA. BLM binds DNA and Fe(II) and hydroxyl radicals are released under the influence of molecular oxygen, causing as a consequence DNA damage and Fe(II) oxidation. BLM is used in the treatment of head and neck squamous cell carcinomas, Hodgkin's disease, non-Hodgkin's lymphoma, testicular carcinomas, ovarian cancer and malignant pleural effusion [16,17]. Drugs containing bleomycin: Bleomycin USP and Blenoxane are available [32,33].

2.3. Doxorubicin

Doxorubicin (DOX) is an anthracycline antibiotic with antitumor activity, originally isolated from *Streptomyces peucetius* var. *caesius*. It is an amphiphilic molecule containing two parts: water-insoluble aglycone (adriamycinone: $C_{21}H_{18}O_9$) and water-soluble, amino-sugar functional group (daunosamine: $C_6H_{13}NO_3$) [20]. DOX acts on the nucleic acids of dividing cells by two main mechanisms: (i) intercalation between the base pairs of the DNA strands and inhibition of the synthesis of DNA and RNA in rapidly growing cells by blocking the replication and transcription processes [34]; and (ii) generation of iron-mediated free radicals, causing oxidative damage to cellular membranes, proteins and DNA [35]. DOX belongs to the most commonly used drugs in chemotherapy. Nowadays, this substance is recommended by the Food and Drug Administration (FDA) in the case of acute lymphoblastic leukaemia, acute myeloblastic leukaemia, Wilms' tumour, neuroblastoma, soft tissue and bone sarcomas, breast carcinoma, ovarian carcinoma, transitional cell bladder carcinoma, thyroid carcinoma, gastric carcinoma, Hodgkin's disease, malignant lymphoma and bronchogenic carcinoma in which the small-cell histologic type is the most responsive compared with other cell types [23]. Preet et al. [36] demonstrated that combining doxorubicin with nisin may improve the treatment efficiency of the skin cancers. Adriblastine PFS, Caelyx, Doxorubicin medac, Doxorubicin-Ebewe, Doxorubicinum Accord and Myocet belong to the drugs containing doxorubicin [37].

2.4. Mitomycin C

Mitomycin C was isolated from a strain of actinomyces, *Streptomyces caespitosus*. Its molecular formula is $C_{15}H_{18}N_4O_5$ and a molecular weight of 334 Da [24]. This antitumor agent inhibits DNA synthesis by binding to DNA on the path of alkylation, which results in crosslinking of strands of double helical DNA [38]. Mitomycin C is utilized in the treatment of cancers of the head and neck, lungs, breast, cervix, bladder, colorectal and anal, hepatic cell carcinoma and melanoma in addition to the stomach and pancreatic cancer [25]. Among others, Mitomycin Accord and Mitomycin C Kyowa are available on the market [39].

3. Bacteriocins

Bacteriocins constitute a heterogeneous group of ribosomally synthesized bacterial peptides or proteins with antimicrobial properties [40]. Some of them also show anticancer activity [41–43]. There are four classes of bacteriocins secreted by Gram-positive bacteria. Group I includes antibiotics or thermostable peptides with a molecular mass below 10 kDa. They come under posttranslational modification and comprise unusual amino acids, including lanthionine (Lan), methyllanthionine (MeLan), dehydroalanine (Dha), dehydrobutyrine (Dhb) and D-alanine (D-Ala). Class II contains thermostable bacteriocins without lanthionine. The molecular weight of these bacteriocins is below 10 kDa. Pediocin-like bacteriocins, dipeptide bacteriocins and cyclic peptides belong to this class. In turn, group III includes thermolabile bacteriocins with a molecular mass above 10 kDa. These substances are subdivided into bacteriolysins and nonlytic proteins. Class IV consists of bacteriocins requiring the presence of lipid or carbohydrate moieties for full activity [40,44,45]. Bacteriocins isolated from Gram-negative bacteria are microcins secreted by Enterobacteriaceae with a molecular weight below 10 kDa and plasmid-encoded colicins with a molecular weight above 20 kDa [40,46]. The origin and biological activity of anticancer bacteriocins are shown in Table 2. Structure models of some anticancer bacteriocins are presented in Figure 3.

Table 2. The origin and biological activity of anticancer bacteriocins.

No.	Protein/Peptide	Source	Biological Target: Human Cancer Cell Lines	IC$_{50}$	References
1	Bovicin HC5	*Streptococcus bovis* HC5	breast adenocarcinoma (MCF-7), liver hepatocellular carcinoma (HepG2)	279.4–289.3 μM	[41,47]
2	Colicins A and E1	*Escherichia coli*	breast carcinoma (MCF7, ZR75, BT549, BT474, MDA-MB-231, SKBR3, T47D), osteosarcoma (HOS), leiomyosarcoma (SKUT-1), fibrosarcoma (HS913T)	n.d.	[41,48]
3	Laterosporulin 10	*Brevibacillus* sp. strain SKDU10	cervical cancer (HeLa), embryonic kidney cancer (HEK293T), fibrosarcoma (HT1080), lung carcinoma (H1299) breast cancer (MCF-7)	n.d.	[49]
4	Microcin E492	*Klebsiella pneumoniae* RYC492	cervical adenocarcinoma (HeLa), acute T cell leukaemia (Jurkat), Burkitt's lymphoma (Ramos), B-lymphoblastoid cells (RJ2.25)	n.d.	[50,51]
5	Nisin A	*Lactococcus lactis*	head and neck squamous cell carcinoma (UM-SCC-17B, UM-SCC-14A, HSC-3), breast adenocarcinoma (MCF-7), liver hepatocellular carcinoma (HepG2), acute T cell leukaemia (Jurkat)	105.5–225 μM	[40,47,52,53]
6	Nisin ZP	*Lactococcus lactis*	head and neck squamous cell carcinoma (UM-SCC-17B, HSC-3)	n.d.	[54]
7	Pediocin CP2	*Pediococcus acidilactici* MTCC 5101	mammary gland adenocarcinoma (MCF-7), hepatocarcinoma (Hep G2), cervical adenocarcinoma (HeLa)	n.d.	[55,56]
8	Pediocin K2a2-3	*Pediococcus acidilactici* K2a2-3	colon adenocarcinoma (HT29)	n.d.	[57]
9	Plantaricin A	*Lactobacillus plantarum* C11	T cell leukaemia (Jurkat)	n.d.	[58]
10	Pyocin S2	*Pseudomonas aeruginosa* 42A	hepatocellular carcinoma (HepG2), multiple myeloma (Im9), cervical adenocarcinoma (HeLa), embryonal ovary carcinoma (AS-II)	n.d.	[59,60]

IC$_{50}$—half maximal inhibitory concentration, n.d.—no data.

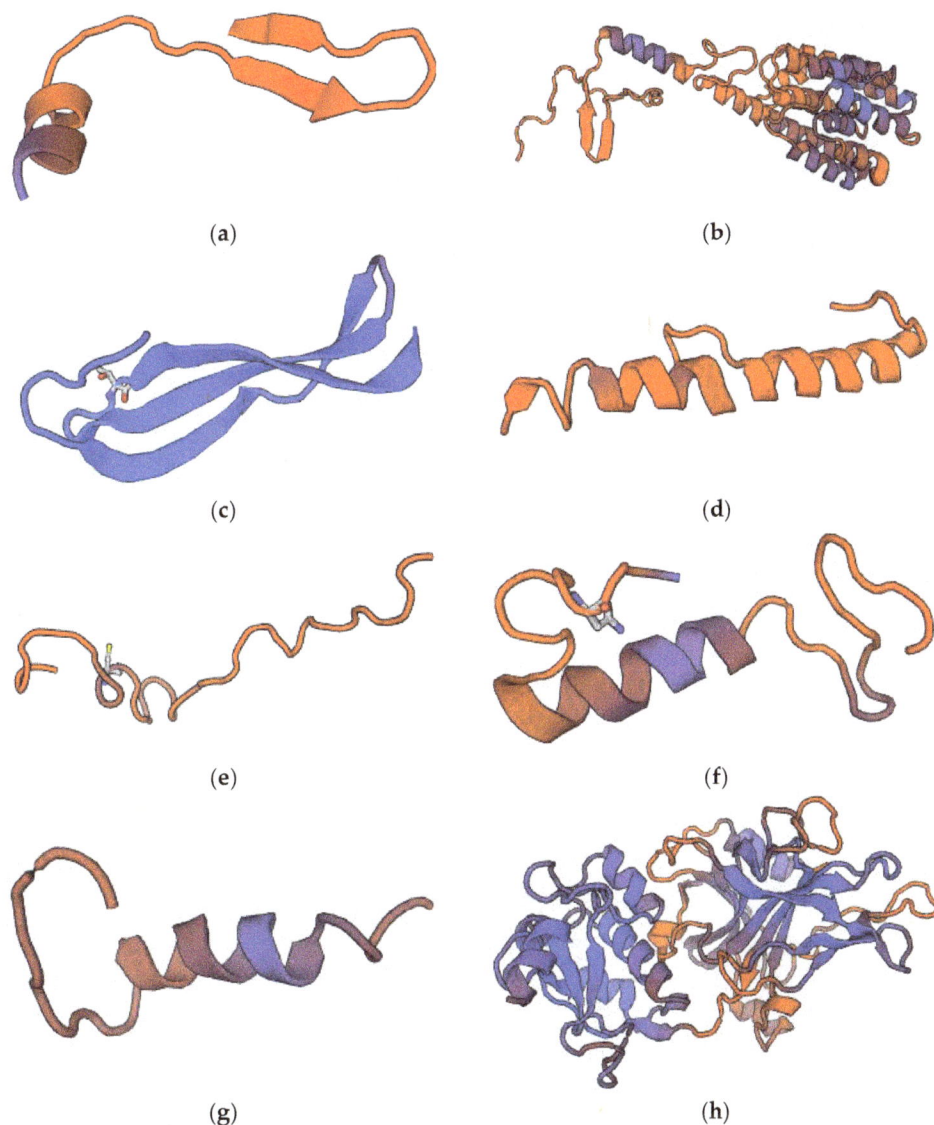

Figure 3. Structure models of anticancer bacteriocins: (**a**) Bovicin HC5; (**b**) Colicin E1; (**c**) Laterosporulin 10; (**d**) Microcin E492; (**e**) Nisin A; (**f**) Pediocin CP2; (**g**) Plantaricin A; (**h**) Pyocin S2 (orig.). Bacteriocin sequences were downloaded from BACTIBASE [61] and UNIPROT [62] and modelling server SWISS-MODEL [63,64] was used to the visualization of the bacteriocin structures.

3.1. Bovicin HC5

The lantibiotic bovicin HC5 is secreted by *Streptococcus bovis* and has a molecular mass of 2.4 kDa. This compound indicates structural and functional similarities to the nisin [41]. Paiva et al. [47] showed in vitro the bovicin HC5 cytotoxicity against human breast adenocarcinoma (MCF-7) and human liver hepatocellular carcinoma (HepG2) with a half maximal inhibitory concentration (IC_{50}) of 279.4 and 289.3 µM, respectively. At the maximum tested dose of bovicin (350 µM), the cell line viability was less than 20% [47].

3.2. Colicins

Colicins A, E1 and E3 are produced by *Escherichia coli* and have molecular sizes: more than 20, 57 and 9.8 kDa, respectively [41]. Colicins E1 and E3 exhibited cytotoxic activity against BM2 cells (chicken monoblasts transformed with the v-myb oncogene of avian myeloblastosis virus). The maximum effect was reached when the cells were exposed to colicin E1 (1.25 µg/mL) for 48 h.

Authors demonstrated that colicin E3 did not result in modifications of cell cycle. It suggests that the above-mentioned substance kills cells on the path of necrosis rather than apoptosis [65]. Chumchalova and Smarda [48] investigated four colicins (A, E1, U, E3) in terms of their inhibition activity against 11 cancer cell lines. Colicin E1 and A inhibited 10 cell lines: breast carcinoma (MCF7, ZR75, BT549, BT474, MDA-MB-231, SKBR3 and T47D), osteosarcoma (HOS), leiomyosarcoma (SKUT-1) and fibrosarcoma (HS913T). Only the colon carcinoma line (HT29) was insensitive to colicin E1. Colicin E1 showed 50% inhibition of fibrosarcoma (HS913T) and 17–40% inhibition of other cancer cell lines. Colicin A indicated from 16 to 56% inhibition of cancer cell lines and 36% inhibition of normal diploid fibroblasts with wild-type p53 (MRC5). Colicin E3 demonstrated no significant inhibition activity against tested cancer cells [48].

3.3. Laterosporulin 10

Laterosporulin 10 (LS10) is a defensin-like peptide of *Brevibacillus* sp. inhibiting microbial pathogens. The anticancer activity of this substance was investigated using normal prostate epithelium cell line (RWPE-1) and five different human cancer cell lines including cervical cancer (HeLa), embryonic kidney cancer (HEK293T), fibrosarcoma (HT1080), lung carcinoma (H1299) and breast cancer (MCF-7). Authors observed a dose-dependent cytotoxic action on all tumour cell lines with maximum activity at 10 μM and the highest activity against MCF-7 cells. Simultaneously, LS10 did not have any cytotoxic properties against normal cells up to 15 μM, whereas significant cytotoxicity was detected against cancer cells at this concentration. At lower doses, this substance caused apoptosis of cancerous cells, while at higher doses it resulted in necrotic death of them [49].

3.4. Microcin E492

Microcin E492 (M-E492) is a bacteriocin produced by *Klebsiella pneumoniae* RYC492 and it has a molecular mass of 7.9 kDa. The cytotoxicity of M-E492 was detected in the case of various malignant human cell lines, including cervical adenocarcinoma (HeLa), acute T cell leukaemia (Jurkat), B cell line originated from Burkitt's lymphoma (Ramos) and B-lymphoblastoid cell lines transformed by infection with Epstein-Barr virus (RJ2.25, a variant of the Raji B-LCL). At the same time, no effect was determined against human endothelial cells from human tonsils (AMG-3) and a monocyte-macrophage cell line (KG-1) [50]. Jurkat cell line was the most sensitive to microcin E492, with 96% viability decrease after 24 h of incubation. At a low concentration (5–10 μg/mL), M-E492 induced apoptosis of cancer cells, while at a higher concentration (20 μg/mL) it caused necrosis of them. It was reported that M-E492 leaded to the morphological and biochemical modifications during apoptosis such as: cell shrinkage, fragmentation of DNA, extracellular exposure of phosphatidylserine, caspase activation, decline of potential of mitochondrial membrane and also release of calcium ions from intracellular stores [50].

3.5. Nisins

Nisin is a 34-amino acid polycyclic antibacterial peptide of *Lactococcus lactis*. Nisin has a broad-spectrum antibacterial effect and inhibits both Gram-positive and Gram-negative bacteria. Additionally, this substance is safe for human consumption, therefore it has been approved for use as a food preservative for over 50 years. Nisin (E 234) is authorized for food preservation in the USA by FDA and in the European Union by Directive 95/2/EC [40]. Joo et al. [53] presented the anticancer activity of this substance and found that nisin A inhibits tumorigenesis of head and neck squamous cell carcinoma (HNSCC). Treatment of three different HNSCC cell lines (UM-SCC-17B, UM-SCC-14A and HSC-3) with increasing concentrations of nisin (from 5 to 80 μg/mL) induced growing level of DNA fragmentation or apoptosis after 24 h of treatment. On the other hand, primary oral keratinocytes did not show higher DNA fragmentation. Nisin has an impact on induction of apoptosis, stopping of cell cycle and reduction of HNSCC cell proliferation, in part, through cation transport regulator homolog 1 (CHAC1), a proapoptotic cation transport regulator and through a concomitant CHAC1-independent influx of extracellular calcium. Nisin also limited HNSCC tumorigenesis in a mouse model [39].

Paiva et al. [47] observed that for human cell lines of breast adenocarcinoma (MCF-7) and liver hepatocellular carcinoma (HepG2) treated with nisin, the obtained IC_{50} value was 105.46 and 112.25 μM, respectively. Also, nisin ZP significantly increased apoptosis of HNSCC cells (UM-SCC-17B and HSC-3). Nisin ZP was suggested by authors for the treatment of HNSCC, through the promotion of apoptosis of HNSCC cells and suppression of their proliferation as well as inhibition of angiogenesis, orasphere formation and tumorigenesis in vivo [54].

3.6. Pediocins

Pediocins belong to the class IIa of bacteriocins. Pediocin CP2 is produced by *Pediococcus acidilactici* MTCC 5101 and it is built from 44 amino acids [55]. Kumar et al. [56] studied cytotoxic effect of native pediocin and recombinant rec-pediocin on several cancerous cell lines. A mouse spleen lymphoblast cell line (Sp2/O-Ag14) exhibited the highest sensitivity to rec-pediocin CP2, while cell lines of mammary gland adenocarcinoma (MCF-7), hepatocarcinoma (HepG2) and cervical adenocarcinoma (HeLa) were sensitive at different degree to the action of native and rec-pediocin. After 48 h of rec-pediocin treatment, epithelial tissue models had only a low level of viability. Total cell viability of Sp2/O-Ag14 decreased to 0% due to acute toxicity of 25 μg/mL of rec-pediocin, whereas cell lines with native pediocin retained 26.7% viability. The viability of cell lines treated with 25 μg/mL of rec-pediocin and native pediocin CP2 was 2.1 and 10.7% for MCF-7 as well as 5.5 and 1.2% for HepG2 cells, respectively. HeLa cells showed lower sensitivity towards rec-pediocin with comparing to other tumour cell lines [56]. In studies of undialyzed (1600 AU/mL) and dialyzed (800 AU/mL) fractions of bacteriocin from *P. acidilactici* K2a2-3, authors observed growth inhibition of 55 and 53.7% of human colon adenocarcinoma cells (HT29), respectively. In turn, undialyzed bacteriocin fraction inhibited the growth of 52.3% of human cervical carcinoma cells (HeLa) and only 15.6% were inhibited by dialyzed fraction [57].

3.7. Plantaricin A

Plantaricin A is a bacteriocin of *Lactobacillus plantarum* C11 and its molecular weight reaches 2.4 kDa. In the case of artificially synthesized plantaricin A, the cytotoxicity against the human T cell leukaemia (Jurkat) was determined in vitro. It was shown that bacteriocin dose of 25 μM at 20 °C caused 75% loss in the cell viability, while at 37 °C it decreased by 55%. Plantaricin A induced apoptosis and necrosis of Jurkat cell line which were observed as a fragmentation of cell nuclei and plasma membrane. Tested substance had also impact on increasing of intracellular concentration of caspase-3 in cancerous cells [58].

3.8. Pyocins

Pyocins are secreted by more than 90% of *Pseudomonas aeruginosa* strains. Additionally, each strain can produce several different compounds from this group [66]. Investigations of Abdi-Ali et al. [59] showed the cytotoxicity of partially purified pyocin and pyocin S2 obtained from *P. aeruginosa* 42A on human hepatocellular carcinoma (HepG2) and human immunoglobulin-secreting cell line derived from multiple myeloma (Im9). Both pyocins were totally non-toxic to normal human foetal foreskin fibroblast cell line (HFFF). Im9 indicated greater sensitivity than HepG2 and the highest inhibition of growth (80%) was determined at a maximum concentration of pyocin (50 U/mL) after 5 days of cell incubation [59]. In turn, Watanabe and Saito [46] presented the cytotoxic action of pyocin S2 on cell lines of cervical adenocarcinoma (HeLa) and embryonal carcinoma of ovary (AS-II) as well as simian virus 40-transformed mouse kidney cells (mKS-A TU-7) and normal mice cells (BALB/3T3). On the other hand, there was no cytotoxic action on cells of metastatic lymph node of gastric cancer (HCG-27) and also normal cells of rat kidney and human lung [60].

4. Enzymes

Some of the bacterial enzymes, like arginine deiminase and L-asparaginase, are utilized in the treatment of selected cancer diseases. The source and biological target of antitumor bacterial enzymes are presented in Table 3 and their structure models are shown in Figure 4.

Table 3. The origin and biological activity of anticancer bacterial enzymes.

No.	Protein/Peptide	Source	Biological Target: Human Cancer Cells/Cell Lines	IC$_{50}$	References
1	Arginine deiminase	*Mycoplasma hominis, M. arginini*	hepatocellular carcinoma (HCC), prostate cancer (CWR22Rv1), glioblastoma (HROG02, HROG05, HROG10, HROG17)	1.95 µg/mL	[67–71]
2	L-asparaginase	*Escherichia coli, Erwinia* sp.	paediatric medulloblastoma (DAOY), glioblastomas (GBM-ES, U87), acute lymphoblastic leukaemia (ALL, HL60, MOLT-3, MOLT-4), myeloblastic leukaemia, acute T cell leukaemia (Jurkat), Hodgkin and non-Hodgkin lymphomas, myelosarcoma, multiple myeloma, extranodal NK/T cell lymphoma, ovarian carcinomas	0.39–90 µg/mL	[72–80]

IC$_{50}$—half maximal inhibitory concentration.

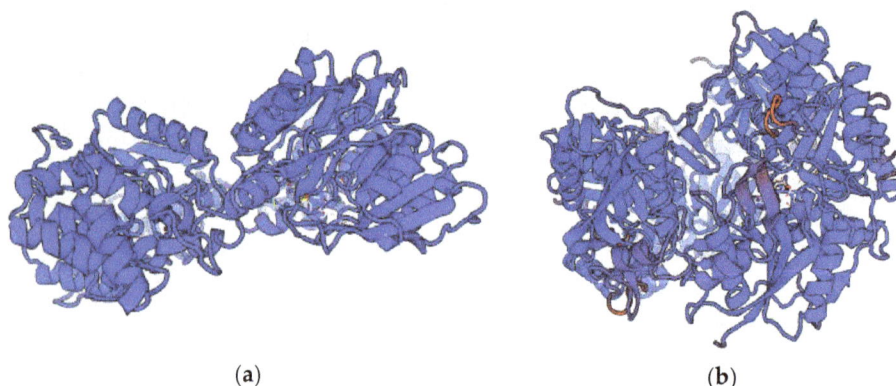

(a)   (b)

Figure 4. Structure models of anticancer antibiotics: (**a**) Arginine deiminase; (**b**) L-asparaginase (orig.). Sequences were downloaded from UNIPROT [62] and modelling server SWISS-MODEL [63,64] was used to visualization of the antibiotic structures.

4.1. Arginine Deiminase

Arginine deiminase (ADI) is an enzyme secreted by *Mycoplasma hominis* or *M. arginini* that degrades arginine to citrulline in vivo, releasing ammonia [67]. Recent studies are based on pegylated arginine deiminase (ADI-PEG20). The efficacy of ADI-PEG20 is directly correlated with the deficiency of argininosuccinate synthetase (ASS) [69]. Arginine deiminase in its native form is strongly antigenic with a half-life of 5 h [81]. ADI-PEG20 (arginine deiminase conjugated to 20,000 mw polyethylene glycol) decreases antigenicity and increases serum half-life [82]. Arginine deiminase may control the growth of argininosuccinate synthase deficient or arginine auxotrophic hepatocellular carcinoma (HCC). The pegylated ADI shows moderate disease-stabilizing activity in HCC and constitutes a promising drug utilizing a high enzymatic deficiency in HCC. This is a safe and well-tolerated therapy, which may benefit patients with unresectable hepatocellular carcinoma. Recently, usage of arginine deiminase as a drug is in the phase II clinical study [68]. Also, prostate cancer cells (CWR22Rv1) are susceptible to ADI-PEG20 in vitro. Apoptosis, observed after 96 h of treatment by 0.3 mg/mL ADI-PEG20 is caspase-independent. The effect of ADIPEG20 in vivo reveals reduced tumour activity and growth. Additionally, authors describe autophagy induced by single amino acid depletion by

ADI-PEG20. Autophagy was reported within 1 to 4 h of 0.3 mg/mL ADI-PEG20 treatment and it was an initial protective response to ADI-PEG20 in CWR22Rv1 cells [69]. A significant reaction, with cytotoxicity up to 50%, was also detected in the case of 4 glioblastoma cell lines (HROG02, HROG05, HROG10 and HROG17). The anticancer effect of ADI was independent of apoptosis, while reduction of cell proliferation was observed [70].

4.2. L-*asparaginase*

L-asparaginase (ASNase) enzyme was obtained from *Escherichia coli* or *Erwinia* species. The anti-tumour action of bacterial ASNases is caused by their ability to reduce asparagine blood concentration causing a selective inhibition of growth of sensitive malignant cells [73]. Panosyan et al. [74] presented that ASNase treatment in vitro resulted in dose-dependent growth inhibition of the following brain tumour cell lines: a paediatric medulloblastoma (DAOY), p53 and PTEN null human glioblastomas (GBM-ES and U87). Recently, ASNase has been utilized in the treatment of acute lymphoblastic leukaemia (ALL), myeloblastic leukaemia, Hodgkin and non-Hodgkin lymphomas, myelosarcoma, multiple myeloma, extranodal NK/T cell lymphoma and ovarian carcinomas [75–77]. *Erwinia* asparaginase should be used for the second- or third-line treatment of acute lymphoblastic leukaemia (ALL), depending upon regulatory requirements, in patients developing hypersensitivity to *E. coli* asparaginase preparations [83].

5. Nonribosomal Peptides (NRPs)

Nonribosomal peptides (NRPs) constitute secondary bioactive metabolites synthesized by an enzyme complex present only in bacteria, cyanobacteria and fungi [84]. NRPs are characterized by a lot of interesting chemical structures including D-amino acids, *N*-terminally attached fatty acid chains, *N*- and *C*-methylated residues, *N*-formylated residues, heterocyclic rings, glycosylated amino acids and phosphorylated residues [85]. Some NRPs exhibit anticancer and/or antimicrobial activity [84]. The source and biological target of anticancer nonribosomal peptides are presented in Table 4, while their chemical structures are shown in Figure 5.

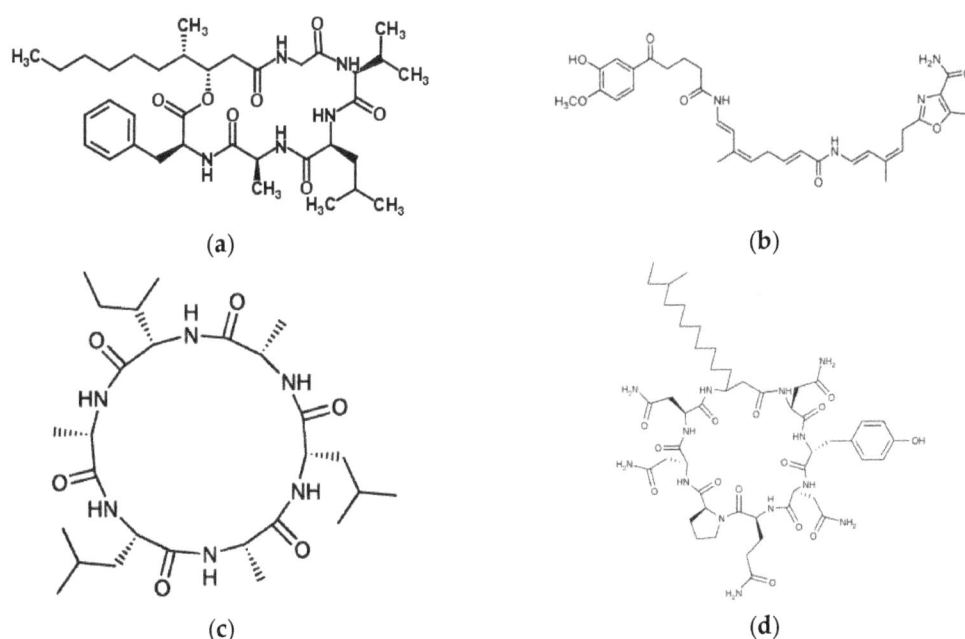

(a) (b) (c) (d)

Figure 5. *Cont.*

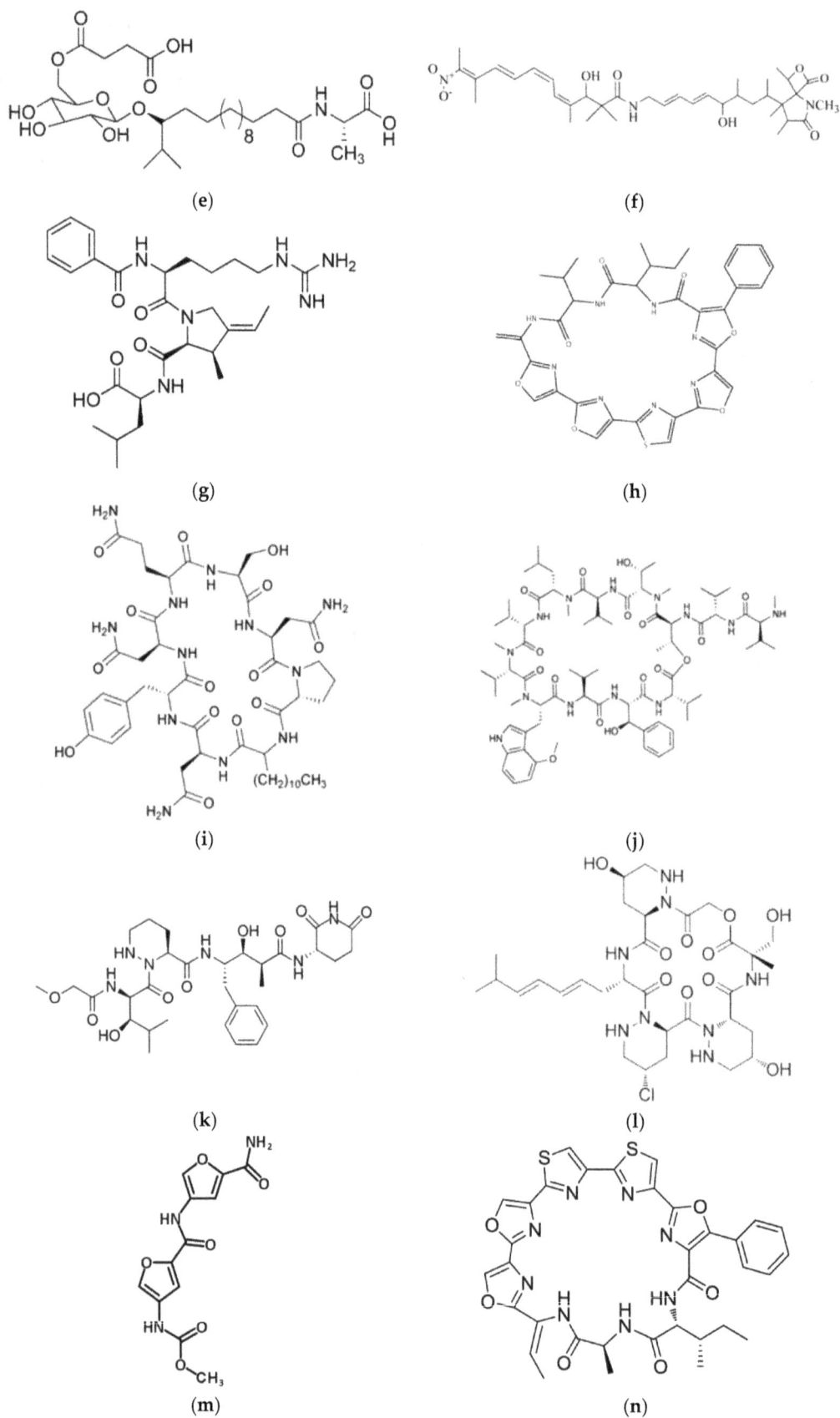

Figure 5.   Chemical structures of anticancer nonribosomal peptides: (**a**) Arenamide A;
(**b**) Ariakemicin A; (**c**) Halolitoralin A; (**d**) Mojavensin A; (**e**) Ieodoglucomide A; (**f**) Lajollamycin;
(**g**) Lucentamycin A; (**h**) Mechercharmycin A; (**i**) Mixirin A; (**j**) Ohmyungsamycin A; (**k**) Padanamide B;
(**l**) Piperazimycin A; (**m**) Proximicin A; (**n**) Urukthapelstatin A.

Table 4. The origin and biological activity of anticancer nonribosomal peptides.

No.	Protein/Peptide	Source	Biological Target: Cancer Cells	IC$_{50}$	References
1	Arenamides A, B	*Salinispora arenicola*	human colon carcinoma (HCT-116)	1.7–3.7 µM	[86]
2	Ariakemicins A, B	*Rapidithrix* sp.	human lung cancer (A549)	25.4–42.3 µM	[87]
3	Halolitoralins A–C	*Halobacillus litoralis* YS3106	human gastric tumour (BGC)	n.d.	[88]
4	Heptapeptide	*Paenibacillus profundus*	human melanoma (SK-MEL-28)	3.07 µM	[89]
5	Ieodoglucomide B	*Bacillus licheniformis*	human lung cancer, human stomach cancer	n.d.	[90]
6	Iso-C16 fengycin B, anteiso-C17 fengycin B, mojavensin A	*Bacillus mojavensis* B0621A	human leukaemia (HL-60)	1.6–100 mM	[91]
7	Lajollamycin	*Streptomyces nodosus* NPS007994	mouse melanoma (B16-F10)	n.d.	[92]
8	Lucentamycins A, B	*Nocardiopsis lucentensis* CNR-712	human colon carcinoma cells (HCT-116)	0.2–11 µM	[93]
9	Mechercharmycin A	*Thermoactinomyces* sp. YM3-251	human lung cancer cells (A549), human leukaemia (Jurkat)	400–460 µM	[94]
10	Mixirins A–C	*Bacillus* sp.	human colon tumour (HCT-116)	0.65–1.6 µM	[95]
11	Ohmyungsamycins A and B	*Streptomyces* sp.	diverse cancer cells	from 359 nM to 16.8 µM	[96]
12	Padanamide A, B	*Streptomyces* sp.	human leukaemia (Jurkat)	30.9–90.7 µM	[97]
13	Piperazimycins A–C	*Streptomyces* sp.	multiple tumour cell lines	n.d.	[98]
14	Proximicins A–C	*Verrucosispora* sp. MG-37 and AB-18-032	human gastric adenocarcinoma (AGS), human hepatocellular carcinoma (HepG2), human breast carcinoma (MCF 7)	n.d.	[99]
15	Urukthapelstatin A	*Mechercharimyces asporophorigenens* YM11-542	human lung cancers (A549, DMS114, NCIH460), ovarian cancers (OVCAR-3, OVCAR-4, OVCAR-5, OVCAR-8, SK-OV3), breast cancer (MCF-7), colon cancer (HCT-116)	12 nM	[100,101]

IC$_{50}$—half maximal inhibitory concentration, n.d.— no data.

5.1. Arenamides

Three new cyclohexadepsipeptides—named arenamides A–C—were obtained from the fermentation broth of *Salinispora arenicola* found in sea sediment (Great Astrolabe Reef, Kandavu Island chain, Fiji). Authors reported that arenamides A and B blocked TNF-induced activation with an IC$_{50}$ value at the level of 3.7 and 1.7 µM, respectively. Moreover, inhibition of nitric oxide and prostaglandin E2 production and also moderate cytotoxic effect on human colon carcinoma (HCT-116) were detected [86].

5.2. Ariakemicins

The culture of the marine gliding bacterium of the *Rapidithrix* genus (Ariake Inland Sea, Japan) yielded two linear hybrid polyketide-nonribosomal peptides (ariakemicins A and B). These proteins show antimicrobial activity and contain threonine, two ω-amino-(ω-3)-methyl carboxylic acids with diene or triene units and δ-isovanilloylbutyric acid. Ariakemicins exhibit low cytotoxicity to human lung tumour cell line (A549) and baby hamster kidney cells with an IC$_{50}$ value at the level of 42.3 and 25.4 µM, respectively [87].

5.3. Halolitoralins

A cyclic hexapeptide (halolitoralin A) and two cyclic tetrapeptides (halolitoralin B and C) were derived from *Halobacillus litoralis* YS3106 found in the marine sediments (Huanghai Sea, China). Halolitoralin A has a molecular mass of 575 Da and a molecular formula of $C_{27}H_{48}O_6N_6$, while halolitoralin B and C appealed as isomers with a chemical formula of $C_{23}H_{42}O_4N_4$. Presented cyclopeptides exhibit moderate activities in vitro against human gastric tumour cells (BGC) [88].

5.4. Heptapeptide from Paenibacillus profundus

A linear glyceryl acid derived heptapeptide (Glyceryl-D-leucyl-D-alanyl-D-leucyl-D-leucyl-L-valyl-D-leucyl-D-alanine) was produced by the culture of marine deep sediment strain SI 79 classified as *Paenibacillus profundus* sp. nov. The peptide is an antibiotic with cytotoxic activity against human melanoma cell line (SK-MEL-28) with IC_{50} = 3.07 μM after 72 h [89].

5.5. Ieodoglucomides

Ieodoglucomide A and B are glycolipopeptides obtained from *Bacillus licheniformis* occurring in marine sediment of Ieodo Reef (South Korea). Both peptides showed low antimicrobial activity in vitro but ieodoglucomide B demonstrated cytotoxicity against lung and stomach cancer cells (50% growth inhibition, GI_{50} = 25.18 and 17.78 μg/mL, respectively) [90].

5.6. Iturinic Lipopeptides

Ma et al. [91] isolated three iturinic lipopeptides from *Bacillus mojavensis* B0621A originated from pearl oyster *Pinctada martensii* in the South China Sea. Mojavensin A has a molecular formula of $C_{50}H_{77}N_{13}O_{14}$ and a molecular weight of 1.1 kDa. Two other isolated substances had singly and doubly-charged molecular ions. Iso-C16 fengycin B possesses a molecular weight of 1.5 kDa and 746 Da, respectively and anteiso-C17 fengycin B has 1.5 kDa and 753 Da, respectively. All three lipopeptides showed weak cytotoxic activities against human leukemia (HL-60) cell line. Mojavensin A, iso-C16 fengycin B and anteiso-C17 fengycin B inhibited the growth of HL-60 with IC_{50} of 100, 100 and 1.6 mM, respectively [91].

5.7. Lajollamycin

Actinomycete *Streptomyces nodosus* NPS007994 obtained from marine sediment of Scripps Canyon, La Jolla, California, USA, was reported as a source of lajollamycin. This peptide, a nitro-tetraene spiro-b-lactone-g-lactam, showed antimicrobial activity. Lajollamycin reduced in vitro the growth of the mouse melanoma cells (B16-F10) with a half maximal effective concentration (EC_{50}) of 9.6 μM [92].

5.8. Lucentamycins

Cho et al. [93] isolated from the broth of a marine-derived actinomycete strain *Nocardiopsis lucentensis* CNR-712 3-methyl-4-ethylideneproline-containing peptides, named as lucentamycins A–D. Among them, lucentamycins A and B exhibited significant in vitro cytotoxicity against human colon carcinoma cells (HCT-116) with IC_{50} values of 0.20 and 11 μM, respectively [93].

5.9. Mechercharmycins

Kanoh et al. [94] obtained mechercharmycins from the *Thermoactinomyces* species YM3-251 originated from mud (Mecherchar, Republic of Palau, North Pacific Ocean). The cyclic peptide mechercharmycin A has a chemical formula of $C_{35}H_{32}N_8O_7S$ and a molecular weight of 708 Da, whereas the linear congener mechercharmycin B has a formula of $C_{35}H_{36}N_8O_{10}$ and a molecular weight of 728 Da. Mechercharmycin A showed relatively strong antitumor activity against human lung cancer cells (A549) and human leukemia (Jurkat cells) with an IC_{50} value of 4.0×10^{-8} M and 4.6×10^{-8} M, respectively. In the case of mechercharmycin B, anticancer activity was not detected [94].

5.10. Mixirins

Three cyclic acylpeptides named as mixirins A-C were isolated by Zhang et al. [95] from marine bacterium *Bacillus* sp., collected from sea mud near the Arctic pole. Mixirin A has a chemical formula of $C_{48}H_{75}N_{12}O_{14}$, mixirin B—$C_{45}H_{69}N_{12}O_{14}$ and mixirin C—$C_{47}H_{73}N_{12}O_{14}$. The molecular weight of all compounds was about 1 kDa. Mixirins A, B and C blocked the growth of human colon tumor cell line (HCT-116) with an IC_{50} value at the level of 0.65, 1.6 and 1.26 µM, respectively [95].

5.11. Ohmyungsamycins

Streptomyces sp. isolated from a volcanic island in the Republic of Korea produced cyclic peptides ohmyungsamycin A and B. These chemical compounds contain amino acid units, such as N-methyl-4-methoxytrytophan, β-hydroxyphenylalanine and N,N-dimethylvaline. Both peptides showed growth inhibition against diverse cancerous cell lines obtaining an IC_{50} value in the range from 359 to 816 nM and from 12.4 to 16.8 µM, respectively. Moreover, ohmyungsamycins exhibited relatively selective anti-proliferative activity against tumor cells in comparison with normal cells [96].

5.12. Padanamides

In the culture of *Streptomyces* sp. isolated from the marine sediment, two highly modified linear tetrapeptides: padanamides A and B were produced. Authors demonstrated that padanamide A inhibits cysteine and methionine biosynthesis and padanamide B is cytotoxic to human leukemia (Jurkat cells) with an IC_{50} value of 30.9 µM [97].

5.13. Piperazimycins

Miller et al. [98] isolated three cyclic hexadepsipeptides piperazimycins A–C from the fermentation broth of *Streptomyces* sp., originated from marine sediments near the island of Guam. These substances contain rare amino acids, such as hydroxyacetic acid, α-methylserine, γ-hydroxypiperazic acid, γ-chloropiperazic acid, 2-amino-8-methyl-4,6-nonadienoic acid and 2-amino-8-methyl-4,6-decadienoic acid. All studied peptides demonstrated cytotoxicity against diverse cancer cells with a mean GI_{50} of 100 nM in the case of piperazimycin A [98].

5.14. Proximicins

Three novel aminofuran antibiotics (proximicins) were extracted by Fiedler et al. [99] from marine member of the rare genus *Verrucosispora*, strain MG-37. Bacterium was isolated from sediment collected in the Raune Fjord, Norway, at a depth of 250 m. Second strain of *Verrucosispora*, AB-18-032 was isolated from sediment obtained from the Sea of Japan at a depth of 289 m. Molecular formulas and weights of proximicins A, B and C are $C_{12}H_{11}N_3O_6$, 293 Da, $C_{20}H_{19}N_3O_7$, 413 Da and $C_{22}H_{20}N_4O_6$, 436 Da, respectively. All compounds demonstrated growth inhibition potential against cell lines of gastric adenocarcinoma (AGS, GI_{50} = 0.25–1.5 µg/mL), hepatocellular carcinoma (HepG2, GI_{50} = 0.78–9.5 µg/mL) and breast carcinoma (MCF-7, GI_{50} = 5.0–9.0 µg/mL). After 24 h of incubation of AGS cells, proximicin C caused cell arrest in the G0/G1 phase, whereas the number of apoptotic cells was increased after 40 h. Additionally, the above-mentioned substance induced upregulation of p53 and of the cyclin kinase inhibitor p21 in AGS cells [99].

5.15. Urukthapelstatin A

A cyclic thiopeptide-urukthapelstatin A was isolated from the cultured mycelia of *Mechercharimyces asporophorigenens* YM11-542 bacterium originated from sediments of marine lake (Urukthapel Island, Palau) [100,101]. The molecular formula of urukthapelstatin A was established as $C_{34}H_{30}N_8O_6S_2$ with weight of 733 Da [101]. Urukthapelstatin A showed dose-dependent growth inhibition of human lung tumor cells (A549) with an IC_{50} value at the level of 12 nM. Presented substance seemed to be the most effective against the ovarian cancer (OVCAR-3, OVCAR-4, OVCAR-5, OVCAR-8 and SK-OV3), breast cancer (MCF-7), colon cancer (HCT-116) and lung cancer (DMS114 and NCIH460) [100].

6. Toxins

Toxins produced by the bacteria damage host tissues directly at the site of bacterial infection or may spread throughout the body. Some toxins are tried to be used for therapeutic purposes [102]. The source and biological target of bacterial toxins with anticancer activity are presented in Table 5 and their structure models in Figure 6.

Table 5. The origin and biological activity of anticancer bacterial toxins.

No.	Protein/Peptide	Source	Biological Target: Human Cancer Cell Lines	IC_{50}	References
1	Botulinum neurotoxin type A	*Clostridium botulinum*	prostate cancer (PC-3, LNCaP), breast cancer (T47D), neuroblastoma (SH-SY5Y)	0.54–300 nM	[103–106]
2	Diphtheria toxin	*Corynebacterium diphtheriae*	adrenocortical carcinoma (H295R), glioblastomas (U118MG, U373MG, U87MG), cutaneous T cell lymphomas (CTCL), breast carcinoma (MCF 7), cervical adenocarcinoma (HeLa)	0.55–2.08 µg/mL	[107–112]
3	Exotoxin A	*Pseudomonas aeruginosa*	pancreatic cancer (PaCa-2), melanomas (FEMX, Melmet-1, Melmet-5, Melmet-44, MelRM, MM200), head and neck squamous carcinomas, Burkitt's lymphoma (Daudi, CA46), leukemias (EHEB, MEC1)	0.3–8.6 ng/mL	[113–117]
4	Listeriolysin O	*Listeria monocytogenes*	breast carcinomas (MCF7, SKBR-3), leukemia T-lymphocytes (Jurkat)	from 50 pM to 0.1 nM, in conjugates	[118–122]

IC_{50}—half maximal inhibitory concentration.

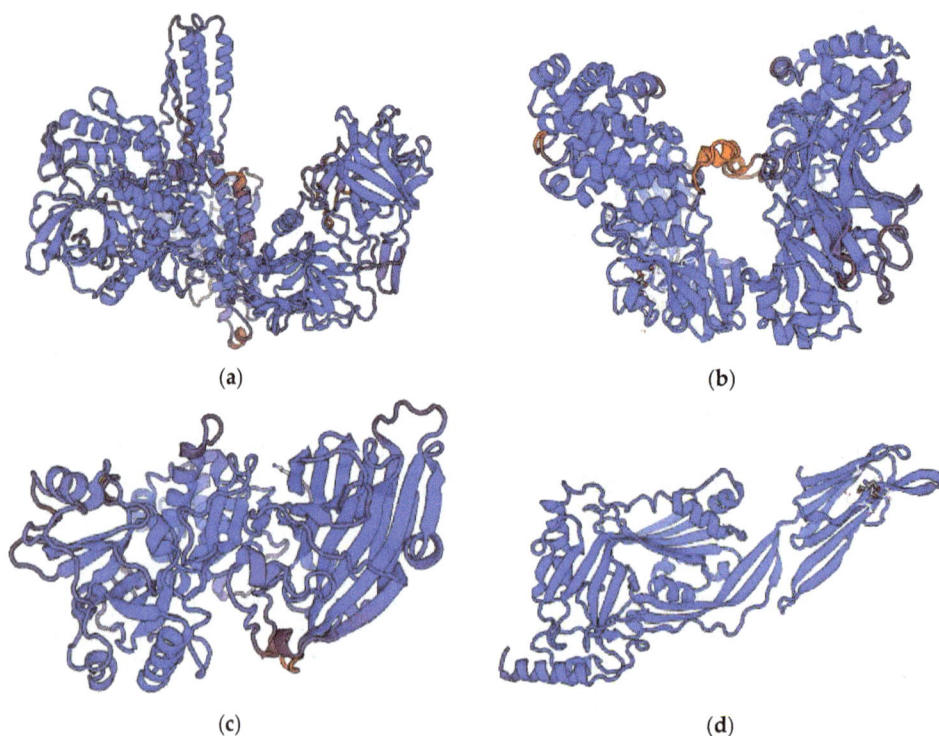

(a)

(b)

(c)

(d)

Figure 6. Structure models of anticancer bacterial toxins: (**a**) Botulinum neurotoxin type A; (**b**) Diphtheria toxin; (**c**) Exotoxin A; (**d**) Listeriolysin O (orig.). Sequences were downloaded from UNIPROT [62], while visualization of the toxin structures was prepared using the SWISS-MODEL modeling server [63,64].

6.1. Botulinum Neurotoxin Type A

Botulinum neurotoxin type A, produced by strains of Clostridium botulinum, is utilized in the treatment of benign prostatic hyperplasia (BPH) due to its apoptotic activity. Toxin reduces also cell growth and proliferation of prostate cancer (PC-3 and LNCaP) cell lines [104,105]. Moreover, botulinum toxin A induces caspase-3 and -7 dependent apoptotic processes in the breast cancer cell line (T47D) [106].

6.2. Diphtheria Toxin

Diphtheria toxin (DT) represents an exotoxin obtained from *Corynebacterium diphtheriae*. This substance has a molecular weight of 60 kDa and its production is caused by the infection of bacteriophage B. DT is encoded by the *tox* gene of some corynebacteriophages, hence only *C. diphtheriae* isolates that contain the *tox*+ phages secrete diphtheria toxin [107]. DT exhibits the anticancer activity but with side effects, so it is utilized in the antitumor therapy in combination with other agents. The cross-reacting material 197 (CRM197) is the nontoxic mutant of diphtheria toxin that binds heparin-binding epidermal growth factor-like growth factor. It was shown that CRM197 inhibited angiogenesis and stimulated cell apoptosis of human adrenocortical carcinoma (H295R) [108]. Other substance, DTAT is DT-based immunotoxin directed to cancer vascular endothelium. DTAT exhibited in vitro strong anticancer action in the case of glioblastoma cell lines (U118MG, U373MG, U87MG) [109]. In turn, denileukin diftitox is a fusion protein designed against cells which express the IL-2 receptor. It is used as a drug named Ontak in cutaneous T cell lymphomas (CTCL) expressing CD25 [110,112].

6.3. Exotoxin A

Exotoxin A belongs to the main toxins produced by *Pseudomonas aeruginosa*. The molecular weight of this peptide is 66 kDa. It inhibits protein synthesis by the inactivation of elongation factor-2 (EF-2). This substance is usually utilized as an immunotoxin with different ligands [114]. Deimmunized *Pseudomonas* exotoxin cloned with human epidermal growth factor (EGF) and interleukin 4 showed activity against pancreatic cancer (PaCa-2) and selectively prevented metastasis [115]. Two exotoxin A-based immunotoxins (9.2.27PE ABT-737) caused synergistic cytotoxicity and death of melanoma cell lines (FEMX, Melmet-1, Melmet-5, Melmet-44, MelRM, MM200) associated with apoptosis [116]. In the case of exotoxin A cloned with an anti-CD133 scFv reactive (dCD133KDEL), the inhibition of cell multiplication of head and neck squamous carcinoma was observed [117].

6.4. Listeriolysin O

Listeriolysin O (LLO) is produced by strains of *Listeria monocytogenes*, a pathogen which develops within the cell cytosol. This chemical compound is crucial to the phagosomal escape of the bacterium into the cytoplasm [119]. The conjugated immunotoxin B3-LLO exhibited high effectiveness in removing the breast carcinoma cell lines MCF7 and SKBR-3, with an EC_{50} value at the level of 2.3 and 12.7 nM, respectively [121]. According to Stachowiak et al. [122], supernatants of *L. monocytogenes* strains showed dose-dependent cytotoxicity against the human leukemia T-lymphocyte cells (Jurkat) and human peripheral blood mononuclear cells (PBMC). Authors suggested that LLO activity is targeted more to T cells than B cells and it may give some therapeutic consequences, including T-cell lymphoma [122].

7. Other Proteins/Peptides

In this part, four bacterial proteins or peptides have been described. The source and biological activity of these anticancer substances are presented in Table 6. In turn, their structure models are shown in Figure 7.

Table 6. The origin and biological activity of other anticancer bacterial proteins/peptides.

No.	Protein/Peptide	Source	Biological Target: Human Cancer Cells/Cell Lines	IC_{50}	References
1	Azurin	*Pseudomonas aeruginosa*	breast cancer (MCF-7, MDA-MB-157), oral squamous carcinoma (YD-9), melanoma (UISO-Mel-2)	32–53 μM	[123–127]
2	p28	*Pseudomonas aeruginosa*	breast cancer (MCF-7, ZR-75-1, T47D), glioblastoma (U87, LN229), melanoma (Mel-29), brain tumors	n.d.	[128–132]
3	Entap	*Enterococcus* sp.	gastric adenocarcinoma (AGS), uterine cervix adenocarcinoma (HeLa), mammary gland adenocarcinoma (MDA-MB-231), prostate carcinoma (22Rv1), colorectal adenocarcinoma (HT-29)	n.d.	[114,133, 134]
4	Pep27anal2	*Streptococcus pneumoniae*	leukemia (AML-2, HL-60, Jurkat), gastric cancer (SNU-601), breast cancer (MCF-7)	10–29 μM	[135,136]

IC_{50}—half maximal inhibitory concentration, n.d.—no data.

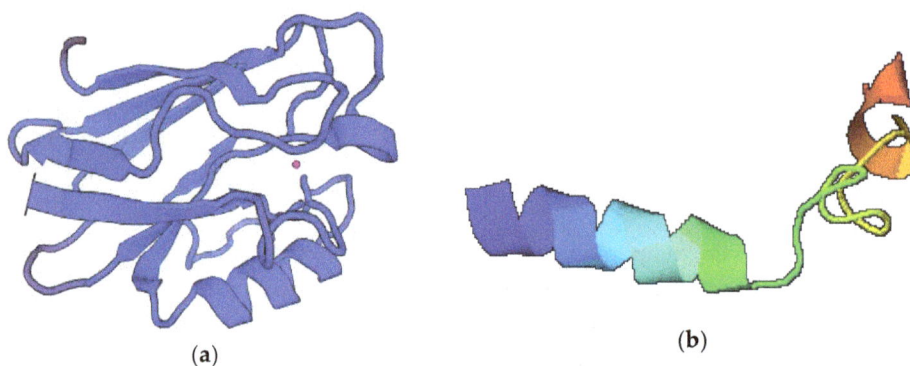

Figure 7. Structure model of: (**a**) Azurin; (**b**) p28 (orig.).

Sequences were downloaded from UNIPROT [62]. Modeling server SWISS-MODEL [63,64] and I-TASSER [137] were used to visualization of the azurin and p28 structure, respectively.

7.1. Azurin

Azurin is a copper-containing protein with a molecular mass of 16 kDa, secreted by *Pseudomonas aeruginosa*. After removing the copper, the cytotoxic apo-azurin is formed [123]. Several different mechanisms of azurin anticancer activity have been proposed: (i) induction of cancer cell apoptosis or growth inhibition by forming complexes with tumor protein p53; (ii) inhibition of cancer cell growth by interfering in the receptor tyrosine kinase EphB2-mediated signaling process; (iii) inhibition of tumor growth by preventing angiogenesis through reducing VEGFR-2 tyrosine kinase activity; (iv) interferention with P-cadherin protein expression and inhibition of the growth of breast cancer cells [124]. Peptide had a strong cytotoxic effect on the breast cancer cell line (MCF-7), resulting in more than 50% increase of apoptosis and poor to other breast cancer cells (MDA-MB-157, MDD2, MDA-MB-231) [125]. In other studies, the azurin showed anticancer activity against oral squamous carcinoma cells (YD-9) [126] and melanoma cells (UISO-Mel-2) [127].

7.2. p28

p28 is a part of azurin (amino acids 50-77) consisting of 28 amino acids. Its molecular mass reaches 2.8 kDa [128]. p28 has an influence on the post-translational increase of p53 and p21 expression, which causes cell arrest in the G2-M phase. Also, p28 showed antiangiogenic effect and preferentially entered the human breast cancer cells (MCF-7, ZR-75-1, T47D) through a caveolin-mediated pathway [129,130]. It is interesting that this substance raised the cytotoxicity of lower doses of DNA-damaging (doxorubicin, dacarbazine, temozolomide) or antimitotic (paclitaxel, docetaxel) drugs in glioblastoma cells (U87 and LN229) and p53wt melanoma (Mel-29). The increased activity of the above-mentioned antitumor medicines in combination with p28 was facilitated through the p53/p21/CDK2 pathway [131]. p28 has recently completed two Phase I clinical trials (brain and solid tumors) [132].

7.3. Entap

Enterococcal anti-proliferative peptide (Entap) is produced by clinical strains of *Enterococcus* genus and has a molecular weight of 6.2 kDa. Entap demonstrated antiproliferative activity against cell lines of human gastric adenocarcinoma (AGS), colorectal adenocarcinoma (HT-29), mammary gland adenocarcinoma (MDA-MB-231), uterine cervix adenocarcinoma (HeLa) and also prostatic carcinoma (22Rv1). The activity of Entap is associated with cancer cell arrest in G1 and induction of autophagous apoptosis [114,133,134].

7.4. Pep27anal2

Pep27anal2, with a molecular weight of 3.3 kDa, constitutes an analogue of the signal peptide of *Streptococcus pneumoniae* (Pep27). This substance activates *S. pneumoniae* death program and exhibits antimicrobial properties [135]. Pep27anal2 gets through the cell membrane inducing caspase- and cytochrome c-independent apoptosis. Pep27anal2 inhibited proliferation of cell lines of leukemia (AML-2, HL-60, Jurkat), gastric cancer (SNU-601) and breast cancer (MCF-7) [136].

8. Final Remarks

In the course of evolution, host defence peptides and proteins developed in various organisms, such as bacteria [138], fungi [139], plants [140], animals [138,141] and human [142]. Some substances exhibit the multifunctional activity, for example, antimicrobial and antitumor properties [51,84,140,143,144]. However, the number of these bioactive compounds known so far is a relatively small. Investigations concerning their isolation, cognition and application are just the tip of the iceberg. In the present review, we described 37 bacterial chemical compounds or groups of compounds with anticancer activity. On the other hand, there are about 30,000 known, cultured bacterial species [145] and about 109,000 of operative taxonomic units of bacteria are found on the basis of the 16S rRNA study [146]. It can be supposed that some of them constitute a potential source of new biologically active agents.

Nowadays, marine organisms are increasingly important in terms of isolated chemical compounds with antibacterial, antiviral and anticancer activity [147]. A large group of anticancer peptides was obtained from bacteria occurring in marine sediments [86–101]. In this work, we presented 15 proteins or groups of them secreted by marine bacteria. However, only the first research conducted by the authors who have isolated these substances are usually available. In most cases, there are no continuations of these studies or other investigations.

Among bacteriocins showing the antitumor action, we reported 8 peptides and proteins (individual compounds or groups of compounds). These substances belong to the better examined constituents. Some of them are produced by fermentation [148] of lactic acid bacteria (LAB) belonging to *Lactobacillus*, *Lactococcus*, *Bifidobacterium*, *Leuconostoc*, *Streptococcus* or *Pediococcus* genera [46]. Nisin is the best known bacteriocin, which in 1969 was approved by the FAO/WHO as a safe food additive. At the present, the above-mentioned bacteriocin is used as a natural preservative in over 50 countries [149]. The literature data show that milk products containing probiotic strains, for example kefir, can inhibit proliferation of cancer cells and induce apoptosis [150].

The combination of Omics techniques with virtual screening and computational methods may contribute to the development of the discussed research direction. These methods can be utilized for modification of the already known anticancer proteins or the selection of new chemical compounds with antitumor activity [151]. The other option is using of the peptide-based drug conjugates that affect the reduction of side effects in cancer patients [152]. It should be added that four described in this review antibiotics (actinomycin D, bleomycin, doxorubicin, mitomycin C) and diphtheria toxin are already utilized as medicines [30,32,33,39,112,114] and p28 has recently completed two Phase I clinical trials [132]. The others have to wait for further investigations.

To sum up, bacteria constitute a valuable and, at the same time, very poorly known source of biologically active substances, including anticancer proteins and peptides. Studies of the majority of bacterial anticancer proteins/peptides end in the in vitro stage and only single ones undergo the entire procedure, from in vitro by clinical trial to registration and use as medicines.

Author Contributions: Both authors shared in the searching for publications, preparation and editing of the manuscript. T.M.K. formatted the tables and supported visualization of the peptide structures. Both authors have approved the final manuscript.

References

1.   Ferlay, J.; Soerjomataram, I.; Ervik, M.; Dikshit, R.; Eser, S.; Mathers, C.; Rebelo, M.; Parkin, D.M.; Forman, D.; Bray, F. *GLOBOCAN 2012 v1.0, Cancer Incidence and Mortality Worldwide: IARC CancerBase No. 11*; International Agency for Research on Cancer: Lyon, France, 2013.

2.   Worldwide Cancer Statistics. Available online: http://www.cancerresearchuk.org/health-professional/cancer-statistics/worldwide-cancer (accessed on 16 January 2018).

3.   Cancer.   Available online: http://www.who.int/mediacentre/factsheets/fs297/en/   (accessed on 16 January 2018).

4.   Cancer Prevention and Control in the Context of an Integrated Approach. WHA70.12. Available online: http://apps.who.int/medicinedocs/documents/s23233en/s23233en.pdf (accessed on 16 January 2018).

5.   Langie, S.A.; Koppen, G.; Desaulniers, D.; Al-Mulla, F.; Al-Temaimi, R.; Amedei, A.; Azqueta, A.; Bisson, W.H.; Brown, D.G.; Brunborg, G.; et al. Causes of genome instability: The effect of low dose chemical exposures in modern society. *Carcinogenesis* **2015**, *36* (Suppl. 1), S61–S88. [CrossRef] [PubMed]

6.   Kuno, T.; Tsukamoto, T.; Hara, A.; Tanaka, T. Cancer chemoprevention through the induction apoptosis by natural compounds. *J. Biophys. Chem.* **2012**, *3*, 156–173. [CrossRef]

7.   Hanahan, D.; Weinberg, R.A. Hallmarks of cancer: The next generation. *Cell* **2011**, *144*, 646–674. [CrossRef] [PubMed]

8.   Raguz, S.; Yagüe, E. Resistance to chemotherapy: New treatments and novel insights into an old problem. *Br. J. Cancer* **2008**, *99*, 387–391. [CrossRef] [PubMed]

9.   Coley, W.B. The treatment of inoperable sarcoma by bacterial toxins (the mixed toxins of the *Streptococcus erysipelas* and *Bacillus prodigiosus*). *Proc. R. Soc. Med. Surg.* **1909**, *3*, 1–48.

10.   Patyar, S.; Joshi, R.; Prasad Byrav, D.S.; Prakash, A.; Medhi, B.; Das, B.K. Bacteria in cancer therapy: A novel experimental strategy. *J. Biomed. Sci.* **2010**, *17*, 21. [CrossRef] [PubMed]

11.   Encyclopaedia Britannica. Available online: http://www.britannica.com/science/antibiotic (accessed on 20 February 2018).

12.   Barret, J.M.; Salles, B.; Provot, C.; Hill, B.T. Evaluation of DNA repair inhibition by antitumor or antibiotic drugs using a chemiluminescence microplate assay. *Carcinogenesis* **1997**, *18*, 2441–2445. [CrossRef] [PubMed]

13.   Wu, C.H.; Pan, J.S.; Chang, W.C.; Hung, J.S.; Mao, S.J. The molecular mechanism of actinomycin D in preventing neointimal formation in rat carotid arteries after balloon injury. *J. Biomed. Sci.* **2005**, *12*, 503–512. [CrossRef] [PubMed]

14.   Koba, M.; Konopa, J. Actinomycin D and its mechanisms of action. *Postepy Hig. Med. Dosw.* **2005**, *59*, 290–298. (In Polish)

15.   Cosmegen® for Injection. Available online: http://www.accessdata.fda.gov/drugsatfda_docs/label/2009/050682s025lbl.pdf (accessed on 20 February 2018).

16.   Segerman, Z.J.; Roy, B.; Hecht, S.M. Characterization of bleomycin-mediated cleavage of a hairpin DNA library. *Biochemistry* **2013**, *52*. [CrossRef] [PubMed]

17. Bayer, R.A.; Gaynor, E.R.; Fisher, R.I. Bleomycin in non-Hodgkin's lymphoma. *Semin. Oncol.* **1992**, *19* (Suppl. 5), 46–53. [PubMed]

18. Chen, J.K.; Yang, D.; Shen, B.; Murray, V. Bleomycin analogues preferentially cleave at the transcription start sites of actively transcribed genes in human cells. *Int. J. Biochem. Cell Biol.* **2017**, *85*, 56–65. [CrossRef] [PubMed]

19. Bleomycin. Genomics of Drug Sensitivity in Cancer. Available online: http://www.cancerrxgene.org/translation/Drug/190 (accessed on 14 April 2018).

20. Abraham, S.A.; Waterhouse, D.N.; Mayer, L.D.; Cullis, P.R.; Madden, T.D.; Bally, M.B. The liposomal formulation of doxorubicin. *Methods Enzymol.* **2005**, *391*, 71–96. [CrossRef] [PubMed]

21. Botlagunta, M.; Kollapalli, B.; Kakarla, L.; Gajarla, S.P.; Gade, S.P.; Dadi, C.L.; Penumadu, A.; Javeed, S. In vitro anti-cancer activity of doxorubicin against human RNA helicase, DDX3. *Bioinformation* **2016**, *12*, 347–353. [CrossRef] [PubMed]

22. Vittorio, O.; Le Grand, M.; Makharza, S.A.; Curcio, M.; Tucci, P.; Iemma, F.; Nicoletta, F.P.; Hampel, S.; Cirillo, G. Doxorubicin synergism and resistance reversal in human neuroblastoma BE(2)C cell lines: An in vitro study with dextran-catechin nanohybrids. *Eur. J. Pharm. Biopharm.* **2018**, *122*, 176–185. [CrossRef] [PubMed]

23. Doxorubicin Hydrochloride for Injection, USP. Available online: http://www.accessdata.fda.gov/drugsatfda_docs/label/2010/050467s070lbl.pdf (accessed on 20 February 2018).

24. Mitomycin C from *Streptomyces caespitosus*. Available online: http://www.sigmaaldrich.com/content/dam/sigma-aldrich/docs/Sigma/Product_Information_Sheet/2/m0503pis.pdf (accessed on 20 February 2018).

25. Bradner, W.T. Mitomycin C: A clinical update. *Cancer Treat. Rev.* **2001**, *27*, 35–50. [CrossRef] [PubMed]

26. Mitomycin-C. Genomics of Drug Sensitivity in Cancer. Available online: http://www.cancerrxgene.org/translation/Drug/136 (accessed on 14 April 2018).

27. Latta, V.D.; Cecchettini, A.; Del Ry, S.; Morales, M.A. Bleomycin in the setting of lung fibrosis induction: From biological mechanisms to counteractions. *Pharmacol. Res.* **2015**, *97*, 122–130. [CrossRef] [PubMed]

28. Farhane, Z.; Bonnier, F.; Byrne, H.J. An in vitro study of the interaction of the chemotherapeutic drug Actinomycin D with lung cancer cell lines using Raman micro-spectroscopy. *J. Biophotonics* **2018**, *11*, e201700112. [CrossRef] [PubMed]

29. D'Arpa, P.; Liu, L.F. Topoisomerase—Targeting antitumor drugs. *Biochim. Biophys. Acta* **1989**, *989*, 163–177. [CrossRef]

30. Dactinomycine. Available online: http://medycyna.anauk.net/101-0-393-.Encyklopedia.Lekow.html (accessed on 20 February 2018).

31. Egger, C.; Cannet, C.; Gérard, C.; Jarman, E.; Jarai, G.; Feige, A.; Suply, T.; Micard, A.; Dunbar, A.; Tigani, B.; et al. Administration of bleomycin via the oropharyngeal aspiration route leads to sustained lung fibrosis in mice and rats as quantified by UTE-MRI and histology. *PLoS ONE* **2013**, *8*, e63432. [CrossRef] [PubMed]

32. Blenoxane. Available online: http://www.accessdata.fda.gov/drugsatfda_docs/label/2010/050443s036lbl.pdf (accessed on 20 February 2018).

33. Bleomycin for Injection USP. Available online: http://oncozine.com/wp-content/uploads/2017/07/Bleomycin-for-Injection-USP.pdf (accessed on 20 February 2018).

34. Thorn, C.F.; Oshiro, C.; Marsh, S.; Hernandez-Boussard, T.; McLeod, H.; Klein, T.E.; Altman, R.B. Doxorubicin pathways: Pharmacodynamics and adverse effects. *Pharmacogenet. Genom.* **2011**, *21*, 440–446. [CrossRef] [PubMed]

35. Cagel, M.; Grotz, E.; Bernabeu, E.; Moretton, M.A.; Chiappetta, D.A. Doxorubicin: Nanotechnological overviews from bench to bedside. *Drug Discov. Today* **2017**, *22*, 270–281. [CrossRef] [PubMed]

36. Preet, S.; Bharati, S.; Panjeta, A.; Tewari, R.; Rishi, P. Effect of nisin and doxorubicin on DMBA-induced skin carcinogenesis—A possible adjunct therapy. *Tumour Biol.* **2015**, *36*, 8301–8308. [CrossRef] [PubMed]

37. Doksorubicyna (Opis Profesjonalny). Available online: http://bazalekow.mp.pl/leki/doctor_subst.html?id=247 (accessed on 20 February 2018).

38. Verweij, J.; Pinedo, H.M. Mitomycin C: Mechanism of action, usefulness and limitations. *Anti-Cancer Drugs* **1990**, *1*, 5–13. [CrossRef] [PubMed]

39. Mitomycin. Available online: http://bazalekow.mp.pl/leki/szukaj.html?item_name=mitomycin (accessed on 20 February 2018).

40. Karpiński, T.M.; Szkaradkiewicz, A.K. Bacteriocins. In *Encyclopedia of Food and Health*; Caballero, B., Finglas, P.M., Toldra, F., Eds.; Elsevier, Academic Press: New York, NY, USA, 2016; Volume 1, pp. 312–319.

41. Kaur, S.; Kaur, S. Bacteriocins as potential anticancer agents. *Front. Pharmacol.* **2015**, *6*, 272. [CrossRef] [PubMed]

42. Mandal, S.M.; Pati, B.R.; Chakraborty, R.; Franco, O.L. New insights into the bioactivity of peptides from probiotics. *Front. Biosci.* **2016**, *8*, 450–459. [CrossRef]

43. Drider, D.; Bendali, F.; Naghmouchi, K.; Chikindas, M.L. Bacteriocins: Not only antibacterial agents. *Probiotics Antimicrob. Proteins* **2016**, *8*, 177–182. [CrossRef] [PubMed]

44. Alvarez-Sieiro, P.; Montalbán-López, M.; Mu, D.; Kuipers, O.P. Bacteriocins of lactic acid bacteria: Extending the family. *Appl. Microbiol. Biotechnol.* **2016**, *100*, 2939–2951. [CrossRef] [PubMed]

45. Gomes, K.M.; Duarte, R.S.; de Freire Bastos, M.D. Lantibiotics produced by Actinobacteria and their potential applications (a review). *Microbiology* **2017**, *163*, 109–121. [CrossRef] [PubMed]

46. Karpiński, T.M.; Szkaradkiewicz, A.K. Characteristic of bacteriocines and their application. *Pol. J. Microbiol.* **2013**, *62*, 223–235. [PubMed]

47. Paiva, A.D.; de Oliveira, M.D.; de Paula, S.O.; Baracat-Pereira, M.C.; Breukink, E.; Mantovani, H.C. Toxicity of bovicin HC5 against mammalian cell lines and the role of cholesterol in bacteriocin activity. *Microbiology* **2012**, *158*, 2851–2858. [CrossRef] [PubMed]

48. Chumchalova, J.; Smarda, J. Human tumor cells are selectively inhibited by colicins. *Folia Microbiol.* **2003**, *48*, 111–115. [CrossRef]

49. Baindara, P.; Gautam, A.; Raghava, G.P.S.; Korpole, S. Anticancer properties of a defensin like class IId bacteriocin Laterosporulin10. *Sci. Rep.* **2017**, *7*, 46541. [CrossRef] [PubMed]

50. Hetz, C.; Bono, M.R.; Barros, L.F.; Lagos, R. Microcin E492, a channel-forming bacteriocin from *Klebsiella pneumoniae*, induces apoptosis in some human cell lines. *Proc. Natl. Acad. Sci. USA* **2002**, *99*, 2696–2701. [CrossRef] [PubMed]

51. Lagos, R.; Tello, M.; Mercado, G.; García, V.; Monasterio, O. Antibacterial and antitumorigenic properties of microcin E492, a pore-forming bacteriocin. *Curr. Pharm. Biotechnol.* **2009**, *10*, 74–85. [CrossRef] [PubMed]

52. Begde, D.; Bundale, S.; Mashitha, P.; Rudra, J.; Nashikkar, N.; Upadhyay, A. Immunomodulatory efficacy of nisin—A bacterial lantibiotic peptide. *J. Pept. Sci.* **2011**, *17*, 438–444. [CrossRef] [PubMed]

53. Joo, N.E.; Ritchie, K.; Kamarajan, P.; Miao, D.; Kapila, Y.L. Nisin, an apoptogenic bacteriocin and food preservative, attenuates HNSCC tumorigenesis via CHAC1. *Cancer Med.* **2012**, *1*, 295–305. [CrossRef] [PubMed]

54. Kamarajan, P.; Hayami, T.; Matte, B.; Liu, Y.; Danciu, T.; Ramamoorthy, A.; Worden, F.; Kapila, S.; Kapila, Y. Nisin ZP a bacteriocin and food preservative, inhibits head and neck cancer tumorigenesis and prolongs survival. *PLoS ONE* **2015**, *10*, e0131008. [CrossRef] [PubMed]

55. Balgir, P.P.; Bhatia, P.; Kaur, B. Sequence analysis and homology based modeling to assess structure-function relationship of pediocin CP2 of *Pediococcus acidilactici* MTCC 5101. *Ind. J. Biotechnol.* **2010**, *9*, 431–434.

56. Kumar, B.; Balgir, P.P.; Kaur, B.; Mittu, B.; Chauhan, A. In vitro cytotoxicity of native and rec-pediocin CP2 against cancer cell lines: A comparative study. *Pharm. Anal. Acta* **2012**, *3*, 1000183. [CrossRef]

57. Villarante, K.I.; Elegado, F.B.; Iwatani, S.; Zendo, T.; Sonomoto, K.; de Guzman, E.E. Purification, characterization and in vitro cytotoxicity of the bacteriocin from *Pediococcus acidilactici* K2a2-3 against human colon adenocarcinoma (HT29) and human cervical carcinoma (HeLa) cells. *World J. Microbiol. Biotechnol.* **2011**, *27*, 975–980. [CrossRef]

58. Zhao, H.; Sood, R.; Jutila, A.; Bose, S.; Fimland, G.; Nissen-Meyer, J.; Kinnunen, P.K. Interaction of the antimicrobial peptide pheromone plantaricin A with model membranes: Implications for a novel mechanism of action. *Biochim. Biophys. Acta* **2006**, *1758*, 1461–1474. [CrossRef] [PubMed]

59. Abdi-Ali, A.; Worobec, E.A.; Deezagi, A.; Malekzadeh, F. Cytotoxic effects of pyocin S2 produced by *Pseudomonas aeruginosa* on the growth of three human cell lines. *Can. J. Microbiol.* **2004**, *50*, 375–381. [CrossRef] [PubMed]

60. Watanabe, T.; Saito, H. Cytotoxicity of pyocin S2 to tumor and normal cells and its interaction with cell surfaces. *Biochim. Biophys. Acta* **1980**, *633*, 77–86. [CrossRef]

61. Bactibase. Available online: http://bactibase.hammamilab.org (accessed on 12 February 2018).

62. Uniprot. Available online: http://www.uniprot.org (accessed on 12 February 2018).

63. Swiss-Model. Available online: http://swissmodel.expasy.org (accessed on 12 February 2018).

64. Kiefer, F.; Arnold, K.; Künzli, M.; Bordoli, L.; Schwede, T. The SWISS-MODEL Repository and associated resources. *Nucleic Acids Res.* **2009**, *37*, D387–D392. [CrossRef] [PubMed]

65. Smarda, J.; Fialova, M.; Smarda, J., Jr. Cytotoxic effects of colicins E1 and E3 on v-myb-transformed chicken monoblasts. *Folia Biol.* **2001**, *47*, 11–13.

66. Michel-Briand, Y.; Baysse, C. The pyocins of *Pseudomonas aeruginosa*. *Biochimie* **2002**, *84*, 499–510. [CrossRef]

67. Ni, Y.; Schwaneberg, U.; Sun, Z.H. Arginine deiminase, a potential anti-tumor drug. *Cancer Lett.* **2008**, *261*, 1–11. [CrossRef] [PubMed]

68. Glazer, E.S.; Piccirillo, M.; Albino, V.; Di Giacomo, R.; Palaia, R.; Mastro, A.A.; Beneduce, G.; Castello, G.; De Rosa, V.; Petrillo, A.; et al. Phase II study of pegylated arginine deiminase for nonresectable and metastatic hepatocellular carcinoma. *J. Clin. Oncol.* **2010**, *28*, 2220–2226. [CrossRef] [PubMed]

69. Kim, R.H.; Coates, J.M.; Bowles, T.L.; McNerney, G.P.; Sutcliffe, J.; Jung, J.U.; Gandour-Edwards, R.; Chuang, F.Y.S.; Bold, R.J.; Kung, H.-J. Arginine deiminase as a novel therapy for prostate cancer induces autophagy and caspase-independent apoptosis. *Cancer Res.* **2009**, *69*, 2. [CrossRef] [PubMed]

70. Fiedler, T.; Strauss, M.; Hering, S.; Redanz, U.; William, D.; Rosche, Y.; Classen, C.F.; Kreikemeyer, B.; Linnebacher, M.; Maletzki, C. Arginine deprivation by arginine deiminase of *Streptococcus pyogenes* controls primary glioblastoma growth in vitro and in vivo. *Cancer Biol. Ther.* **2015**, *16*, 1047–1055. [CrossRef] [PubMed]

71. Kaur, B.; Kaur, R. Purification of a dimeric arginine deiminase from *Enterococcus faecium* GR7 and study of its anti-cancerous activity. *Protein Expr. Purif.* **2016**, *125*, 53–60. [CrossRef] [PubMed]

72. Pritsa, A.A.; Papazisis, K.T.; Kortsaris, A.H.; Geromichalos, G.D.; Kyriakidis. Antitumor activity of L-asparaginase from *Thermus thermophilus*. *Anticancer Drugs* **2001**, *12*, 137–142. [CrossRef] [PubMed]

73. Avramis, V.I.; Sencer, S.; Periclou, A.P.; Sather, H.; Bostrom, B.C.; Cohen, L.J.; Ettinger, A.G.; Ettinger, L.J.; Franklin, J.; Gaynon, P.S.; et al. A randomized comparison of native *Escherichia coli* asparaginase and polyethylene glycol conjugated asparaginase for treatment of children with newly diagnosed standard-risk acute lymphoblastic leukemia: A Children's Cancer Group study. *Blood* **2002**, *99*, 1986–1994. [CrossRef] [PubMed]

74. Panosyan, E.H.; Wang, Y.; Xia, P.; Lee, W.N.; Pak, Y.; Laks, D.R.; Lin, H.J.; Moore, T.B.; Cloughesy, T.F.; Kornblum, H.I.; et al. Asparagine depletion potentiates the cytotoxic effect of chemotherapy against brain tumors. *Mol. Cancer Res.* **2014**, *12*, 694–702. [CrossRef] [PubMed]

75. Jaccard, A.; Gachard, N.; Marin, B.; Rogez, S.; Audrain, M.; Suarez, F.; Tilly, H.; Morschhauser, F.; Thieblemont, C.; Ysebaert, L.; et al. Efficacy of L-asparaginase with methotrexate and dexamethasone (AspaMetDex regimen) in patients with refractory or relapsing extranodal NK/T-cell lymphoma, a phase 2 study. *Blood* **2011**, *117*, 1834–1839. [CrossRef] [PubMed]

76. Covini, D.; Tardito, S.; Bussolati, O.; Chiarelli, L.R.; Pasquetto, M.V.; Digilio, R.; Valentini, G.; Scotti, C. Expanding targets for a metabolic therapy of cancer: L-asparaginase. *Recent Pat. Anti-Cancer Drug Discov.* **2012**, *7*, 4–13. [CrossRef]

77. Yu, M.; Henning, R.; Walker, A.; Kim, G.; Perroy, A.; Alessandro, R.; Virador, V.; Kohn, E.C. L-asparaginase inhibits invasive and angiogenic activity and induces autophagy in ovarian cancer. *J. Cell. Mol. Med.* **2012**, *16*, 2369–2378. [CrossRef] [PubMed]

78. Oza, V.P.; Parmar, P.P.; Kumar, S.; Subramanian, R.B. Anticancer properties of highly purified L-asparaginase from *Withania somnifera* L. against acute lymphoblastic leukemia. *Appl. Biochem. Biotechnol.* **2010**, *160*, 1833–1840. [CrossRef] [PubMed]

79. Meghavarnam, A.K.; Salah, M.; Sreepriya, M.; Janakiraman, S. Growth inhibitory and proapoptotic effects of L-asparaginase from *Fusarium culmorum* ASP-87 on human leukemia cells (Jurkat). *Fundam. Clin. Pharmacol.* **2017**, *31*, 292–300. [CrossRef] [PubMed]

80. Arjun, J.K.; Aneesh, B.P.; Kavitha, T.; Harikrishnan, K. Characterization of a novel asparaginase from soil metagenomic libraries generated from forest soil. *Biotechnol. Lett.* **2018**, *40*, 343–348. [CrossRef] [PubMed]

81. Takaku, H.; Takase, M.; Abe, S.; Hayashi, H.; Miyazaki, K. In vivo anti-tumor activity of arginine deiminase purified from *Mycoplasma arginini*. *Int. J. Cancer* **1992**, *51*, 244–249. [CrossRef] [PubMed]

82. Holtsberg, F.W.; Ensor, C.M.; Steiner, M.R.; Bomalaski, J.S.; Clark, M.A. Poly(ethylene glycol) (PEG) conjugated arginine deiminase: Effects of PEG formulations on its pharmacological properties. *J. Controll. Release* **2002**, *80*, 259–271. [CrossRef]

83. Pieters, R.; Hunger, S.P.; Boos, J.; Rizzari, C.; Silverman, L.; Baruchel, A.; Goekbuget, N.; Schrappe, M.; Pui, C.H. L-asparaginase treatment in acute lymphoblastic leukemia: A focus on *Erwinia* asparaginase. *Cancer* **2011**, *117*, 238–249. [CrossRef] [PubMed]

84. Agrawal, S.; Acharya, D.; Adholeya, A.; Barrow, C.J.; Deshmukh, S.K. Nonribosomal peptides from marine microbes and their antimicrobial and anticancer potential. *Front. Pharmacol.* **2017**, *8*, 828. [CrossRef] [PubMed]

85. Sieber, S.A.; Marahiel, M.A. Learning from nature's drug factories: Nonribosomal synthesis of macrocyclic peptides. *J. Bacteriol.* **2003**, *185*, 7036–7043. [CrossRef] [PubMed]

86. Asolkar, R.N.; Freel, K.C.; Jensen, P.R.; Fenical, W.; Kondratyuk, T.P.; Park, E.-J.; Pezzuto, J.M. Arenamides A–C, cytotoxic NFκB inhibitors from the marine actinomycete *Salinispora arenicola*. *J. Nat. Prod.* **2009**, *72*, 396–402. [CrossRef] [PubMed]

87. Oku, N.; Adachi, K.; Matsuda, S.; Kasai, H.; Takatsuki, A.; Shizuri, Y. Ariakemicins A and B, novel polyketide-peptide antibiotics from a marine gliding bacterium of the genus *Rapidithrix*. *Org. Lett.* **2008**, *10*, 2481–2484. [CrossRef] [PubMed]

88. Yang, L.; Tan, R.-X.; Wang, Q.; Huang, W.-Y.; Yin, Y.-X. Antifungal cyclopeptides from *Halobacillus litoralis* YS3106 of marine origin. *Tetrahedron Lett.* **2002**, *43*, 6545–6548. [CrossRef]

89. Kalinovskaya, N.I.; Romanenko, L.A.; Kalinovsky, A.I.; Dmitrenok, P.S.; Dyshlovoy, S.A. A new antimicrobial and anticancer peptide producing by the marine deep sediment strain "*Paenibacillus profundus*" sp. nov. Sl 79. *Nat. Prod. Commun.* **2013**, *8*, 381–384. [PubMed]

90. Tareq, F.S.; Kim, J.H.; Lee, M.A.; Lee, H.-S.; Lee, Y.-J.; Lee, J.S.; Shin, H.J. Ieodoglucomides A and B from a marine-derived bacterium *Bacillus licheniformis*. *Org. Lett.* **2012**, *14*, 1464–1467. [CrossRef] [PubMed]

91. Ma, Z.; Wang, N.; Hu, J.; Wang, S. Isolation and characterization of a new ituriniclipopeptide, mojavensin A produced by a marine-derived bacterium *Bacillus mojavensis* B0621A. *J. Antibiot.* **2012**, *65*, 317–322. [CrossRef] [PubMed]

92. Rama, M.R.; Teisan, S.; White, D.J.; Nicholson, B.; Grodberg, J.; Neuteboom, S.T.C.; Lam, K.S.; Mosca, D.A.; Lloyd, K.G.; Potts, B.C.M. Lajollamycin, a nitro-tetraene spiro-β-lactone-γ-lactam antibiotic from the marine actinomycete *Streptomyces nodosus*. *J. Nat. Prod.* **2005**, *68*, 240–243. [CrossRef]

93. Cho, J.Y.; Williams, P.G.; Kwon, H.C.; Jensen, P.R.; Fenical, W. Lucentamycins A-D, cytotoxic peptides from the marine-derived actinomycete *Nocardiopsis lucentensis*. *J. Nat. Prod.* **2007**, *70*, 1321–1328. [CrossRef] [PubMed]

94. Kanoh, K.; Matsuo, Y.; Adachi, K.; Imagawa, H.; Nishizawa, M.; Shizuri, Y. Mechercharmycins A and B, cytotoxic substances from marine-derived *Thermoactinomyces* sp. YM3-251. *J. Antibiot.* **2005**, *58*, 289–292. [CrossRef] [PubMed]

95. Zhang, H.L.; Hua, H.M.; Pei, Y.H.; Yao, X.S. Three new cytotoxic cyclic acylpeptides from marine *Bacillus* sp. *Chem. Pharm. Bull.* **2004**, *52*, 1029–1030. [CrossRef] [PubMed]

96. Um, S.; Choi, T.J.; Kim, H.; Kim, B.Y.; Kim, S.-H.; Lee, S.K.; Oh, K.-B.; Shin, J.; Oh, D.-C. Ohmyungsamycins A and B: Cytotoxic and antimicrobial cyclic peptides produced by *Streptomyces* sp. from a volcanic island. *J. Org. Chem.* **2013**, *78*, 12321–12329. [CrossRef] [PubMed]

97. Williams, D.E.; Dalisay, D.S.; Patrick, B.O.; Matainaho, T.; Andrusiak, K.; Deshpande, R.; Myers, C.L.; Piotrowski, J.S.; Boone, C.; Yoshida, M.; et al. Padanamides A and B, highly modified linear tetrapeptides produced in culture by a *Streptomyces* sp. isolated from a marine sediment. *Org. Lett.* **2011**, *13*, 3936–3939. [CrossRef] [PubMed]

98. Miller, E.D.; Kauffman, C.A.; Jensen, P.R.; Fenical, W. Piperazimycins: Cytotoxic hexadepsipeptides from a marine-derived bacterium of the genus *Streptomyces*. *J. Org. Chem.* **2007**, *72*, 323–330. [CrossRef] [PubMed]

99. Fiedler, H.-P.; Bruntner, C.; Riedlinger, J.; Bull, A.T.; Knutsen, G.; Goodfellow, M.; Jones, A.; Maldonado, L.; Pathom-aree, W.; Beil, W.; et al. Proximicin A, B and C, novel aminofuran antibiotic and anticancer compounds isolated from marine strains of the actinomycete *Verrucosispora*. *J. Antibiot.* **2008**, *61*, 158–163. [CrossRef] [PubMed]

100. Matsuo, Y.; Kanoh, K.; Yamori, T.; Kasai, H.; Katsuta, A.; Adachi, K.; Shin-Ya, K.; Shizuri, Y. Urukthapelstatin A, a novel cytotoxic substance from marine-derived *Mechercharimyces asporophorigenens* YM11-542. I. Fermentation, isolation and biological activities. *J. Antibiot.* **2007**, *60*, 251–255. [CrossRef] [PubMed]

101. Matsuo, Y.; Kanoh, K.; Imagawa, H.; Adachi, K.; Nishizawa, M.; Shizuri, Y. Urukthapelstatin A, a novel cytotoxic substance from marine-derived *Mechercharimyces asporophorigenens* YM11-542. II. Physico-chemical properties and structural elucidation. *J. Antibiot.* **2007**, *60*, 256–260. [CrossRef] [PubMed]

102. Henkel, J.S.; Baldwin, M.R.; Barbieri, J.T. Toxins from bacteria. *EXS* **2010**, *100*, 1–29. [PubMed]

103. Purkiss, J.R.; Friis, L.M.; Doward, S.; Quinn, C.P. *Clostridium botulinum* neurotoxins act with a wide range of potencies on SH-SY5Y human neuroblastoma cells. *Neurotoxicology* **2001**, *22*, 447–453. [CrossRef]

104. Karsenty, G.; Rocha, J.; Chevalier, S.; Scarlata, E.; Andrieu, C.; Zouanat, F.Z.; Rocchi, P.; Giusiano, S.; Elzayat, E.A.; Corcos, J. Botulinum toxin type A inhibits the growth of LNCaP human prostate cancer cells in vitro and in vivo. *Prostate* **2009**, *69*, 1143–1150. [CrossRef] [PubMed]

105. Proietti, S.; Nardicchi, V.; Porena, M.; Giannantoni, A. Botulinum toxin type-A toxin activity on prostate cancer cell lines. *Urologia* **2012**, *79*, 135–141. [CrossRef] [PubMed]

106. Bandala, C.; Perez-Santos, J.L.; Lara-Padilla, E.; Delgado Lopez, G.; Anaya-Ruiz, M. Effect of botulinum toxin A on proliferation and apoptosis in the T47D breast cancer cell line. *Asian Pac. J. Cancer Prev.* **2013**, *14*, 891–894. [CrossRef] [PubMed]

107. Holmes, R.K. Biology and molecular epidemiology of diphtheria toxin and the *tox* gene. *J. Infect. Dis.* **2000**, *181* (Suppl. 1), S156–S167. [CrossRef] [PubMed]

108. Martarelli, D.; Pompei, P.; Mazzoni, G. Inhibition of adrenocortical carcinoma by diphtheria toxin mutant CRM197. *Chemotherapy* **2009**, *55*, 425–432. [CrossRef] [PubMed]

109. Vallera, D.A.; Li, C.; Jin, N.; Panoskaltsis-Mortari, A.; Hall, W.A. Targeting urokinase-type plasminogen activator receptor on human glioblastoma tumors with diphtheria toxin fusion protein DTAT. *J. Natl. Cancer Inst.* **2002**, *94*, 597–606. [CrossRef] [PubMed]

110. Lutz, M.B.; Baur, A.S.; Schuler-Thurner, B.; Schuler, G. Immunogenic and tolerogenic effects of the chimeric IL-2-diphtheria toxin cytocidal agent Ontak® on CD25+ cells. *Oncoimmunology* **2014**, *3*, e28223. [CrossRef] [PubMed]

111. Shafiee, F.; Rabbani, M.; Jahanian-Najafabadi, A. Production and evaluation of cytotoxic effects of DT386-BR2 fusion protein as a novel anti-cancer agent. *J. Microbiol. Methods* **2016**, *130*, 100–105. [CrossRef] [PubMed]

112. Lewis, D.J.; Dao, H., Jr.; Nagarajan, P.; Duvic, M. Primary cutaneous anaplastic large-cell lymphoma: Complete remission for 13 years after denileukin diftitox. *JAAD Case Rep.* **2017**, *3*, 501–504. [CrossRef] [PubMed]

113. Alderson, R.F.; Kreitman, R.J.; Chen, T.; Yeung, P.; Herbst, R.; Fox, J.A.; Pastan, I. CAT-8015: A second-generation *Pseudomonas* exotoxin A-based immunotherapy targeting CD22-expressing hematologic malignancies. *Clin. Cancer Res.* **2009**, *15*, 832–839. [CrossRef] [PubMed]

114. Karpiński, T.M.; Szkaradkiewicz, A.K. Anticancer peptides from bacteria. *Bangladesh J. Pharmacol.* **2013**, *8*, 343–348. [CrossRef]

115. Oh, S.; Todhunter, D.A.; Panoskaltsis-Mortari, A.; Buchsbaum, D.J.; Toma, S.; Vallera, D.A. A deimmunized bispecific ligand-directed toxin that shows an impressive anti-pancreatic cancer effect in a systemic nude mouse orthotopic model. *Pancreas* **2012**, *41*, 789–796. [CrossRef] [PubMed]

116. Risberg, K.; Fodstad, O.; Andersson, Y. Synergistic anticancer effects of the 9.2.27PE immunotoxin and ABT-737 in melanoma. *PLoS ONE* **2011**, *6*, e24012. [CrossRef] [PubMed]

117. Waldron, N.N.; Kaufman, D.S.; Oh, S.; Inde, Z.; Hexum, M.K.; Ohlfest, J.R.; Vallera, D.A. Targeting tumor-initiating cancer cells with dCD133KDEL shows impressive tumor reductions in a xenotransplant model of human head and neck cancer. *Mol. Cancer Ther.* **2011**, *10*, 1829–1838. [CrossRef] [PubMed]

118. Kerr, D.E.; Wu, G.Y.; Wu, C.H.; Senter, P.D. Listeriolysin O potentiates immunotoxin and bleomycin cytotoxicity. *Bioconjug. Chem.* **1997**, *8*, 781–784. [CrossRef] [PubMed]

119. Provoda, C.J.; Stier, E.M.; Lee, K.D. Tumor cell killing enabled by listeriolysin O-liposome-mediated delivery of the protein toxin gelonin. *J. Biol. Chem.* **2003**, *278*, 35102–35108. [CrossRef] [PubMed]

120. Vázquez-Boland, J.A.; Kuhn, M.; Berche, P.; Chakraborty, T.; Domínguez-Bernal, G.; Goebel, W.; González-Zorn, B.; Wehland, J.; Kreft, J. *Listeria* pathogenesis and molecular virulence determinants. *Clin. Microbiol. Rev.* **2001**, *14*, 584–640. [CrossRef] [PubMed]

121. Bergelt, S.; Frost, S.; Lilie, H. Listeriolysin O as cytotoxic component of an immunotoxin. *Protein Sci.* **2009**, *18*, 1210–1220. [CrossRef] [PubMed]

122. Stachowiak, R.; Lyzniak, M.; Budziszewska, B.K.; Roeske, K.; Bielecki, J.; Hoser, G.; Kawiak, J. Cytotoxicity of bacterial metabolic products, including listeriolysin *O*, on leukocyte targets. *J. Biomed. Biotechnol.* **2012**, *2012*, 954375. [CrossRef] [PubMed]

123. Goto, M.; Yamada, T.; Kimbara, K.; Horner, J.; Newcomb, M.; Gupta, T.K.; Chakrabarty, A.M. Induction of apoptosis in macrophages by *Pseudomonas aeruginosa* azurin: Tumour-suppressor protein p53 and reactive oxygen species, but not redox activity, as critical elements in cytotoxicity. *Mol. Microbiol.* **2003**, *47*, 549–559. [CrossRef] [PubMed]

124. Gao, M.; Zhou, J.; Su, Z.; Huang, Y. Bacterial cupredoxin azurin hijacks cellular signaling networks: Protein-protein interactions and cancer therapy. *Protein Sci.* **2017**, *26*, 2334–2341. [CrossRef] [PubMed]

125. Punj, V.; Bhattacharyya, S.; Saint-Dic, D.; Vasu, C.; Cunningham, E.A.; Graves, J.; Yamada, T.; Constantinou, A.I.; Christov, K.; White, B.; et al. Bacterial cupredoxin azurin as an inducer of apoptosis and regression in human breast cancer. *Oncogene* **2004**, *23*, 2367–2378. [CrossRef] [PubMed]

126. Choi, J.-H.; Lee, M.-H.; Cho, Y.-J.; Park, B.S.; Kim, S.; Kim, G.C. The bacterial protein azurin enhances sensitivity of oral squamous carcinoma cells to anticancer drugs. *Yonsei Med. J.* **2011**, *52*, 773–778. [CrossRef] [PubMed]

127. Yamada, T.; Goto, M.; Punj, V.; Zaborina, O.; Chen, M.L.; Kimbara, K.; Majumdar, D.; Cunningham, E.; Das Gupta, T.K.; Chakrabarty, A.M. Bacterial redox protein azurin, tumor suppressor protein p53, and regression of cancer. *Proc. Natl. Acad. Sci. USA* **2002**, *99*, 14098–14103. [CrossRef] [PubMed]

128. Bernardes, N.; Chakrabarty, A.M.; Fialho, A.M. Engineering of bacterial strains and their products for cancer therapy. *Appl. Microbiol. Biotechnol.* **2013**, *97*, 5189–5199. [CrossRef] [PubMed]

129. Yamada, T.; Mehta, R.R.; Lekmine, F.; Christov, K.; King, M.L.; Majumdar, D.; Shilkaitis, A.; Green, A.; Bratescu, L.; Beattie, C.W.; et al. A peptide fragment of azurin induces a p53-mediated cell cycle arrest in human breast cancer cells. *Mol. Cancer Ther.* **2009**, *8*, 2947–2958. [CrossRef] [PubMed]

130. Mehta, R.R.; Yamada, T.; Taylor, B.N.; Christov, K.; King, M.L.; Majumdar, D.; Lekmine, F.; Tiruppathi, C.; Shilkaitis, A.; Bratescu, L.; et al. A cell penetrating peptide derived from azurin inhibits angiogenesis and tumor growth by inhibiting phosphorylation of VEGFR-2, FAK and Akt. *Angiogenesis* **2011**, *14*, 355–369. [CrossRef] [PubMed]

131. Yamada, T.; Das Gupta, T.K.; Beattie, C.W. p28-mediated activation of p53 in G2-M phase of the cell cycle enhances the efficacy of DNA damaging and antimitotic chemotherapy. *Cancer Res.* **2016**, *76*, 2354–2365. [CrossRef] [PubMed]

132. CDG. Available online: http://www.cdgti.com/clinical-trials/ (accessed on 14 February 2018).

133. Karpiński, T.M. New Peptide (Entap) with Anti-Proliferative Activity Produced by Bacteria of *Enterococcus* Genus. Habilitation Thesis, Scientific Publisher of Poznań University of Medical Sciences, Poznan, Poland, 2012. (In Polish)

134. Karpiński, T.M.; Szkaradkiewicz, A.; Gamian, A. New enterococcal anticancer peptide. In Proceedings of the 23rd European Congress of Clinical Microbiology and Infectious Diseases, Berlin, Germany, 27–30 April 2013.

135. Sung, W.S.; Park, Y.; Choi, C.H.; Hahm, K.S.; Lee, D.G. Mode of antibacterial action of a signal peptide, Pep27 from *Streptococcus pneumoniae*. *Biochem. Biophys. Res. Commun.* **2007**, *363*, 806–810. [CrossRef] [PubMed]

136. Lee, D.G.; Hahm, K.-S.; Park, Y.; Kim, H.Y.; Lee, W.; Lim, S.C.; Seo, Y.K.; Choi, C.H. Functional and structural characteristics of anticancer peptide Pep27 analogues. *Cancer Cell Int.* **2005**, *5*, 21. [CrossRef] [PubMed]

137. I-TASSER. Available online: http://zhanglab.ccmb.med.umich.edu/I-TASSER/ (accessed on 16 February 2018).

138. Pangestuti, R.; Kim, S.-K. Bioactive peptide of marine origin for the prevention and treatment of non-communicable diseases. *Mar. Drugs* **2017**, *15*, 67. [CrossRef] [PubMed]

139. Vijaya, T. Anticancer, antimicrobial and antioxidant bioactive factors derived from marine fungal endophytes; a review. *Indo Am. J. Pharm. Res.* **2017**, *7*, 7313–7321.

140. Guzmán-Rodríguez, J.J.; Ochoa-Zarzosa, A.; López-Gómez, R.; López-Meza, J.E. Plant antimicrobial peptides as potential anticancer agents. *BioMed Res. Int.* **2015**, *2015*, 735087. [CrossRef] [PubMed]

141. Negi, B.; Kumar, D.; Rawat, D.S. Marine peptides as anticancer agents: A remedy to mankind by nature. *Curr. Protein Pept. Sci.* **2017**, *18*, 885–904. [CrossRef] [PubMed]

142. Karpiński, T.M.; Szkaradkiewicz, A.K. Human defensins. *Arch. Biomed. Sci.* **2013**, *1*, 1–5.

143. Deslouches, B.; Di, P.Y. Antimicrobial peptides with selective antitumor mechanisms: Prospect for anticancer applications. *Oncotarget* **2017**, *8*, 46635–46651. [CrossRef] [PubMed]

144. Huang, L.; Chen, D.; Wang, L.; Lin, C.; Ma, C.; Xi, X.; Chen, T.; Shaw, C.; Zhou, M. Dermaseptin-PH: A novel peptide with antimicrobial and anticancer activities from the skin secretion of the south american orange-legged leaf frog, *Pithecopus (Phyllomedusa) hypochondrialis*. *Molecules* **2017**, *22*, 1805. [CrossRef] [PubMed]

145. Dykhuizen, D. Species numbers in bacteria. *Proc. Calif. Acad. Sci.* **2005**, *56* (Suppl. 1), 62–71. [PubMed]

146. Schloss, P.D.; Girard, R.A.; Martin, T.; Edwards, J.; Thrash, J.C. Status of the archaeal and bacterial census: An update. *mBio* **2016**, *7*, E00201-16. [CrossRef] [PubMed]

147. Cheung, R.C.; Ng, T.B.; Wong, J.H. Marine peptides: Bioactivities and applications. *Mar. Drugs* **2015**, *13*, 4006–4043. [CrossRef] [PubMed]

148. Daliri, E.B.-M.; Oh, D.H.; Lee, B.H. Bioactive peptides. *Foods* **2017**, *6*, 32. [CrossRef] [PubMed]

149. Shin, J.M.; Gwak, J.W.; Kamarajan, P.; Fenno, J.C.; Rickard, A.H.; Kapila, Y.L. Biomedical applications of nisin. *J. Appl. Microbiol.* **2016**, *120*, 1449–1465. [CrossRef] [PubMed]

150. Sharifi, M.; Moridnia, A.; Mortazavi, D.; Salehi, M.; Bagheri, M.; Sheikhi, A. Kefir: A powerful probiotics with anticancer properties. *Med. Oncol.* **2017**, *34*, 183. [CrossRef] [PubMed]

151. Ruiz-Torres, V.; Encinar, J.A.; Herranz-López, M.; Pérez-Sánchez, A.; Galiano, V.; Barrajón-Catalán, E.; Micol, V. An updated review on marine anticancer compounds: The use of virtual screening for the discovery of small-molecule cancer drugs. *Molecules* **2017**, *22*, 1037. [CrossRef] [PubMed]

152. Gilad, Y.; Firer, M.; Gellerman, G. Recent innovations in peptide based targeted drug delivery to cancer cells. *Biomedicines* **2016**, *4*, 11. [CrossRef] [PubMed]

14

Extended Duration Vascular Endothelial Growth Factor Inhibition in the Eye: Failures, Successes, and Future Possibilities

Michael W. Stewart

Department of Ophthalmology, Mayo Clinic School of Medicine, 4500 San Pablo Rd., Jacksonville, FL 32224, USA; stewart.michael@mayo.edu

Abstract: Vascular endothelial growth factor (VEGF) plays a pivotal role in the development of neovascularization and edema from several common chorioretinal vascular conditions. The intravitreally injected drugs (aflibercept, bevacizumab, conbercept, pegaptanib, and ranibizumab) used to treat these conditions improve the visual acuity and macular morphology in most patients. Monthly or bimonthly injections were administered in the phase III pivotal trials but physicians usually individualize therapy with *pro re nata* (PRN) or treat and extend regimens. Despite these lower frequency treatment regimens, frequent injections and clinic visits are still needed to produce satisfactory outcomes. Newly developed drugs and refillable reservoirs with favorable pharmacokinetic profiles may extend durations of action and require fewer office visits. However, we have learned from previous experiences that the longer durations of action seen in strategically designed phase III trials often do not translate to less frequent injections in real-life clinical practice. Unfortunately, long-acting therapies that produce soluble VEGF receptors (encapsulated cell technology and adenovirus injected DNA) have failed in phase II trials. The development of longer duration therapies remains a difficult and frustrating process, and frequent drug injections are likely to remain the standard-of-care for years to come.

Keywords: age-related macular degeneration; diabetic macular edema; extended duration therapy; intravitreal injections; vascular endothelial growth factor

---

1. Introduction

The discovery of vascular endothelial growth factor (VEGF) [1,2] and the subsequent recognition of its critical role in the pathogenesis of several chorioretinal vascular conditions constitute the most important advances in ophthalmology over the past 30 years. Strong evidence correlates the development of both neovascularization and macular edema in the two most common causes of blindness in industrialized nations—neovascular age-related macular degeneration (nAMD) and diabetic retinopathy (DR)—with the upregulation of VEGF [3]. Furthermore, disease severity frequently correlates with intraocular VEGF concentrations, thereby making VEGF a logical target for therapeutic intervention.

Soon after VEGF was discovered and sequenced, the production of inhibitory molecules began [4]. Thus far, five VEGF-neutralizing molecules (pegaptanib, Macugen®, Bausch & Lomb, Bridgewater, NJ, USA; ranibizumab, Lucentis®, Genentech, S. San Francisco, CA, USA/Roche, Basel, Switzerland; aflibercept, Eylea®, Regeneron, Tarrytown, NY, USA; conbercept, Chengdu Kanghong Pharmaceutical Group, Chengdu, China; and bevacizumab, Avastin®, Genentech, S. San Francisco, CA, USA/Roche, Basel, Switzerland) have been used to treat ophthalmologic conditions, though only the first three have received United States Food and Drug Administration (US FDA) approval for intraocular use. Intravitreal therapy usually begins with monthly injections (in accordance with package labeling) but most physicians will attempt to extend the time between injections as much as possible with either monthly *pro re nata* (PRN) or treat and extend strategies [5]. Treatment intervals for many patients cannot be extended beyond eight weeks [6], resulting in a large group of patients who require frequent injections for long periods of time. This large number of intravitreal injections burdens physicians and their staffs, and challenges patients' compliance. Therefore, new, longer acting anti-VEGF medications and drug delivery systems are needed to improve outcomes, optimize compliance, and reduce the total cost of care.

This manuscript discusses extended duration anti-VEGF therapies that have been recently introduced, as well as those that are in various stages of development.

2. Vascular Endothelial Growth Factor (VEGF) Physiology and Pharmacokinetics

VEGF was discovered independently by two research groups in 1989 [1,2] and its important role in both physiologic angiogenesis and pathological neovascularization was realized almost immediately. VEGF is actually a group of molecules that segregate into seven closely related families: VEGF-A, VEGF-B, VEGF-C, VEGF-D, VEGF-E, VEGF-F, and placental growth factor (PlGF) [7]. Each of the families is characterized by common, critical binding sequences, and most families contain multiple isoforms that share similar binding properties and biological actions.

VEGF-A synthesis is upregulated in eyes with chorioretinal vascular conditions, including nAMD, diabetic macular edema (DME), and retinal vein occlusion (RVO) [3], and is believed to play a central role in the development of these conditions. Several in vivo models show that VEGF-A promotes the growth of choroidal neovascular membranes [8] and produces retinal vascular lesions that resemble DR [9]. Evidence suggests that $VEGF_{165}$ may be the most biologically active isoform because of its high tissue concentrations and 10-fold potentiation of activity through its interaction with the transmembrane co-receptor neuropilin-1 [10]. Most VEGF inhibitory molecules block the receptor binding region (amino acids 81–92) of VEGF-A isoforms, whereas pegaptanib interacts with the heparin binding region (amino acids 110–165) of $VEGF_{165}$. Research suggests that VEGF-B, VEGF-C, VEGF-D, and PlGF may also contribute to pathologic ocular angiogenesis in humans but their relative contribution is not known [11,12].

Increased VEGF synthesis by vascular endothelial cells, glia, pericytes, Müller cells, retinal pigment epithelium (RPE) cells, and invading leukocytes [13,14] results from tissue ischemia and inflammation [15,16]. Cells throughout the retina and choroid respond to increased VEGF concentrations but the primary targets are retinal and choroidal vascular endothelial cells [17].

VEGF-A has a short half-life of 30 min in the eye and serum, and homeostatic concentrations are generally low (approximately 9 ng/mL) [18]. Some systemic conditions increase serum VEGF concentrations but chorioretinal vascular conditions produce insufficient VEGF to meaningfully change serum levels.

3. Currently Available Therapies

Several anti-VEGF drugs have been developed exclusively for ocular use or, in the case of bevacizumab, are used off-label for chorioretinal vascular conditions. Peak clinical efficacies of these drugs (except for pegaptanib) are similar and though product labels describe different injection intervals (monthly or every two months) the differences in their duration of action are on the order of only days. Currently available drugs, recently failed therapies, and drugs and systems under development are listed in Table 1.

Table 1. This table lists the currently available anti-VEGF drugs, several that have failed clinical trials, and others that are in various stages of development. Additional information includes regulatory approvals and comments on drug characteristics, pharmacokinetics, preclinical studies, and clinical trials. AMD: age-related macular degeneration; DME: diabetic macular edema; DR: diabetic retinopathy; RVO: retinal vein occlusion; VEGF: vascular endothelial growth factor; PlGF: placental growth factor; CNVM: choroidal neovascular membrane; RPE: retinal pigment epithelium; BCVA: best corrected visual acuity.

Currently Available Drugs		
Drug	**Approvals**	**Comments**
Pegaptanib	Neovascular AMD	• Binds to $VEGF_{165}$ • Poor efficacy [19], used rarely
Bevacizumab	Advanced carcinomas [20] Off-label for all ophthalmic use	• Recombinant, humanized, murine antibody to VEGF-A • National Eye Institute sponsored studies have established effectiveness for neovascular AMD [6], DME [21], and RVOs • Inexpensive dose cost after compounding • Most commonly used intraocular anti-VEGF drug in the United States
Ranibizumab	Neovascular AMD, DME, DR, Macular edema due to RVOs, Myopic CNVM [22]	• Recombinant, humanized, murine antibody fragment (Fab) to VEGF-A [4] • Most thoroughly studied anti-VEGF drug
Aflibercept	Neovascular AMD [23], DME, DR, Macular edema due to RVOs	• Completely human, fusion protein, soluble receptor [24] • High affinity for VEGF-A, VEGF-B, and PlGF
Conbercept	Neovascular AMD (China only)	• Similar structure and binding affinity as aflibercept [24,25] • In phase III DME trial • United States trials being planned
Therapies Under Development or Recently Failed		
Drug	**Technology**	**Comments**
Abicipar	Designed Ankyrin Repeat Protein (DARPin)	• Pegylation may extend intravitreal half-life (estimated as 13.4 days in humans) [26] • Phase III CEDAR and SEQUOIA nAMD trials have completed enrollment • q8week and q12week experimental arms; control is q4week ranibizumab
Brolucizumab	Single strand, antibody fragment	• Small size (26 kDa) allows for injection of large quantity of drug [27] • Phase III nAMD trials recently completed • 57% and 52% of eyes sustained with q12week injection intervals [28]
Ranibizumab Port Delivery System	Trans-scleral refillable drug reservoir	• Reservoir is refilled via trans-conjunctival injection • Phase I study showed +10 letter improvement in BCVA with average of 4.8 refills [29] • Phase II LADDER trial underway with three different dose treatment arms [30]

Table 1. *Cont.*

Therapies Under Development or Recently Failed		
Drug	Technology	Comments
AVA-101	Adenovirus vector Insertion of soluble VEGF-receptor DNA	• Injected subretinally after vitrectomy • BCVA changes were better than ranibizumab in phase II trial but both arms performed poorly with minimal decrease in edema [31]
NT-503	Encapsulated Cell Technology using immortalized RPE cells	• Ciliary neurotrophic eluting device failed in dry AMD and retinitis pigmentosa trials [32] • High dose (NT-503) device failed in phase II neovascular AMD trial [33] • Currently being tested in patients with macular telangiectasia
Colloidal Carriers	Liposomal formulated ranibizumab	• Liposomal formulation delays drug release • Ranibizumab can cross sclera after subconjunctival depot [34]
Posterior Micropump Delivery System	Microelectromechanical Systems (MEMS) Technology	• Same technology as in insulin pumps • Safely delivered 100 injections in animal models [35,36] • Three-month DME trial in humans was well tolerated [37]
PAN-90806	Small molecular weight drug	• Formulated for eye drop delivery • In animal models, found to produce high retinal concentrations 17 h later • Judged to show therapeutic promise in small human nAMD study [38]

3.1. Pegaptanib

Pegaptanib (molecular weight (MW) of 50 kDa), an aptamer to VEGF, was the first ocular drug approved for the intravitreal treatment of neovascular age-related macular degeneration (nAMD). Clinicians hoped that q6week treatment with pegaptanib would improve best corrected visual acuity (BCVA) but in most eyes it only decreased the rate of vision loss by approximately one half [19]. Its use dropped significantly when more potent anti-VEGF drugs were introduced and pegaptanib is rarely used today.

3.2. Bevacizumab

Bevacizumab is a full-length, recombinant, humanized, monoclonal antibody (MW of 149 kDa) that binds all isoforms of VEGF-A. It was developed and approved for the intravenous treatment of several advanced solid tumors (colorectal carcinoma, non-small cell lung carcinoma, renal cell carcinoma, glioblastoma, and breast cancer, though this approval was rescinded in 2011) [20].

Single injections of bevacizumab were first given to patients with nAMD and macular edema due to a central retinal vein occlusion (CRVO) in 2005 [39,40], and within six months off-label use of bevacizumab had become the accepted standard-of-care treatment of chorioretinal vascular conditions. Hundreds of ocular disease studies have established bevacizumab's efficacy and safety, though the best evidence comes from the Comparison of Age-related Macular Degeneration Treatment Trials (CATT) for nAMD and the Diabetic Retinopathy Clinical Research Network Protocol T trial for DME [6,21].

The use of bevacizumab varies among countries due to regulatory restrictions, reimbursement policies, and availability of safely compounded drug. Because physicians have accumulated extensive clinical experience with bevacizumab and are able to acquire it inexpensively, bevacizumab remains the most commonly used anti-VEGF drug in the United States.

3.3. Ranibizumab

Ranibizumab is a recombinant, humanized, monoclonal antibody fragment (Fab with MW of 48 kDa) that binds all isoforms of VEGF-A [4]. It has been approved by the United States Food and Drug Administration (USFDA) for the treatment of nAMD (2006), DME, DR, macular edema due to vein occlusions, and choroidal neovascular membranes (CNVM) associated with high myopia [22].

Following completion of the phase III MARINA and ANCHOR trials, ranibizumab was approved for the monthly treatment of nAMD and subsequently for PRN treatment. The CATT trial reported that PRN treatment is non-inferior to monthly treatment for nAMD [6] though pooled data from CATT and IVAN suggest that PRN is inferior to monthly injections. Ranibizumab is approved for the monthly treatment of DME, but after one year of intensive treatment in the Diabetic Retinopathy Clinical Research (DRCR).net Protocol I trial, less frequent injections are needed during subsequent years [41].

Because ranibizumab was the first approved intravitreal anti-VEGF drug (after pegaptanib), it became the standard against which other drugs have been compared in most randomized, controlled trials. These trials have included CATT [6], IVAN [42], and the other national AMD trials; the VIEW 1 and 2 trials (nAMD) [43]; CEDAR and SEQUOIA (nAMD); and DRCR.net Protocol T (DME) [21].

3.4. Aflibercept

Aflibercept is a recombinant fusion protein (MW of 115 kDa) consisting of the natural (all human) extracellular ligand binding sequences of VEGFR1 (domain 2) and VEGFR2 (domain 3) attached to the Fc portion of an IgG molecule [24]. Aflibercept is approved for the treatment of nAMD, DME, DR, and macular edema due to RVO [23].

The three-dimensional configuration of aflibercept enables it to simultaneously bind both sides of the VEGF dimer in a "two-fisted grasp". This results in a higher binding affinity for $VEGF_{165}$ ($k_D = 0.45$ pM) compared to ranibizumab ($k_D = 46$–172 pM) and bevacizumab ($k_D = 58$–1100 pM) [44]. Rabbit studies suggest that aflibercept has a slightly longer intravitreal half-life that either bevacizumab or ranibizumab but head-to-head human studies have not been performed [45].

Peak efficacy of aflibercept in patients with nAMD is similar to that of ranibizumab but the duration of action is slightly longer [46]. Though aflibercept is approved for q8week dosing (compared to monthly for ranibizumab), its duration of action exceeds that of ranibizumab by only five to seven days. So despite the fact that the phase III trials suggested that aflibercept could be equally effective with only half the dosing frequency of ranibizumab, clinical use suggests that the difference is considerably shorter.

Ziv-aflibercept (Zaltrap®, Regeneron, Tarrytown, NY, USA) is the intravenous formulation of aflibercept that is used to treat advanced colorectal carcinoma. Small series of patients with nAMD, DME, and RVOs have responded well to intravitreal ziv-aflibercept with excellent improvements in macular morphology and visual acuity [47]. Head-to-head studies with aflibercept have not been performed, but the two molecules will likely perform comparably, though the lower dose of ziv-aflibercept (1.25 mg vs. 2 mg) may provide a slightly shorter duration of action.

3.5. Conbercept

Conbercept (KH902, Chengdu Kanghong Biotech Co., Sichuan, China) is a recombinant, fusion protein (MW of 143 kDa) that contains the second immunoglobulin (Ig) binding domain from VEGFR1, the third and the fourth binding domains from VEGFR2, and the Fc region of human IgG. Like aflibercept, conbercept acts as a soluble, decoy receptor [24,25] that binds all isoforms of VEGF-A, VEGF-B, and placental growth factor. Conbercept has a high affinity for $VEGF_{165}$ ($k_D = 0.77$ pM) because the fourth Ig domain of VEGFR2 enhances the association rate of VEGF to the receptor [25].

At concentrations between 100 ng/mL and 100 μg/mL, conbercept is not cytotoxic to cultured human retinal vascular endothelial cells (hRVACs). Conbercept significantly suppresses glucose-induced migration and sprouting of hRVACs by downregulating the expression of phosphoinositide 3-kinase and inhibiting the activation of Src, Akt1, and Erk1/2 [48]. Four weeks after intravitreal injection, conbercept-treated diabetic rats had better retinal electrophysiological function, less retinal vessel leakage, and lower levels of PlGF, VEGFR2, PI3K, Akt, p-Akt, p-ERK and p-SRC than did Pbs or bevacizumab-treated rats [49]. The distribution of claudin-5 and occludin in the retinal vessels of diabetic rats treated with conbercept was smoother and more uniform than those of diabetic rats treated by Pbs or bevacizumab.

Conbercept is approved in China for the treatment of nAMD and a phase III trial evaluating the efficacy of conbercept for the treatment of DME is currently enrolling patients. Conbercept trials within the United States are now being planned.

4. Therapies under Development

The currently available anti-VEGF drugs have significantly advanced our treatment of chorioretinal vascular conditions and have benefitted hundreds of thousands of patients, but injections must usually be administered every four to eight weeks and treatment often continues for years. The extended durations of action that were promised by the newer drugs have not concretized, since a wealth of clinical experience shows us that the differences among the drugs are far shorter than are suggested by the packaging labels.

Nevertheless, research continues with new drugs and delivery methods that developers hope will extend the clinical duration of action. Several of the most promising drugs and some of the recent failures are discussed below.

4.1. Abicipar Pegol

Abicipar pegol is a designed ankyrin repeat protein (DARPin) that binds all isoforms of VEGF-A. Its small size (MW = 34 kDa) would suggest a brief intraocular half-life, but pegylation (binding to a poly(ethylene) glycol moiety) may give it the pharmacokinetic characteristics of a much larger molecule (approximately 250–350 kDa) [50]. Abicipar has an intravitreal half-life of six days in rabbits and, in a small DME study of four eyes, of 13.4 days in humans [26]. Its strong binding affinity to $VEGF_{165}$ ($k_D = 2$ pM) also favors a long duration of action.

In dose escalation trials, a maximum tolerated dose of 4.2 mg was found, so investigators elected to develop the two-milligram dose. In the phase II PALM DME trial, abicipar injections every 8 or 12 weeks were non-inferior to monthly ranibizumab [51]. In the ongoing phase III nAMD CEDAR (NCT02462928) and SEQUOIA (NCT02462486) trials, q8week and q12week abicipar is being compared to monthly ranibizumab.

4.2. Brolucizumab

Brolucizumab is a single-chain, high binding affinity (k_D for $VEGF_{165}$ = 1.6 pM), antibody fragment currently being developed by Alcon/Novartis (Ft. Worth, TX; Basel, Switzerland) for the treatment of nAMD [52]. Its small size (MW = 26 kDa) allows for the injection (six milligrams) of 12–24 times as many molecules as with the other anti-VEGF drugs [27].

A phase II clinical trial compared brolucizumab to aflibercept in patients with nAMD. The trial's primary objective was to compare the efficacy of six-milligram brolucizumab against two-milligram aflibercept with the primary endpoint being the mean change in BCVA from baseline to 12 weeks. Patients continued receiving q8week treatment until week 40, though brolucizumab patients were eligible for two q12week cycles. At week 12, BCVA gains with brolucizumab (+5.75 letters) were similar to those with aflibercept (+6.89 letters). Approximately 50% of brolucizumab patients were stable during the q12week cycles [53].

The phase III nAMD clinical trials, HAWK and HARRIER, were initiated in December 2014, with an enrollment goal of 1700 patients in more than 50 countries. These two-year, double-masked, multi-center trials randomize patients with untreated nAMD to one of two dosage intervals of brolucizumab, or aflibercept bimonthly. At the 48-week primary endpoint, mean BCVA gains in both brolucizumab arms were non-inferior to aflibercept. The majority of patients receiving six milligrams brolucizumab (57% and 52%) were maintained exclusively on q12week dosing [28].

4.3. Ranibizumab Port Delivery System

A refillable ranibizumab port delivery system is being co-developed by Genentech and ForSight Vision 4 to reduce the need for repeated intravitreal anti-VEGF injections. The preloaded implant is surgically implanted beneath the conjunctiva through a 3.2 mm scleral incision over the pars plana. The reservoir tip can be accessed easily in the office and refilled through the conjunctiva as needed. The device continuously releases ranibizumab into the vitreous between refills.

A phase I trial for patients with nAMD was performed in Latvia [29]. At baseline, the reservoir was implanted and eyes were given 500 µg of ranibizumab, 250 µg into the vitreous and 250 µg into the reservoir for sustained release. Additional refills were performed when indicated by optical coherence tomography (OCT) evaluation of disease activity. The primary endpoint was 12 months with an observation period that extended through 36 months. The primary objective of the study was safety assessment, with secondary objectives that included functional measurements.

Four of the patients suffered significant or serious adverse events (endophthalmitis, vitreous hemorrhage (2), and traumatic cataract) but three of these four had improved vision by the study's endpoint. The average visual acuity gains for the cohort were +10 letters, 10 eyes (50%) gained at least three lines, and two (10%) lost at least three lines. The mean number of refills through 12 months was 4.8 per patient.

The multicenter, randomized, treatment-control, phase II LADDER trial will include 220 patients at 55 U.S. sites. Patients will be randomized 3:3:3:2 to receive one of three different ranibizumab implant doses or monthly 0.5 mg ranibizumab injections. Study enrollment was completed in October 2017 [30].

4.4. Gene Therapy

Avalanche Biotechnologies developed a viral delivery system (AVA-101) to induce long-term anti-VEGF receptor synthesis by the outer retina. An adenovirus vector inserts the DNA for a naturally occurring sFLT-1 (soluble VEGF receptor-1) into RPE cells. Infected cells synthesize and excrete the soluble VEGF inhibitory protein into the outer retina and choriocapillaris.

In a phase IIa trial, 21 patients with nAMD received AVA-101, with 0.5 mg ranibizumab injected both at baseline and one month, and as rescue therapy when needed. Patients underwent core vitrectomy and subretinal injection of AVA-101 adjacent to the macula at day seven. Evaluations were performed monthly and patients were eligible for rescue ranibizumab therapy based on pre-specified criteria. Eleven control patients received only 0.5 mg ranibizumab monthly.

At the 52-week endpoint, mean improvement in BCVA was +2.2 letters in the AVA-101 group compared to −9.3 letters in the control group [31]. These differences were statistically significant. Mean center point thickness improved by −27 µm in the AVA-101 group and −85 µm in the control group. There were no serious ocular adverse events in the AVA-101 group and no systemic safety signals were noted. All patients in the AVA-101 group that were phakic at baseline developed cataracts and three (14%) developed moderate vitreous hemorrhages. Gene therapy was well tolerated by patients but the technology failed to provide a complete or durable anti-VEGF response.

Though AVA-101 produced superior BCVA changes compared to the control group, the overall performance of the AVA-101 group was disappointing. Soon after the phase IIa trial results were announced, Avalanche decided not to proceed with phase IIb trials [54].

4.5. Encapsulated Cell Technology

Encapsulated cell technology (ECT) uses immortalized RPE cells that have been programmed to over-synthesize a specified biochemical product, and packages them in a cylinder lined by semi-permeable membranes that allow ingress of nutrients and egress of the synthesized product. The membrane prevents outward migration of the modified cells while shielding them from the body's immune system. The 10 mm long cylinder is surgically implanted through the pars plana and is sutured to the sclera.

Trials with ciliary neurotrophic factor (CNF) production have been completed in eyes with retinitis pigmentosa and atrophic AMD [32]. Pharmacokinetic analyses showed that the half-life of CNF production was 54 months and the ECT cylinder was well tolerated. Unfortunately, the trials failed to meet their primary therapeutic endpoints.

Phase I trials with a cylinder that produces a high-affinity VEGF binding protein similar to aflibercept have been completed. A multi-center phase II trial compared a higher dose, anti-VEGF implant against ranibizumab therapy. The trial was discontinued early because a larger number of patients than expected required intravitreal rescue injections [33]. No further nAMD trials have been announced but Neurotech continues to develop the platform for other retinal vascular conditions such as macular telangiectasia.

4.6. Colloidal Carriers

Injections of some liposomal drug formulations have shown promise including early work with anti-VEGF agents. In experimental models, in vitro release of ranibizumab from negatively charged liposomes was exhausted at two days, whereas ex vivo transport across sclera (simulating a subconjunctival injection) occurred in a linear manner for seven days [34]. This suggests that sclera acts as a classic membrane that allows the diffusion of liposomal-formulated ranibizumab and raises the possibility that subconjunctival injections could serve as long-acting depots. These results differ from those reported by Kim et al. [55] in which poly lactic-co-glycolic acid nanoparticles and liposomes do not facilitate drug diffusion across sclera. A steep concentration gradient created by the thick sclera, Bruch's membrane-choroid, and retinal pigment epithelium results in low drug concentrations within the retina.

4.7. Pump Delivery

Microelectromechanical system (MEMS) technology is a miniaturized system that is currently used in insulin pumps to deliver drug to tissues. The Posterior MicroPump Drug Delivery System (PMP, Replenish Inc., Pasadena, CA, USA) using MEMS technology is implanted on the sclera, similar to placement of a glaucoma drainage device, to deliver drug into the eye. Long-term safety after implantation into animal eyes has been demonstrated [35,36] as the PMP reliably delivered 100 programmed doses of an anti-VEGF drug (equivalent to over eight years of therapy). The PMP was well tolerated by 11 patients with DME over three months, with no cases of endophthalmitis or strabismus [37].

4.8. Topical Therapy

PanOptica, Inc. is developing a topical anti-VEGF medication (PAN-90806) for the treatment of nAMD and proliferative diabetic retinopathy (PDR). In animal models, pharmacokinetic measurements show excellent drug concentrations in the central retina and choroid as long as 17 h after administration. Control of leakage and bleeding from choroidal neovascular membranes was comparable to that achievable with intravitreal anti-VEGF antibodies, but with minimal systemic exposure to the drug.

In a phase II trial with 50 treatment-naïve nAMD patients, an independent panel of experts judged that PAN-90806 showed promise as a therapeutic agent [38]. Approximately 45–50% of treated patients experienced improvements in vascular leakage, retinal morphology, and vision. No systemic adverse events were noted and ocular surface irritation due to the eye drops reversed when therapy was discontinued. PanOptica plans to investigate higher doses in a phase I/II nAMD trial, and a phase I trial for the treatment of PDR is underway.

5. Discussion

The quest for longer duration anti-VEGF therapies continues along several fronts with the injectable drugs abicipar and brolucizumab most likely to achieve US FDA approval. Each drug may be shown to be effective as q12week therapy—roughly half of the brolucizumab patients were sustained on q12week injections—but the importance of such a finding is not clear. Control groups in the phase III trials were treated with q4week ranibizumab and q8week aflibercept but neither of these drugs was tested in a q12week arm. Therefore, true head-to-head comparisons of these control drugs to abicipar and brolucizumab have not been performed with similar injection frequencies.

In the VIEW trials, q4week ranibizumab was compared to q8week aflibercept during the first year. Aflibercept-treated patients experienced comparable improvements in BCVA and edema at 52 weeks compared to ranibizumab and was approved for q8week therapy (compared to q4week for ranibizumab). However, when patients received PRN (with 12-week cap) injections in the second year of the trials, aflibercept-treated patients received a mean of 4.2 injections, compared to 4.7 for ranibizumab. This difference in durations of action has been estimated to be five to seven days and post-approval experience also suggests that the difference is small. It is reasonable to suspect that post-approval differences with abicipar and brolucizumab will also be disappointingly small.

The quest for a single application, long-term anti-VEGF therapy has been disappointing. Encapsulated cell technology and adenovirus-mediated gene therapy are exciting technologies, but both failed to perform adequately in phase II trials and neither developer will pursue phase III anti-VEGF trials.

The ranibizumab port delivery system allows for trans-conjunctival (as opposed to intravitreal) injections as needed. However, since the phase I trial required a mean of 4.8 refills over the course of 12 months, this does little to decrease the frequency of clinic visits or injections. Unless the new dosing arms in the phase II trials decrease the number of refills, many physicians will likely continue with PRN and treat and extend regimens since they have comparable treatment burdens.

The use of eye drops does not constitute long-duration therapy but some patients will prefer self-administering drops when coupled with infrequent visits to the clinic. Eye drops effectively treat many anterior segment conditions and experimental CNVM in rats, but drops do not effectively treat retinal disorders in humans. Because topically delivered medications must pass through cornea, conjunctiva, sclera, uvea, and vitreous to reach the retina, the molecule must be small. Therefore, antibody-related macromolecules would be ineffective in eye drop form.

We have been fortunate in identifying VEGF as a pivotal molecule in the pathogenesis of chorioretinal vascular conditions, but just as the search for additional molecular targets has been disappointing, our attempts to significantly extend the duration of action of anti-VEGF therapy has met with more failures than successes. Despite ongoing research, it remains likely that frequent injection of anti-VEGF drugs will remain the standard-of-care for several years to come.

Author Contributions: Michael W. Stewart was solely responsible for the production of this manuscript.

References

1. Connolly, D.T.; Heuvelman, D.M.; Nelson, R.; Olander, J.V.; Eppley, B.L.; Delfino, J.J.; Siegel, N.R.; Leimgruber, R.M.; Feder, J. Tumor vascular permeability factor stimulates endothelial cell growth and angiogenesis. *J. Clin. Investig.* **1989**, *84*, 1470–1478. [CrossRef] [PubMed]
2. Ferrara, N.; Henzel, W.J. Pituitary follicular cells secrete a novel heparin-binding growth factor specific for vascular endothelial cells. *Biochem. Biophys. Res. Commun.* **1989**, *161*, 851–858. [CrossRef]

3.   Aiello, L.P.; Avery, R.L.; Arrigg, P.G.; Keyt, B.A.; Jampel, H.D.; Shah, S.T.; Pasquale, L.R.; Thieme, H.;
      Iwamoto, M.A.; Park, J.E.; et al. Vascular endothelial growth factor in ocular fluid of patients with diabetic
      retinopathy and other retinal disorders. *N. Engl. J. Med.* **1994**, *131*, 1480–1487. [CrossRef] [PubMed]

4.   Ferrara, N.; Damico, L.; Shams, N.; Lowman, H.; Kim, R. Development of ranibizumab, an anti-vascular
      endothelial growth factor antigen binding fragment, as therapy for neovascular age-related macular
      degeneration. *Retina* **2006**, *26*, 859–870. [CrossRef] [PubMed]

5.   American Academy of Ophthalmology. Available online: https://www.aao.org/eyenet/article/treat-
      extend-strategy-is-there-consensus (accessed on 11 December 2017).

6.   The CATT Research Group; Martin, D.F.; Maguire, M.G.; Ying, G.S.; Grunwald, J.E.; Fine, S.L.; Jaffe, G.J.
      Ranibizumab and bevacizumab for neovascular age-related macular degeneration. *N. Engl. J. Med.* **2011**,
      364, 1897–1908. [CrossRef] [PubMed]

7.   Ferrara, N.; Gerber, H.P.; LeCouter, J. The biology of VEGF and its receptors. *Nat. Med.* **2003**, *9*, 669–676.
      [CrossRef] [PubMed]

8.   Nork, T.M.; Dubielzig, R.R.; Christian, B.J.; Miller, P.E.; Miller, J.M.; Cao, J.; Zimmer, E.P.; Wiegand, S.J.
      Prevention of experimental choroidal neovascularization and resolution of active lesions by VEGF trap in
      nonhuman primates. *Arch. Ophthalmol.* **2011**, *129*, 1042–1052. [CrossRef] [PubMed]

9.   Tolentino, M.J.; Miller, J.W.; Gragoudas, E.S.; Chatzistefanou, K.; Ferrara, N.; Adamis, A.P. Vascular
      endothelial growth factor is sufficient to produce iris neovascularization and neovascular glaucoma in
      a nonhuman primate. *Arch. Ophthalmol.* **1996**, *114*, 964–970. [CrossRef] [PubMed]

10.   Fujisawa, H.; Kitsukawa, T.; Kawakami, A.; Takagi, S.; Shimizu, M.; Hirata, T. Roles of a neuronal cell-surface
      molecule, neuropilin, in nerve fiber fasciculation and guidance. *Cell Tissue Res.* **1997**, *90*, 465–470. [CrossRef]

11.   Zhong, X.; Huang, H.; Shen, J.; Zacchigna, S.; Zentilin, L.; Giacca, M.; Vinores, S.A. Vascular endothelial
      growth factor-B gene transfer exacerbates retinal and choroidal neovascularization and vasopermeability
      without promoting inflammation. *Mol. Vis.* **2011**, *17*, 492–507. [PubMed]

12.   Rakic, J.M.; Lambert, V.; Devy, L.; Luttun, A.; Carmeliet, P.; Claes, C.; Nguyen, L.; Foidart, J.M.; Noël, A.;
      Munaut, C.; et al. Placental growth factor, a member of the VEGF family, contributes to the development of
      choroidal neovascularization. *Investig. Ophthalmol. Vis. Sci.* **2003**, *44*, 3186–3193. [CrossRef]

13.   Adamis, A.P.; Miller, J.W.; Bernal, M.T.; D'Amico, D.J.; Folkman, J.; Yeo, T.K.; Yeo, K.T. Increased vascular
      endothelial growth factor levels in the vitreous of eyes with proliferative diabetic retinopathy. *Am. J. Ophthalmol.*
      1994, *118*, 445–450. [CrossRef]

14.   Nomura, M.; Yamagishi, S.I.; Harada, S.I.; Hayashi, Y.; Yamashima, T.; Yamashita, J.; Yamamoto, H. Possible
      participation of autocrine and paracrine vascular endothelial growth factors in hypoxia-induced proliferation
      of endothelial cells and pericytes. *J. Biol. Chem.* **1995**, *270*, 28316–28324. [PubMed]

15.   Semenza, G. Signal transduction to hypoxia-inducible factor 1. *Biochem. Pharmacol.* **2002**, *64*, 993–998. [CrossRef]

16.   Ben-Av, P.; Crofford, L.J.; Wilder, R.L.; Hla, T. Induction of vascular endothelial growth factor expression
      in synovial fibroblasts by prostaglandin E and interleukin-1: A potential mechanism for inflammatory
      angiogenesis. *FEBS Lett.* **1995**, *372*, 83–87. [CrossRef]

17.   Yuan, F.; Chen, Y.; Dellian, M.; Safabakhsh, N.; Ferrara, N.; Jain, R.K. Time-dependent vascular regression
      and permeability changes in established human tumor xenografts induced by an anti-vascular endothelial
      growth factor-vascular permeability factor antibody. *Proc. Natl. Acad. Sci. USA* **1996**, *93*, 14765–14770.
      [CrossRef] [PubMed]

18.   De Vries, C.; Escobedo, J.A.; Ueno, H.; Houck, K.; Ferrara, N.; Williams, L.T. The fms-like tyrosine kinase, a
      receptor for vascular endothelial growth factor. *Science* **1992**, *255*, 989–991. [CrossRef] [PubMed]

19.   Gragoudas, E.S.; Adamis, A.P.; Cunningham, E.T., Jr.; Feinsod, M.; Guyer, D.R. VEGF Inhibition Study
      in Ocular Neovascularization Clinical Trial Group. Pegaptanib for neovascular age-related macular
      degeneration. *N. Engl. J. Med.* **2004**, *351*, 2805–2816. [CrossRef] [PubMed]

20.   Bevacizumab Product Label. Available online: https://www.accessdata.fda.gov/drugsatfda_docs/label/
      2011/125085s225lbl.pdf (accessed on 11 December 2017).

21.   Diabetic Retinopathy Clinical Research Network; Wells, J.A.; Glassman, A.R.; Ayala, A.R.; Jampol, L.M.;
      Aiello, L.P.; Antoszyk, A.N.; Arnold-Bush, B.; Baker, C.W.; Bressler, N.M.; et al. Aflibercept, bevacizumab, or
      ranibizumab for diabetic macular edema. *N. Engl. J. Med.* **2015**, *372*, 1193–1203. [CrossRef] [PubMed]

22. Ranibizumab Product Label. Available online: https://www.google.com/search?source=hp&ei=HjcvWtyCI5KgjwSIx43wBg&q=ranibizumab+product+label&oq=ranibizumab+product+la&gs_l=psy-ab.1.0.33i160k1l3.1532.6084.0.8731.22.19.0.3.3.0.313.2540.0j7j5j1.13.0....0...1c.1.64.psy-ab.7.15.2345...0j46j0i131k1j0i46k1j0i3k1j0i10k1j0i22i30k1.0.XaF7BcYR0Ig (accessed on 11 December 2017).

23. Aflibercept Product Label. Available online: https://www.accessdata.fda.gov/drugsatfda_docs/label/2011/125387lbl.pdf (accessed on 12 December 2017).

24. Holash, J.; Davis, S.; Papadopoulos, N.; Croll, S.D.; Ho, L.; Russell, M.; Boland, P.; Leidich, R.; Hylton, D.; Burova, E.; et al. VEGF-Trap: A VEGF blocker with potent antitumor effects. *Proc. Natl. Acad. Sci. USA* **2002**, *99*, 11393–11398. [CrossRef] [PubMed]

25. Zhang, M.; Zhang, J.; Yan, M.; Luo, D.; Zhu, W.; Kaiser, P.K.; Yu, D.C. KH902 Phase 1 Study Group. A phase 1 study of KH902, a vascular endothelial growth factor receptor decoy, for exudative age-related macular degeneration. *Ophthalmology* **2011**, *118*, 672–678. [CrossRef] [PubMed]

26. Campochiaro, P.A.; Channa, R.; Berger, B.B.; Heier, J.S.; Brown, D.M.; Fiedler, U.; Hepp, J.; Stumpp, M.T. Treatment of Diabetic Macular Edema with a Designed Ankyrin Repeat Protein That Binds Vascular Endothelial Growth Factor: A Phase I/II Study. *Am. J. Ophthalmol.* **2013**, *155*, 697–704. [CrossRef] [PubMed]

27. Tietz, J.; Spohn, G.; Schmid, G.; Konrad, J.; Jampen, S.; Maurer, P.; Schmidt, A.; Escher, D. Affinity and potency of RTH258 (ESBA1008), a novel inhibitor of vascular endothelial growth factor a for the treatment of retinal disorders. *Investig. Ophthalmol. Vis. Sci.* **2015**, *56*, 1501.

28. Novartis Media Release. Available online: https://www.novartis.com/news/media-releases/novartis-brolucizumab-rth258-demonstrates-superiority-versus-aflibercept-key (accessed on 10 December 2017).

29. Retina Today Website. Available online: http://retinatoday.com/2014/08/long-acting-anti-vegf-delivery (accessed on 15 January 2016).

30. Healio Online News. Available online: https://www.healio.com/ophthalmology/retina-vitreous/news/online/%7Bd94023a0-da11-4e37-94a0-ab173941d238%7D/genentech-completes-enrollment-in-ranibizumab-port-delivery-system-trial (accessed on 10 December 2017).

31. Heier, J. Top line results from the phase I and IIa clinical trials of AVA-101. In Proceedings of the 2015 American Academy of Ophthalmology Annual Meeting, Las Vegas, NV, USA, 15 November 2015.

32. Kauper, K.; McGovern, C.; Sherman, S.; Heatherton, P.; Rapoza, R.; Stabila, P.; Dean, B.; Lee, A.; Borges, S.; Bouchard, B.; et al. Two-year intraocular delivery of ciliary neurotrophic factor by encapsulated cell technology implants in patients with chronic retinal degenerative diseases. *Investig. Ophthalmol. Vis. Sci.* **2012**, *53*, 7484–7491. [CrossRef] [PubMed]

33. Neurotech Press Release. Available online: http://www.neurotechusa.com/nc-503-ect.html (accessed on 10 December 2017).

34. Joseph, R.R.; Tan, D.W.N.; Ramon, M.R.M.; Natarajan, J.V.; Agrawal, R.; Wong, T.T.; Venkatraman, S.S. Characterization of liposomal carriers for the trans-scleral transport of Ranibizumab. *Sci. Rep.* **2017**, *7*, 16803. [CrossRef] [PubMed]

35. Gutiérrez-Hernándes, J.-C.; Caffey, S.; Abdallah, W.; Cavillo, P.; González, R.; Shih, J.; Brennan, J.; Zimmerman, J.; Martínez-Camarillo, J.C.; Rodriguez, A.R.; et al. One-Year Feasibility Study of Replenish MicroPump for Intravitreal Drug Delivery: A Pilot Study. *Transl. Vis. Sci. Technol.* **2014**, *3*, 8. [CrossRef] [PubMed]

36. Saati, S.; Lo, R.; Li, P.Y.; Meng, E.; Varma, R.; Humayan, M.S. Mini drug pump for ophthalmic use. *Trans. Am. Ophthalmol. Soc.* **2009**, *107*, 60–70. [CrossRef] [PubMed]

37. Humayan, M.; Santos, A.; Altamirano, J.C.; Ribeiro, R.; Gonzalez, R.; de la Rosa, A.; Shih, J.; Pang, C.; Jiang, F.; Calvillo, P.; et al. Implantable micropump for drug delivery in patients with diabetic macular edema. *Trans. Vis. Sci. Technol.* **2014**, *3*, 5. [CrossRef] [PubMed]

38. Chemdiv. Available online: http://www.chemdiv.com/panoptica-reports-positive-results-phase-12-clinical-trial-pan-90806-novel-topical-anti-vegf-eye-drop/ (accessed on 10 December 2017).

39. Rosenfeld, P.J.; Moshfeghi, A.A.; Puliafito, C.A. Optical coherence tomography findings after an intravitreal injection of bevacizumab (avastin) for neovascular age-related macular degeneration. *Ophthalmic Surg. Lasers Imaging Retina* **2005**, *36*, 331–335.

40. Rosenfeld, P.J.; Fung, A.E.; Puliafito, C.A. Optical coherence tomography findings after an intravitreal injection of bevacizumab (avastin) for macular edema from central retinal vein occlusion. *Ophthalmic Surg. Lasers Imaging Retina* **2005**, *36*, 336–339.

41. Diabetic Retinopathy Clinical Research Network Writing Committee; Elman, M.J.; Qin, H.; Aiello, L.P.; Beck, R.W.; Bressler, N.M.; Ferris, F.L.; Glassman, A.R.; Maturi, R.K.; Melia, M. Intravitreal ranibizumab for diabetic macular edema with prompt versus deferred laser treatment. Three-year randomized trial results. *Ophthalmology* **2012**, *119*, 2312–2318. [CrossRef] [PubMed]

42. IVAN Study Investigators; Chakravarthy, U.; Harding, S.P.; Rogers, C.A.; Downes, S.M.; Lotery, A.J.; Wordsworth, S.; Reeves, B.C. Ranibizumab versus bevacizumab to treat neovascular age-related macular degeneration: One-year findings from the IVAN randomized trial. *Ophthalmology* **2012**, *119*, 1399–1411. [CrossRef] [PubMed]

43. Heier, J.S.; Brown, D.M.; Chong, V.; Korobelnik, J.F.; Kaiser, P.K.; Nguyen, Q.D.; Kirchhof, B.; Ho, A.; Ogura, Y.; Yancopoulos, G.D.; et al. Intravitreal aflibercept (VEGF trap-eye) in wet age-related macular degeneration. *Ophthalmology* **2012**, *119*, 2537–2548. [CrossRef] [PubMed]

44. Papadopoulos, N.; Martin, J.; Ruan, Q.; Rafique, A.; Rosconi, M.P.; Shi, E.; Pyles, E.A.; Yancopoulos, G.D.; Stahl, N.; Wiegand, S.J. Binding and neutralization of vascular endothelial growth factor (VEGF) and related ligands by VEGF Trap, ranibizumab and bevacizumab. *Angiogenesis* **2012**, *15*, 171–185. [CrossRef] [PubMed]

45. Furfine, E.; Coppi, A.; Koehler-Stec, E.; Zimmer, E.; Tu, W.; Struble, C. Pharmacokinetics and ocular tissue penetration of VEGF Trap after intravitreal injections in rabbits. *Investig. Ophthalmol. Vis. Sci.* **2006**, *47*, 1430.

46. Schmidt-Erfurth, U.; Kaiser, P.K.; Korobelnik, J.F.; Brown, D.M.; Chong, V.; Nguyen, Q.D.; Ho, A.C.; Ogura, Y.; Simader, C.; Jaffe, G.J.; et al. Intravitreal aflibercept injection for neovascular age-related macular degeneration: Ninety-six-week results of the VIEW studies. *Ophthalmology* **2014**, *121*, 193–201. [CrossRef] [PubMed]

47. Singh, S.R.; Dogra, A.; Stewart, M.; Das, T.; Chhablani, J. Intravitreal Ziv-Aflibercept: Clinical Effects and Economic Impact. *Asia. Pac. J. Ophthalmol.* **2017**, *6*, 561–568.

48. Chen, X.; Li, J.; Li, M.; Zeng, M.; Li, T.; Xiao, W.; Wu, Q.; Ke, X.; Luo, D.; Tang, S.; et al. KH902 suppresses high glucose-induced migration and sprouting of human retinal endothelial cells by blocking VEGF and PlGF. *Diabetes Obes. Metab.* **2013**, *15*, 224–233. [CrossRef] [PubMed]

49. Huang, J.; Li, X.; Li, M.; Li, S.; Xiao, W.; Chen, X.; Cai, M.; Wu, Q.; Luo, D.; Tang, S.; et al. Effects of intravitreal injection of KH902, a vascular endothelial growth factor receptor decoy, on the retina of streptozotocin-induced diabetic rats. *Diabetes Obes. Metab.* **2012**, *14*, 644–653. [CrossRef] [PubMed]

50. Sennhauser, G.; Grütter, M.G. Chaperone-Assisted Crystallography with DARPins. *Structure* **2008**, *16*, 1443–1453. [CrossRef] [PubMed]

51. Retinal Physician Website. Available online: https://www.retinalphysician.com/issues/2017/june-2017/allergan-seeks-durable-response-in-phase-3-darpin (accessed on 12 December 2017).

52. Gaudreault, J.; Gunde, T.; Floyd, H.S.; Ellis, J.; Tietz, J.; Binggeli, D.; Keller, B.; Schmidt, A.; Escher, D. Preclinical pharmacology and safety of ESBA1008, a single-chain antibody fragment, investigated as potential treatment for age related macular degeneration. *Investig. Ophthalmol. Vis. Sci.* **2012**, *53*, 3025.

53. Dugel, P.U.; Jaffe, G.J.; Sallstig, P.; Warburton, J.; Weichselberger, A.; Wieland, M. Brolucizumab versus aflibercept in participants with neovascular age-related macular degeneration: A randomized trial. *Ophthalmology* **2017**, *124*, 1296–1304. [CrossRef] [PubMed]

54. Bioterppartners Announcement. Available online: http://www.bioterppartners.com/single-post/2015/08/17/Is-There-ANYTHING-Left-at-Avalanche-AAVL (accessed on 10 December 2017).

55. Kim, S.H.; Lutz, R.J.; Wang, N.S.; Robinson, M.R. Transport Barriers in Transscleral Drug Delivery for Retinal Diseases. *Ophthalmic Res.* **2007**, *39*, 44–254. [CrossRef] [PubMed]

Permissions

List of Contributors

Caifu Xue, Xunjie Zhang and Weimin Cai
Department of Clinical Pharmacy and Pharmaceutical Management, School of Pharmacy, Fudan University, 826 Zhangheng Road, Shanghai 201203

Chung-Wei Kao, Po-Ting Wu
Department of Chemical Engineering, National Taiwan University, Taipei 10617, Taiwan

Jiashing Yu
Department of Chemical Engineering, National Taiwan University, Taipei 10617, Taiwan
Molecular Imaging Center, National Taiwan University, Taipei 10617, Taiwan

Mei-Yi Liao
Department of Applied Chemistry, National Pingtung University, Pingtung 90003, Taiwan

I-Ju Chung
Department and Graduate Institute of Pharmacology College of Medicine, National Taiwan University, Taipei 10617, Taiwan

Wen-Yih Isaac Tseng
Department and Graduate Institute of Pharmacology College of Medicine, National Taiwan University, Taipei 10617, Taiwan
Molecular Imaging Center, National Taiwan University, Taipei 10617, Taiwan

Kai-Chien Yang
Institute of Medical Device and Imaging, National Taiwan University, Taipei 10617, Taiwan

Parijat Kanaujia and Yin Yani
Institute of Chemical and Engineering Sciences, 1, Pesek Road Jurong Island, Singapore 627833, Singapore

Poovizhi Ponnammal and Reginald B. H. Tan
Institute of Chemical and Engineering Sciences, 1, Pesek Road Jurong Island, Singapore 627833, Singapore
Department of Chemical and Biomolecular Engineering, National University of Singapore, Singapore 117585, Singpore

Wai Kiong Ng
Institute of Chemical and Engineering Sciences, 1, Pesek Road Jurong Island, Singapore 627833, Singapore

Department of Pharmacy, National University of Singapore, Singapore 117559, Singpore

Feng Zhang and Robert O. Williams III
College of Pharmacy, The University of Texas at Austin, 2409 University Avenue, Austin, TX 78712, USA

Michael B. Lowinger
College of Pharmacy, The University of Texas at Austin, 2409 University Avenue, Austin, TX 78712, USA
MRL, Merck and Co., Inc., 126 E. Lincoln Ave, Rahway, NJ 07065, USA

Stephanie E. Barrett
MRL, Merck and Co., Inc., 126 E. Lincoln Ave, Rahway, NJ 07065, USA

Yuri Park, Nahye Kim, Jangmi Choi, Min-Ho Park, Byeong ill Lee, Seok-Ho Shin, Jin-Ju Byeon and Young G. Shin
College of Pharmacy and Institute of Drug Research and Development, Chungnam National University, Daejeon 34134, Korea

Virginia Campani, Laura Mayol and Giuseppe De Rosa
Department of Pharmacy, Università degli Studi di Napoli Federico II, Via D. Montesano 49, 80131 Naples, Italy

Eliana Pagnozzi and Ilaria Mataro
M.D. Department of Plastic and Reconstructive Surgery and Burn Unit, Hospital Hospital "A. Cardarelli", Via A. Cardarelli 9, 80131 Naples, Italy

Alessandra Perna
First Division of Nephrology, Department of Cardio-thoracic and Respiratory Sciences, Second University of Naples, School of Medicine, via Pansini 5, Ed. 17, 80131 Naples, Italy

Floriana D'Urso, Antonietta Carillo and Maria Cammarota
U.O.S.C Farmacia, U.O.S.S. Galenica Clinica e Preparazione Farmaci Antiblastici, Hospital "A. Cardarelli", Via A. Cardarelli 9, 80131 Naples, Italy

Maria Chiara Maiuri
U.M.R.S. 1138, Centre de Recherche des Cordeliers, 15, rue de l'Ecole de Médecine, 75006 Paris, France

Sushma V. Lute, Ranjit M. Dhenge and Agba D. Salman
Department of Chemical and Biological Engineering, University of Sheffield, Mappin Street, Sheffield S1 3JD, UK

M. Danaei, M. Dehghankhold, S. Ataei, F. Hasanzadeh Davarani, R. Javanmard, A. Dokhani, S. Khorasani and M. R. Mozafari
Australasian Nanoscience and Nanotechnology Initiative, 8054 Monash University LPO, Clayton, Victoria 3168, Australia

Yuki Shirosaki
Faculty of Engineering, Kyushu Institute of Technology, 1-1 Sensui-cho, Tobata-ku, Kitakyushu 804-8550, Japan

Motomasa Furuse and Toshihiko Kuroiwa
Department of Neurosurgery, Osaka Medical College, 2-7 Daigaku-machi, Takatsuki, Osaka 569-8686, Japan

Takuji Asano and Yoshihiko Kinoshita
Nikkiso Co., Ltd., Ebisu, Shibuya-ku, Tokyo 150-6022, Japan

Nivesh K. Mittal, Bivash Mandal and Dileep R. Janagam
Plough Center for Sterile Drug Delivery Solutions, University of Tennessee Health Science Center, Memphis, TN 38163, USA

Pavan Balabathula
Plough Center for Sterile Drug Delivery Solutions, University of Tennessee Health Science Center, Memphis, TN 38163, USA
Department of Pharmaceutical Sciences, College of Pharmacy, University of Tennessee Health Science Center, Memphis, TN 38163, USA

Saini Setua, Laura A. Thoma and George C. Wood
Department of Pharmaceutical Sciences, College of Pharmacy, University of Tennessee Health Science Center, Memphis, TN 38163, USA

Leonard Lothstein
Department of Pathology, College of Medicine, University of Tennessee Health Science Center, Memphis, TN 38163, USA

Marion Dubald
Univ Lyon, Université Claude Bernard Lyon 1, Centre National de la Recherche Scientifique (CNRS), Laboratoire d'Automatique et de GEnie des Procédés (LAGEP) Unité Mixte de Recherche UMR 5007, 43 boulevard du 11 novembre 1918, F-69100, Villeurbanne, France
Horus Pharma, Cap Var, 148 avenue Georges Guynemer, F-06700 Saint Laurent du Var, France

Sandrine Bourgeois and Hatem Fessi
Univ Lyon, Université Claude Bernard Lyon 1, Centre National de la Recherche Scientifique (CNRS), Laboratoire d'Automatique et de GEnie des Procédés (LAGEP) Unité Mixte de Recherche UMR 5007, 43 boulevard du 11 novembre 1918, F-69100, Villeurbanne, France
Univ Lyon, Université Claude Bernard Lyon 1, Institut des Sciences Pharmaceutiques et Biologiques (ISPB) — Faculté de Pharmacie de Lyon, 8 avenue Rockefeller, F-69008, Lyon, France

Véronique Andrieu
Unité de Recherche sur les Maladies Infectieuses et Tropicales Émergentes (URMITE), Unité Mixte de Recherche 6236 Centre National de la Recherche Scientifique (CNRS), Aix Marseille Université, Faculté de Médecine et de Pharmacie, F-13005 Marseille, France

Ian P. Harrison and Fabrizio Spada
Department of Research and Development, Ego Pharmaceuticals Pty Ltd., 21-31 Malcolm Road, Braeside, VIC 3195, Australia

Tomasz M. Karpiński
Department of Genetics and Pharmaceutical Microbiology, Poznań University of Medical Sciences, Święcickiego 4, 60-781 Poznań, Poland

Artur Adamczak
Department of Botany, Breeding and Agricultural Technology of Medicinal Plants, Institute of Natural Fibres and Medicinal Plants, Kolejowa 2, 62-064 Plewiska, Poland

Michael W. Stewart
Department of Ophthalmology, Mayo Clinic School of Medicine, 4500 San Pablo Rd., Jacksonville, FL 32224, USA

Index

www.ingramcontent.com/pod-product-compliance
Lightning Source LLC
Chambersburg PA
CBHW080248230326

41458CB00097B/4083